Surgical Pathology
of the
Mediastinum

Second Edition

Surgical Pathology
of the
Mediastinum

Second Edition

Alberto M. Marchevsky, M.D.
Director, Division of Anatomic Pathology
Department of Pathology and Laboratory Medicine
Cedars-Sinai Medical Center
Los Angeles, California

Mamoru Kaneko, M.D.
Director of Surgical Pathology
The Mount Sinai Medical Center
New York, New York

with contributions by

Burton A. Cohen, M.D.
New York, New York

Jonathan W. Said, M.D.
Department of Pathology
and Laboratory Medicine
Cedars-Sinai Medical Center
Los Angeles, California

Raven Press   New York

Raven Press, 1185 Avenue of the Americas, New York, New York 10036

Made in the United States of America

Library of Congress Cataloging-in-Publication Data

Marchevsky, Alberto M.
    Surgical pathology of the mediastinum / Alberto M. Marchevsky,
Mamoru Kaneko ; contributions by Burton A. Cohen, Jonathan Said.—
2nd ed.
        p.   cm.
    Includes bibliographical references and index.
    ISBN 0-88167-818-X
    1. Mediastinum—Diseases—Cytodiagnosis.   2. Pathology, Surgical.
I. Kaneko, Mamoru.   II. Title.
    [DNLM: 1. Mediastinal Diseases—pathology.   2. Mediastinal
Diseases—surgery.   WF 900 M317s]
    RC754.M37   1991
    617.5′45—dc20
    DNLM/DLC
    for Library of Congress   91-23675
                                                                          CIP

9 8 7 6 5 4 3 2 1

Contents

Preface to the First Edition

The mediastinum, an area of great interest to pathologists, surgeons, internists, and radiologists, is the site of origin of numerous pathologic processes. Surprisingly, there are no recent reviews of the pathology of this area. This book is intended to provide a concise, clearly written, and thoroughly illustrated monograph on the surgical pathology of the mediastinum. We have selected cases from over 1,000 mediastinal lesions from our files at the Mount Sinai Hospital, New York, and discuss the basic anatomic aspects of the area, diagnostic techniques used for the localization and diagnosis of mediastinal masses, and the clinicopathologic aspects of mediastinal inflammatory conditions and endocrine, lymphoid, soft tissue, and neurogenic tumors. Three chapters are devoted to the study of the thymus, thymic neoplasms and nontumoral conditions, and include an up-to-date discussion of the newly discovered thymic hormones, immunologic functions of the gland, and recent biochemical findings in thymomas and thymic carcinomas. Mediastinal cysts also are reviewed in detail, and over 1,000 references are provided. Various specific diagnostic problems are addressed in a practical manner.

This volume will be useful as a reference for pathologists with the difficult task of diagnosing mediastinal diseases in daily practice, as well as for clinical specialists interested in the study of thoracic diseases.

Preface

We were gratified at the renewed interest in the pathology of the mediastinum and the thymus gland since the publication of our first edition in 1984. At least two excellent volumes on the surgery of the thymus and surgical pathology of the mediastinum have been published, and our literature search yielded several thousand original publications dealing with the pathology, biology, surgery, and other aspects of the thymus gland and mediastinal organs.

In this new edition, we have incorporated the materials from this vast body of information that are relevant for pathologists faced with the diagnosis of mediastinal lesions and for clinical specialists with an interest in the area.

The chapter on the histology, physiology, and other aspects of the normal thymus gland has been extensively revised incorporating new concepts about the nature of the lymphoid and epithelial cells of the gland. New hypotheses about the role of the thymus in the development of myasthenia gravis and about the pathology of thymic hyperplasia and dysplasia are now discussed in Chapter 5. Chapter 6, which describes the pathology of thymomas, also has been extensively revised. The number of references is markedly increased, new classification schemes are discussed, and recent concepts about the immunopathology of these interesting tumors are reviewed. There are similar changes in Chapter 7, which deals with other thymic neoplasms. Chapter 9, which details mediastinal lymphadenopathies, has been completely rewritten by Dr. Jonathan Said, who has had a long-standing interest in the pathology of malignant lymphomas and of T-cell lymphomas in particular. New information about the pathology of other mediastinal neoplasms has been incorporated. A few color photographs are included as well.

These changes were introduced while trying to remain faithful to the original concept of a concise, yet comprehensive, monograph about the surgical pathology of the mediastinum that reflects our interest in this fascinating area of the thorax.

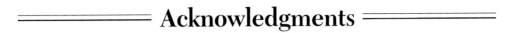

Acknowledgments

Kim Moore and Carolyn Campbell provided excellent secretarial help. Miriam Marchevsky performed the additional photographic work. The authors are very grateful to them for their valuable contribution.

1

The Mediastinum

The mediastinum is the portion of the chest cavity located as a "septum" between the two pleural cavities. It is an area of great interest to internists, radiologists, thoracic surgeons, and pathologists because it can be the site of origin of numerous pathologic processes. Indeed, this portion of the chest cavity has been compared to a "Pandora's box" full of surprises for physicians concerned with chest diseases.

Many interesting clinical problems related to the mediastinum have become apparent in the last few decades with the development of very sensitive new radiologic techniques such as computerized tomography and the extensive use of invasive diagnostic procedures such as mediastinoscopy, limited thoracotomy, and fine needle aspiration biopsy. These techniques enable chest physicians to detect and localize mediastinal lesions hitherto located in "blind spots" of other radiologic procedures. Not infrequently, however, "the buck stops" at the surgical pathology bench, as the surgical pathologist has the responsibility of establishing a definitive diagnosis. This task is often not simple, as the mediastinum contains numerous organs such as the thymus, lymph nodes, ganglia, soft tissues, and others that can become involved in various pathologic processes.

The aim of this volume is to review the clinicopathologic aspects of all mediastinal lesions of interest to the surgical pathologist, with the exception of pathologic processes in the esophagus, pericardium, heart, and major vessels: Although the latter organs are located in the mediastinum, a detailed description of their pathology is well beyond the scope of this volume.

ANATOMY OF THE MEDIASTINUM

The mediastinum extends anteroposteriorly from the sternum to the spine and sagitally from the thoracic inlet to the diaphragm. Its boundaries include the sternum anteriorly, the thoracic vertebra posteriorly, the first thoracic rib, first thoracic vertebra, and manubrium superiorly, and the diaphragm inferiorly (1,2).

ANATOMIC CLASSIFICATIONS OF THE MEDIASTINUM

It has become customary in clinical practice to divide the mediastinum into anatomic compartments separated by arbitrary lines (3). There are several anatomic classifications of the area, but the most widely used scheme is a simple one that divides the mediastinum into four compartments: superior, anterior, middle, and posterior (1). This classification is useful in that certain pathologic lesions are found most frequently in certain compartments. For example, thymic and thyroid tumors are usually in the anterior mediastinum, whereas most neurogenic lesions are found in the posterior compartment (3). This scheme, however, has several drawbacks such as the fact that there is no agreement in the literature on whether the posterior mediastinum should extend backward only to the anterior margins of the vertebral bodies or more posteriorly into what some authors term the paraspinal area (3).

Heitzman tried to overcome the limitations of this oversimplified view of the mediastinum and proposed a much more detailed classification of the area based on anatomic landmarks that can be recognized on chest roentgenograms (3). In his scheme, the mediastinum can be divided into thoracic inlet, anterior mediastinum, supraaortic area, infraaortic area, supraazygous area, infraazygous area, and hila.

The *thoracic inlet* is the area above and below a plane drawn transversely through the first rib. It marks the cervicothoracic junction. The *anterior mediastinum* is the region extending from the thoracic inlet to the diaphragm in front of the pericardium, ascending aorta, and superior vena cava. The *supraaortic area* is the region located behind the left side of the anterior mediastinum. It extends from the aortic arch to the thoracic inlet. The *infraaortic area* is the region located behind the left side of the anterior mediastinum. It extends from below the aortic arch to the diaphragm. The *supraazygous area* is the region located behind the right side of the anterior mediastinum. It extends from the arch of the azygous vein to the thoracic inlet. The *infraazygous area* is the region extending behind the right side of the anterior mediastinum from below the arch of the azygous vein to the diaphragm. The *hila* include both major bronchi and surrounding bronchopulmonary structures.

This classification is very practical from the radiologic point of view because it enables radiologists to localize lesions with accuracy, facilitates the learning of structural relationships, and aids in suggesting differential diagnosis.

This somewhat complicated scheme, however, is of relatively little value to a surgical pathologist faced with the task of establishing the pathologic diagnosis of mediastinal lesions. Therefore, throughout this volume we utilize the simpler and more widely used classification of the mediastinum into four compartments.

ANATOMIC COMPARTMENTS

The *superior mediastinum* extends above a line drawn from the manubrium of the sternum through the lower edge of the fourth thoracic vertebral body (1). The *anterior mediastinum* lies below the superior compartment, between the sternum and the pericardium. The *posterior mediastinum* extends behind a coronal plane through the posterior aspect of the pericardium. The *middle compartment* lies between the anterior and posterior divisions of the mediastinum.

The superior and middle mediastina contain a large number of structures that can be explored with the mediastinoscope (4–6). These structures are usually classified according to their relationship to the trachea, as the mediastinoscopist follows its pathway in order to explore the paratracheal areas. They include (a) anterior to the trachea, thyroid isthmus and blood vessels (superior vena cava, pulmonary artery, aortic arch, anterior communicating jugular vein, thyroid veins, and thyroidea ima artery and vein); (b) to the right of the trachea, blood vessels (right carotid artery, right subclavian artery, azygous vein, pulmonary artery, and superior division of the right pulmonary artery), nerves (right recurrent laryngeal nerve, vagus nerve), and bronchi (right main bronchus and right upper lobe bronchus); (c) to the left of the trachea, blood vessels (thoracic duct, aortic arch, bronchial artery, pulmonary arteries), left recurrent laryngeal nerve, esophagus, and left main bronchus; and (d) inferior to the trachea, carinal lymph nodes, esophagus, and tracheal bifurcation (4–6).

In addition, the superior mediastinum contains the phrenic nerves and the superficial and deep cardiac plexuses (1).

The middle mediastinum strictly should include only the pericardium and its contents. For convenience, however, most anatomy textbooks describe the hila of the lungs in this compartment and include in the middle mediastinum important bronchopulmonary lymph nodes classified by Nagaishi as follows: bronchopulmonary, pulmonary ligament, Botallo's ligament, tracheal bifurcation, tracheobronchial, paratracheal, pretracheal, aortic arch, and innominate vein angle nodes (1,2,7).

The anterior mediastinum merges at its upper end with the superior compartment and reaches inferiorly to the diaphragm (8–10). It contains the thymus gland, blood vessels (e.g., the internal mammary artery and vein), lymph nodes (internal mammary and diaphragmatic lymph nodes), connective tissue, and fat. Occasionally it can contain thyroid and parathyroid tissue.

The posterior mediastinum is the space located behind the pericardium and the diaphragm (1). It merges directly with the superior mediastinum and includes important structures such as the descending portion of the thoracic aorta, esophagus, veins of the azygous system (azygous and superior and inferior hemiazygous veins), thoracic duct, lymph nodes (preaortic, paraaortic, posterior intercostal, middle diaphragmatic, and descending intercostal nodes), and ganglia and nerves of the thoracic sympathetic trunk.

REFERENCES

1. Last RJ: *Anatomy, Regional and Applied.* Edinburgh, New York, Churchill Livingstone, 1978.
2. Warwick R, Williams PL: *Gray's Anatomy,* ed. 35. Philadelphia, WB Saunders, 1973.
3. Heitzman ER: *The Mediastinum. Radiologic Correlations with Anatomy and Pathology.* St. Louis, CV Mosby, 1977.
4. Carter DR: The anatomy of the mediastinum. *Ear Nose Throat J* 1981;60:153–157.
5. Mast WR, Jafek BW: Mediastinal anatomy for the mediastinoscopist. *Arch Otolaryngol* 1975;101:596–599.
6. Foster ED, Munro DD, Dobell ARC: Mediastinoscopy. A review of anatomical relationships and complications. *Ann Thorac Surg* 1972;13:273–286.
7. Nagaishi C: *Functional Anatomy and Histology of the Lung.* Baltimore, University Park Press, 1972.
8. Masaoka A, Nagaoka Y, Kotake Y: Distribution of thymic tissue at the anterior mediastinum. Current procedures in thymectomy. *J Thorac Cardiovasc Surg* 1975;70:747–754.
9. Oliphant M, Wiot JF, Whalen JP: The cervicothoracic continuum. *Radiology* 1976;120:257–262.
10. Sone S, Higashihara T, Morimoto S, et al: Normal anatomy of thymus and anterior mediastinum by pneumomediastinography. *Am J Roentgenol* 1980;134:81–89.

2

Diagnostic Techniques

Burton A. Cohen, M.D.

Prior to the last four decades, the mediastinum was considered an inaccessible area to study because many mediastinal lesions were difficult to detect and localize utilizing plain film examination of the thorax (1). However, with the development of mediastinoscopy in the 1950s, the advent of sophisticated new imaging techniques in the 1960s and 1970s, and improvement in surgical techniques, it has become possible to detect, localize, and surgically remove lesions previously overlooked or considered inaccessible (2). The purpose of this chapter is to review briefly some of the diagnostic techniques utilized for the diagnosis of mediastinal lesions. Although surgical pathologists are interested mainly in establishing pathologic diagnosis based on the use of strict morphologic criteria, it is important for them to have a basic familiarity with diagnostic clinical procedures. This will assist the pathologist in interacting effectively with his or her clinical colleagues and in playing a more active role in helping patients with mediastinal lesions.

RADIOLOGIC EXAMINATION OF THE MEDIASTINUM

The mediastinum can be examined roentgenographically with a variety of techniques including standard chest X-rays; conventional, angled, and computed tomography; angiography; studies of the esophagus; and fluoroscopy (3).

Radiologic evaluation of the mediastinum has been revolutionized by the use of computed body tomography (CT) (3–6). With its cross-sectional images and its increased contrast resolution, CT and magnetic resonance imaging (MRI) are now the procedures of choice for studying the region. Indeed, it has changed the diagnostic approach to mediastinal disease.

Posteroanterior and Lateral Chest Radiographs

Conventional chest X-rays taken in posteroanterior and lateral projections are the most commonly used radiologic techniques for the evaluation of the thorax (7,8). They function as an effective screening tool in evaluating thoracic diseases. Mediastinal disease is, in fact, most frequently detected initially by conventional X-rays. Accurate localization of a mass can also be accomplished with conventional films.

The location of a mediastinal mass is important for a radiologic diagnosis. For example, a lesion in the anterior mediastinum or prevascular space anterior to the ascending aorta most likely represents a thymoma, goiter, teratoma, or enlarged lymph node. A lesion in the middle mediastinal or vascular space most likely rep-

resents a vascular abnormality, lymph node, or bronchogenic, pericardial, or mediastinal cyst. A lesion in the posterior mediastinum or postvascular space is most
likely neurogenic or esophageal in origin.

Conventional chest X-rays have several pitfalls. They often fail to demonstrate
small mediastinal lesions because they rely on either an alteration of the mediastinal
contour with displacement of air–soft tissue interfaces or increased density as a result of the presence of a mass. Thus, the many overlying mediastinal structures often
hide abnormalities. Conventional chest X-rays also offer little information about the
relative density of a lesion. It must be stressed, however, that carefully performed
and interpreted chest X-rays are an effective screening tool in mediastinal disease.

Conventional Tomography of the Mediastinum

Conventional tomography of the mediastinum utilizes posteroanterior and lateral
views and offers more information regarding mediastinal masses than conventional
roentgenograms (5,6). However, the radiation dose is larger, and it has been almost
totally replaced by computed tomography, which better demonstrates the normal
anatomy and pathology of the mediastinum.

Angled Tomography of the Hila

The hila are often best studied radiologically by tomography performed in the 55°
posterior oblique position (9–11). This technique differentiates enlarged hilar lymph
nodes from blood vessels and demonstrates the major bronchi in profile, simplifying
the evaluation of endobronchial lesions.

Angled tomography and CT scanning are the two modalities currently used for the
evaluation of hilar pathology (Figs. 2-1, 2-2).

The Esophagram

The esophagram, utilized primarily for the study of esophageal lesions, is also
useful to evaluate the interaction between the esophagus and contiguous mediastinal
structures. It is helpful, for example, in the detection of mediastinal tumors that
compress the esophagus extrinsically.

Fluoroscopy

Fluoroscopy is seldom utilized, although it may be helpful to evaluate mediastinal
densities by demonstrating changes in the shape of soft, cystic, or vascular lesions
with respiration. It can also be utilized to determine whether a lesion is intrapulmonary or mediastinal, as the former usually moves with respiration.

Angiography

Superior vena cavagrams with injections of contrast material in one or both arms
are occasionally performed to evaluate the venous structures of the superior me-

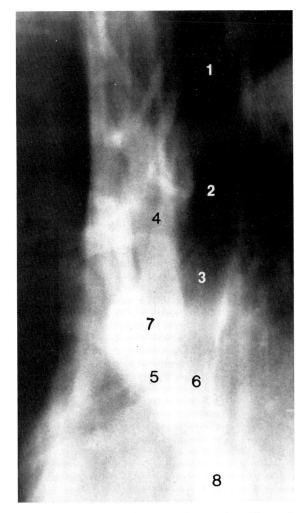

FIG. 2–1. Tomogram of the right hilum taken at 55° posterior oblique demonstrates (*1*) the trachea, (*2*) the right mainstem bronchus, (*3*) the bronchus intermedius, (*4*) the right upper lobe bronchus, (*5*) the right middle lobe bronchus, (*6*) the right lower lobe bronchus, (*7*) the pulmonary artery, and (*8*) inferior pulmonary veins.

diastinum (8). Aortography is the standard technique for evaluation of the aorta and other major arteries of the chest (3,4).

Computed Tomography

Computed tomography has revolutionized radiology. Indeed, this technique is far superior to any other modality in evaluating mediastinal masses (12–20). It has two basic advantages: (a) it provides cross-sectional images that obviate the problem of superimposition of overlapping structures, and (b) it allows high-contrast resolution of mediastinal masses. With CT the replacement of mediastinal fatty tissue by a tumor mass or an enlarged mediastinal structure can be easily and accurately stud-

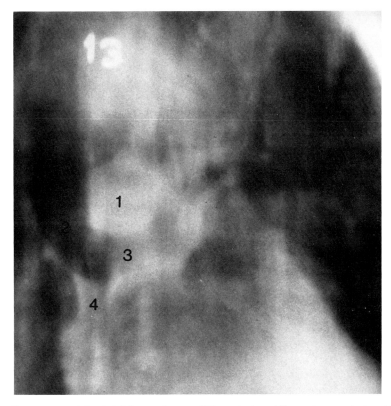

FIG. 2–2. Tomogram of the left hilum taken at 55° posterior oblique demonstrates (*1*) the left pulmonary artery, (*2*) the left mainstem bronchus, (*3*) the left upper lobe bronchus, and (*4*) the left lower lobe bronchus.

ied. The size, density, contours, and anatomical relationships of a lesion can be accurately defined.

Computed tomographic scanning is currently utilized at our institution for (a) the staging of malignancy, (b) the investigation of questionable mediastinal abnormalities detected on conventional studies, (c) the evaluation of tissue density—that is, whether a lesion is cystic or solid, (d) the evaluation of the hila to rule out lymphadenopathy, (e) the evaluation of paraspinal widening, and (f) the detection of thymic lesions.

Technique of CT Scan

A survey view of the chest, which resembles a conventional chest X-ray, is initially performed (Fig. 2-3). With this view used as a reference, a scanning sequence for the axial views is then prescribed using 10-mm contiguous images of the entire chest from the lung apices through the adrenal glands. The multiple cross-sectional images obtained at these levels (Fig. 2-4) provide very accurate information on all mediastinal structures. Intravenous contrast material may be useful to better delineate vascular structures.

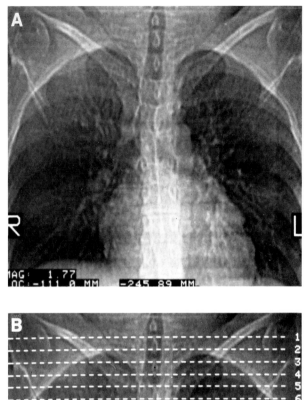

FIG. 2–3. A: Computed tomographic "scout" view of the mediastinum performed prior to axial CT scans. **B:** "Scout" view of the mediastinum. Images that are taken during a routine CT scan have been superimposed on this "scout" view to demonstrate the multiple mediastinal levels that are studied with the procedure.

RADIONUCLIDE IMAGING

Radionuclide scanning with different isotopes is also a very useful technique for the study of mediastinal disease (21). Isotope venography is utilized to determine whether mediastinal masses are vascular (i.e., aneurysm) or not (21). Iodinated and pertechnetate radionuclide scans are useful to evaluate intrathoracic goiters (22).

Gallium scanning is widely used to assess malignant lymphomas and tumors metastatic to mediastinal lymph nodes (23). It is a sensitive technique to detect abnormalities, but it is not a very specific one, as many inflammatory conditions of the mediastinum such as sarcoidosis and tuberculosis can take up the tracer (24,25).

PERCUTANEOUS NEEDLE BIOPSY

Percutaneous needle biopsy has proven to be a useful technique for the diagnosis of lung lesions (25). However, the method has not yet been applied extensively to the study of mediastinal disease, in part because of a reluctance to place a needle in areas close to major vessels or the pericardium (25–27).

Techniques for the biopsy of anterior and posterior mediastinal lesions have been described using cannula, guidewire, and catheter systems, but they have not been accepted widely (25). The biopsy procedure that appears to have gained increased acceptance consists of the use of a fluoroscopically guided percutaneous needle biopsy utilizing 18-gauge or finer needles (26). This procedure results in a high rate of accuracy in patients with carcinomas, and it is a convenient means of establishing a diagnosis of metastatic tumor in patients with superior vena cava obstruction when bronchoscopic biopsies are negative. It has also proven useful in the evaluation of other benign and malignant mediastinal lesions such as teratomas, thymomas, and lymphomas. The diagnostic interpretation of aspirated materials from these lesions is difficult and requires ample experience for an accurate and reliable interpretation (27).

MEDIASTINOSCOPY

Mediastinoscopy was introduced by Harken and associates (28) in 1954 and further developed by Carlens in 1959 (29). It was originally conceived as a tool for the diagnosis of resectability of primary lung cancer, but it is now utilized for the exploration and biopsy of many other mediastinal lesions including enlarged lymph nodes, primary and metastatic tumors, cysts, and soft tissue tumors (30–35).

The procedure allows the thoracic surgeon to explore the peritracheal portions of the superior and middle compartments of the mediastinum and is performed under general or local anesthesia (32,33). The patient is placed in a supine position with the neck fully extended, and a mediastinoscope is inserted through a transverse incision in the suprasternal notch area (30).

The instrument is placed beneath the innominate artery and the aorta and in a position anterior to the trachea. Biopsies are taken under direct visualization with a laryngeal cup or tissue forceps. Small structures such as lymph nodes are resected *in toto,* a procedure that usually yields better tissue specimens with fewer artifactual changes. The tissue samples are submitted for frozen-section examination.

Mediastinoscopy is a safe diagnostic procedure, with an incidence of complications of 1% to 3%. These complications include: perforation of the trachea, main stem bronchi, or esophagus; subcutaneous emphysema; pneumothorax; hemorrhage; air embolism; tumor seeding; mediastinitis; and wound infection (30–34). Several large series, however, report no mortality from the procedure (30–35). It is now accepted in clinical practice that the potential benefits of mediastinoscopy far outweigh its risk of complications (35).

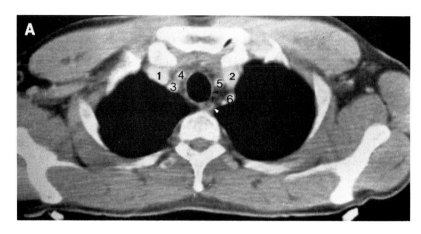

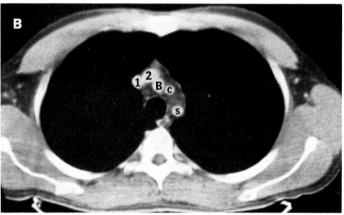

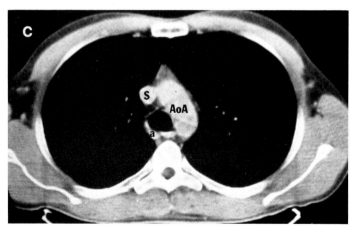

FIG. 2–4. Selected axial views of the chest area. **A:** Computed tomographic scan taken at the level of the manubrium showing the brachiocephalic veins (*1,2*) as the most anterolateral structures, the right subclavian artery (*3*), right common carotid artery (*4*), left common carotid artery (*5*), and left subclavian artery (*6*). In addition, the *arrow* indicates the trachea, and the *arrowheads* the esophagus. **B:** Computed tomographic scan taken at a level above the aortic arch showing the right brachiocephalic vein (*1*), left brachiocephalic vein (*2*), right brachiocephalic artery (*B*), left common carotid artery (*c*), and left subclavian artery (*s*). **C:** Computed tomographic scan taken at the level of the aortic arch showing the superior vena cava (*S*), aortic arch (*AoA*), and azygous vein (*a*).

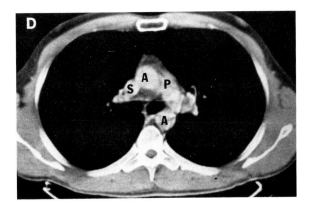

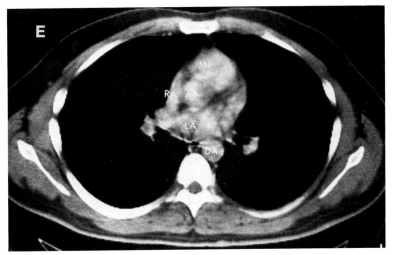

FIG. 2–4. *Continued.* **D:** Computed tomographic scan taken at the level of the pulmonary arteries showing the ascending and descending aorta (*A*), left pulmonary artery (*P*), and superior vena cava (*S*). **E:** Computed tomographic scan taken at the level of the left atrium showing the ascending aorta (*AA*), descending aorta (*DA*), right atrium (*RA*), left atrium (*LA*), and main pulmonary artery (*MP*).

REFERENCES

1. Rose JS: Radiologic analysis of the mediastinum. *Ear Nose Throat J* 1981;60:170–184.
2. Jones R Jr, Bitter M: Pathology of the mediastinum. *Ear Nose Throat J* 1981;60:158–169.
3. Fraser RG, Pare JAP: *Diagnosis of Diseases of the Chest*, ed 2. Philadelphia, WB Saunders, 1977.
4. Heitzman ER: *The Mediastinum. Radiologic Correlations with Anatomy and Pathology.* St. Louis, CV Mosby, 1977.
5. Lee JHT, Sagel SS, Stanley RJ: *Computed Body Tomography*. New York, Raven Press, 1983.
6. Solomon EH, Haaga JR: The mediastinum, in Haaga JR, Alfidi RJ (eds): *Computed Tomography of the Whole Body*. St. Louis, CV Mosby, 1983.
7. Felson B: *Chest Roentgenology*. Philadelphia, WB Saunders, 1973.
8. Berne AS, Gerle RD, Mitchell GE: The mediastinum—normal roentgen anatomy and radiologic techniques. *Semin Roentgenol* 1969;4:3–21.
9. Favez G, Willa C, Heinzer F: Posterior oblique tomography at an angle of 55 degrees in chest roentgenology. *Am J Roentgenol* 1974;120:907–915.

10. McLeod RA, Brown LR, Miller WE, et al: Evaluation of the pulmonary hilar by tomography. *Radiol Clin North Am* 1976;14:51–84.

11. Janower ML: 55° Posterior oblique tomography of the pulmonary hilum. *J Can Assoc Radiol* 1978;29:158–160.

12. Heitzman ER: Computed tomography of the thorax. Current perspectives. *Am J Roentgenol* 1981;136:2–12.

13. Heitzman ER, Goldwin RL, Proto AV: Radiologic analysis of the mediastinum utilizing computed tomography. *Radiol Clin North Am* 1977;15:309–329.

14. Crowe JK, Brown LR, Muhm JR: Computed tomography of the mediastinum. *Radiology* 1978;128:75–87.

15. Baron RL, Levitt RG, Sagel SS, et al: Computed tomography in the evaluation of mediastinal widening. *Radiology* 1981;138:107–113.

16. Baron RL, Gutierrez FR, Sagel SS, et al: CT of anomalies of mediastinal vessels. *Am J Roentgenol* 1981;137:571–576.

17. Baron RL, Lee JKT, Sagel SS, et al: Computed tomography of the normal thymus. *Radiology* 1982;142:121–125.

18. Baron RL, Lee JKT, Sagel SS, et al: Computed tomography of the abnormal thymus. *Radiology* 1982;142:127–134.

19. Pugatch RD, Faling LJ, Robbins AH, et al: CT diagnosis of benign mediastinal abnormalities. *Am J Roentgenol* 1980;134:685–694.

20. Efremidis SC, Dan SJ, Cohen BA, et al: The displaced paraspinal line. Role of computed tomography and lymphangiography. *Am J Roentgenol* 1981;136:505–509.

21. Bonte FJ, Curry TS: III. Radionuclide scanning in the diagnosis of mediastinal masses. *Semin Roentgenol* 1969;4:33–40.

22. Irwin RS, Braman SS, Arvanitidis AN, et al: 131-I Thyroid scanning in preoperative diagnosis of mediastinal goiter. *Ann Intern Med* 1978;89:73–74.

23. Turner DA, Fordham EW, Ali A, et al: Gallium-67 imaging in the management of Hodgkin's disease and other malignant lymphomas. *Semin Nucl Med* 1978;8:205–218.

24. Fosburg RG, Hopkins GB, Kan MW: Evaluation of the mediastinum by gallium-67 scintigraphy in lung cancer. *J Thorac Cardiovasc Surg* 1979;77:76–82.

25. House AJS: Biopsy techniques in the investigation of diseases of the lung, mediastinum and chest wall. *Radiol Clin North Am* 1979;17:393–412.

26. Westcott JL: Percutaneous needle aspiration of hilar and mediastinal masses. *Radiology* 1981;141:323–329.

27. Jereb M, US-Krašovec M: Transthoracic needle biopsy of mediastinal and hilar lesions. *Cancer* 1977;40:1354–1357.

28. Harken DE, Black H, Clauss R, et al: A simple cervicomediastinal exploration for tissue diagnosis of intrathoracic disease. *N Engl J Med* 1954;251:1041–1044.

29. Carlens E: Mediastinoscopy: a method for inspection and tissue biopsy in the superior mediastinum. *Dis Chest* 1959;36:343–352.

30. Kinzler D, Jafek BW: The technique of mediastinoscopy. *Ear Nose Throat J* 1981;60:185–190.

31. Widstrom A, Schnurer L-B: The value of mediastinoscopy—experience of 374 cases. *J Otolaryngol* 1978;7:103–109.

32. Ward PH, Jafek B, Harris P: Interesting and unusual lesions encountered during mediastinoscopy. *Ann Otol Rhinol Laryngol* 1971;80:487–491.

33. Ward PH: Mediastinoscopy under local anesthesia: a valuable diagnostic technique. *Calif Med* 1970;112:15–22.

34. Tucker JA: Mediastinoscopy: 300 cases reported and literature reviewed. *Laryngoscope* 1972;82:2226–2248.

35. Nohl-Oser HC: The evolution and present status of mediastinoscopy. *Endoscopy* 1979;11:1–4.

3

Inflammatory Diseases of
the Mediastinum

A variety of etiologic factors can contribute to acute and chronic inflammation of the mediastinum. Although many of these conditions can be diagnosed clinically, the surgical pathologist is called on to describe the type of mediastinitis present (i.e., acute, chronic nonspecific, granulomatous), to identify specific infectious agents (i.e., fungi and mycobacteria), and to carry out special studies (i.e., immunopathologic evaluation of such poorly understood conditions as fibrosing mediastinitis). The inflammatory conditions of the mediastinum can be classified according to their clinical course and histologic characteristics into acute and chronic mediastinitis.

ACUTE MEDIASTINITIS

Etiology

Acute mediastinitis is an uncommon and potentially lethal clinical condition that is almost always a complication of other clinical problems such as sternal osteomyelitis, dental abscess, esophageal perforation, or thoracic surgery (1–11). Esophageal perforation is the most common contributing factor and frequently results from postoperative dehiscence of intrathoracic esophageal anastomoses (1,5). Perforation can also follow endoscopy and/or therapeutic dilatation of the esophagus, blunt or penetrating trauma, ingestion of foreign body, emesis (Mallory–Weiss syndrome), radiation-associated necrosis, or erosion of the esophageal wall by malignant tumors (3,4,6) (Table 1). The development of infection following esophageal perforation is potentiated by the dynamics of respiration, as the fluctuations in negative intrathoracic pressures tend to suck esophageal contents including air, saliva, enzymes, bile, acid food, and bacteria into the mediastinum. The usual result is a highly virulent necrotizing mediastinitis (2,7).

Infrequently, acute necrotizing mediastinitis develops as the result of direct penetration through soft tissue planes, usually anterior to the prevertebral fascia, or lymphatic spread of infections present in structures such as the neck, pleura, lung, subphrenic spaces, and vertebrae adjacent to the mediastinum (1–3). The complication of cellulitis secondary to odontogenic infections, tonsillitis, pharyngitis, vertebral osteomyelitis, subphrenic abscess, and empyema is seldom seen today, as these underlying conditions are treated early with antibiotics.

TABLE 1. *Etiologic factors in acute mediastinitis*

Esophageal perforation caused by
    Postoperative dehiscence of esophageal anastomoses
    Endoscopy
    Therapeutic dilatation of esophagus
    Blunt or penetrating trauma
    Ingestion of foreign body
    Mallory–Weiss syndrome
    Tumors
Extension of infectious processes in adjacent areas
    Cervical cellulitis caused by odontogenic and other infections
    Lung abscess
    Vertebral osteomyelitis
    Sternal osteomyelitis
    Subphrenic abscess

Clinical Findings

Patients with acute mediastinitis present with fever to 102°F, pain that varies in location according to the area of inflammation, respiratory distress, and dysphagia (1). Respiratory distress occurs when the pleura is involved by extension of the acute inflammatory process from the mediastinum. Pain is usually present at the site of perforation. This lateralization is often useful in defining the site of esophageal perforation.

Severe dyspnea appears in patients with severe necrotizing mediastinitis, usually as a result of airway compression by the inflammatory process or because of massive pleural effusions and/or pneumothorax. Dysphagia accompanies perforation of the esophagus or the pharynx and is manifested by pain and distress while swallowing that can also help to localize the site of perforation.

The physical examination is usually not diagnostic, but there may be cervical tenderness in patients with cervical cellulitis and subcutaneous emphysema in cases of esophageal perforation. Chest roentgenograms are essential for the diagnosis of acute mediastinitis. They usually show mediastinal widening with ill-defined borders and pleural effusion that can be best demonstrated in lateral decubitus views. Occasionally the chest roentgenogram may be normal. Esophagoscopy is contraindicated except when necessary to remove a foreign body (1).

Pathology

The pathology of acute mediastinitis is that of severe inflammation in the mediastinal soft tissues, often with abscess formation. These findings are seldom a diagnostic problem for the surgical pathologist. Aerobic and anaerobic bacteria such as β-hemolytic *Streptococcus, Staphylococcus aureus,* anaerobic *Streptococcus,* and *Bacteroides* can be isolated from resected tissues (1).

Treatment

The treatment of acute mediastinitis includes surgery for the correction of the pathogenetic factors and drainage of abscesses as well as appropriate antibiotic therapy and electrolyte, ventilatory, and nutritional support (1–7).

CHRONIC MEDIASTINITIS—GRANULOMATOUS MEDIASTINITIS WITH FIBROSIS

A number of infectious and noninfectious diseases can lead to the development of chronic mediastinal inflammation accompanied in most instances by granuloma formation (12–32).

Dense fibrosis is frequent and can be visualized on chest roentgenograms as mass densities that compress various mediastinal structures and simulate a malignant process.

This syndrome has been reported with various names, such as fibrous mediastinitis, sclerosing mediastinitis, granulomatous mediastinitis, mediastinal fibrosis complicating healed primary histoplasmosis and tuberculosis, as well as others (12–32).

Etiology

The etiology and pathogenesis of chronic mediastinitis remain enigmatic in many instances. Oulmont (33) described the first patient with this syndrome in 1855 and classified it as idiopathic fibrous mediastinitis. Osler (34) in 1903 described several additional patients with mediastinal fibrosis of unclassified etiology and superior vena cava obstruction. The disease was thought to be secondary to tuberculosis or syphilis until 1925, when Knox (35) reported cases associated with fungal infections. Among the various etiologies currently proposed are infections by fungi (histoplasmosis, aspergillosis, mucormycosis, and cryptococcosis) and mycobacteria (tuberculous and nontuberculous) and noninfectious factors such as autoimmune disease, sarcoidosis, rheumatic fever, neoplasms, traumatic hemorrhage, and drugs (methysergide) (Table 2) (36–52). In rare instances, the disease is familial and multifocal, and patients present with retroperitoneal and mediastinal fibrosis, sclerosing cholangitis, Riedel's thyroiditis, and pseudotumor of the orbit (30,53).

Histoplasmosis is the most frequently implicated etiologic factor of granulomatous mediastinitis with fibrosis in the United States, but in many instances the cause of

TABLE 2. *Etiologic factors of granulomatous mediastinitis with fibrosis*

Fungal infections
  Histoplasmosis
  Aspergillosis
  Mucormycosis
  Cryptococcosis
Mycobacterial infections
  Tuberculosis
  Nontuberculous infections
Bacterial infections
  Nocardiosis
  Actinomycosis
Autoimmune disease
Sarcoidosis
Rheumatic fever
Neoplasms
Trauma
Drugs
Idiopathic

the disease remains undetermined, and the process is classified as idiopathic sclerosing mediastinitis (12–52).

Patients with bacterial infections caused by *Nocardia* or *Actinomyces* have been cited as examples of chronic mediastinitis with granuloma formation but usually develop extensive areas of mediastinal fibrosis and present with clinical manifestations similar to other instances of sclerosing mediastinitis (54–56). They should be included in this syndrome.

Pathogenesis

The pathogenesis of the development of extensive, progressive fibrosis in some patients with mediastinal granulomas remains unclear, and several theories have been proposed to explain this complication.

Kunkel and associates (15) suggested that mediastinal fibrosis resulted from traumatic rupture of granulomatous lymph nodes with spread of their irritating contents into adjacent soft tissues. However, there are reported instances of accidental spillage of granulomatous tissues into the mediastinum at surgery without any evidence of subsequent dissemination of the disease (51). Mathisen and Holta (57) demonstrated lymph stasis and vein obstruction in patients with retroperitoneal fibrosis and suggested that the transudation of protein-rich fluid resulted in progressive fibrous organization. This theory fails to explain why chronic edema in other parts of the body does not result in fibrosis that extends progressively into adjacent tissues.

Baum and associates (58) and Goodwin and collaborators (14) proposed the most interesting and currently accepted hypothesis. They suggested that sclerosing mediastinitis results from a delayed hypersensitivity reaction. They demonstrated the development of progressive fibrosis in granulomas caused by histoplasmosis and postulated the presence of an unidentified antigen that stimulated fibroblastic activity at the periphery of the granulomas. This antigen, in their concept, could diffuse into adjacent tissues and stimulate the development of an enlarging histoplasmoma that extends from areas of caseous necrosis in mediastinal lymph nodes into adjacent soft tissues. Known findings that support this hypothesis include the presence of strongly positive skin reactivity and serologic reactivity to histoplasma in some patients with sclerosing mediastinitis and hypergammaglobulinemia and hypercomplementemia in others. The infiltration of the fibrous mass by extensive aggregates of plasma cells also suggests an immunologic reaction.

Moreover, antinuclear antibodies and deposits of IgA, IgG, and IgM have been demonstrated on the surface of collagen fibers of patients with retroperitoneal fibrosis, a disorder thought to be related to sclerosing mediastinitis (22,50,52).

Clinical Findings

Sclerosing mediastinitis is usually self-limiting and tends to regress with time, but it can be a serious clinical problem resulting in permanent incapacity or even death. All age groups may be affected, but the condition is found most often in white (90%), young (average age 19 to 25 years) females (female/male ratio of 3:1) (8,52).

The clinical manifestations of this disorder vary considerably depending on the presence of an infectious process or the development of an expanding fibrous mass that can slowly infiltrate, surround, and compress various mediastinal structures such as blood vessels, trachea, esophagus, heart, and nerves. Thin-walled veins are most commonly affected, and superior vena cava obstruction is a common complication. Indeed, mediastinal granuloma with fibrosing mediastinitis is the most common benign cause of superior vena cava obstruction (Fig. 3-1) (8,59).

About 40% of patients with sclerosing mediastinitis are asymptomatic at the time of the initial diagnosis and are found to have abnormal chest roentgenograms with mediastinal densities suggesting the presence of a neoplasm (Fig. 3-2) (12). Most patients, however, present with nonspecific complaints such as cough, dyspnea, chest pain, fever, wheezing, dysphagia, and/or hemoptysis.

Roentgenographic findings in sclerosing mediastinitis include asymmetric widening of the mediastinum with distortion and obliteration of the tissue planes, recognizable in frontal and lateral chest roentgenographs (Fig. 3-3). The process may also be seen as a diffuse mass with lobular contours. Calcification of mediastinal lymph nodes, particularly in endemic areas, is a strong indication of histoplasmosis. A small number of patients also have pulmonary reticular and nodular interstitial infiltrates that appear to originate from the hilar areas and are related to congestion, lymphatic

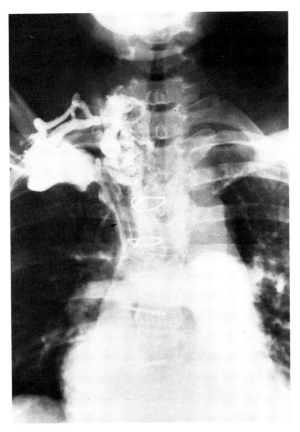

FIG. 3–1. Sclerosing mediastinitis. Superior venacavagram taken post-insertion of a graft between the right subclavian vein and the proximal superior vena cava (*arrow*) and showing marked collateral circulation consistent with partial obstruction of the superior vena cava and the graft. (Courtesy of Dr. Jack Rabinowitz, New York.)

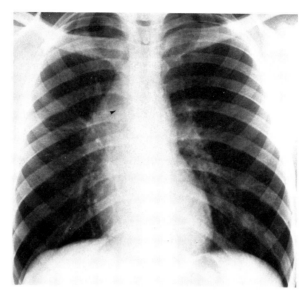

FIG. 3–2. Sclerosing mediastinitis. Anterior/posterior view of the chest demonstrating a widened mediastinum that extends upward from the right hilar region (*arrowhead*). (Courtesy of Dr. Jack Rabinowitz, New York.)

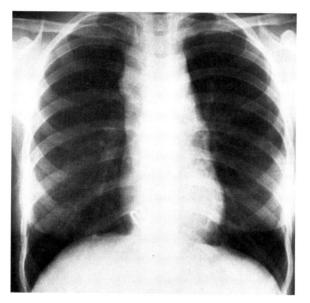

FIG. 3–3. Sclerosing mediastinitis. Anterior/posterior view of the chest showing asymmetrical mediastinal widening. (Courtesy of Dr. Jack Rabinowitz, New York.)

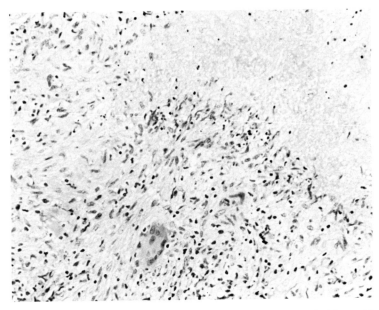

FIG. 3–4. Sclerosing mediastinitis. Granuloma with necrosis surrounded by epithelioid cells and multinucleated giant cells. (H&E × 100, original)

stasis, and/or interstitial fibrosis. Rarely, wedge-shaped areas of consolidation suggestive of pulmonary infarcts have been seen (23). Tomograms and CT scans are useful in order to study airways and to demonstrate areas of narrowing of the trachea and/or bronchi. Angiograms and venograms are helpful to detect compression of arteries and veins by the fibrosing process. Upper gastrointestinal X-ray studies can demonstrate esophageal narrowing.

Pathology

Sclerosing mediastinitis is characterized by a diffuse and ill-defined infiltration of mediastinal structures by dense fibrous tissue with varying degrees of infiltration by chronic inflammatory cells (Color figs. 1 and 2*). Epithelioid granulomas with or without central caseous necrosis are often seen (Fig. 3-4). They may be encountered, however, only in focal areas encased by dense fibrous tissue, and their detection may require the study of multiple histologic sections. Special stains such as methenamine silver and PAS are useful for the detection and morphologic characterization of fungi such as *Histoplasma* (Fig. 3-5), *Aspergillus* (Fig. 3-6), *Cryptococcus* (Fig. 3-7), and others. Acid-fast bacilli, either *Mycobacterium tuberculosis* or atypical mycobacteria, may be found.

Lymph nodes with active granulomatous infections may also be present (Fig. 3-8). These lymph nodes as well as other areas of caseating necrosis are ideal sites to

---

*Color figures 1, 2, and 3 appear following page 64.

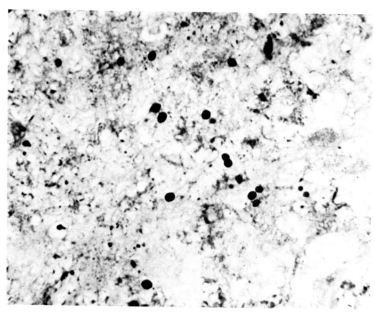

FIG. 3–5. Sclerosing mediastinitis secondary to histoplasmosis. Oval and round forms of *Histoplasma capsulatum*. (Methenamine silver, ×400, original)

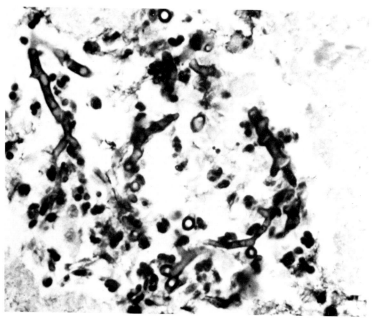

FIG. 3–6. Sclerosing mediastinitis caused by aspergillosis. Hyphae of *Aspergillus* sp. (Methenamine silver, ×400, original)

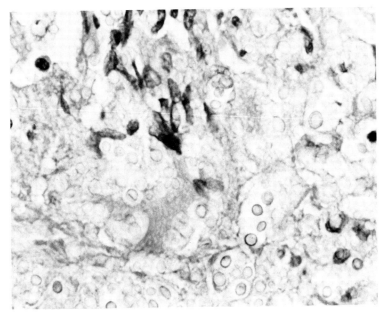

FIG. 3–7. Sclerosing mediastinitis caused by cryptococcosis. Oval forms of *Cryptococcus neoformans* with mucinous capsule. (Mucicarmine, × 400, original)

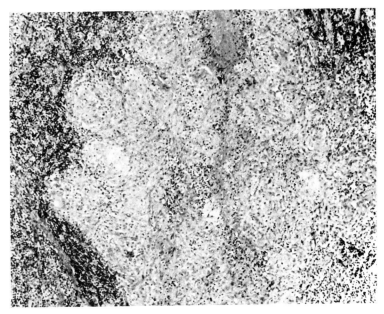

FIG. 3–8. Sclerosing mediastinitis caused by tuberculosis. Lymph node showing multiple, confluent, caseating epithelioid cell granulomas. (H&E × 40, original)

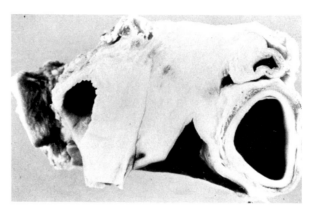

FIG. 3–9. Sclerosing mediastinitis. Cross section of aorta, trachea, esophagus, and superior vena cava showing compression by dense fibrous mass. (Courtesy of Dr. Jack Rabinowitz, New York.)

biopsy and should be looked for by thoracic surgeons at the time of thoracotomy (47).

The infiltration of mediastinal structures in patients with sclerosing mediastinitis can be massive and simulate a malignant neoplasm (Color fig. 1). Infiltration of the superior vena cava results in superior vena cava syndrome, which can worsen considerably when secondary thrombosis of the stenosed vein ensues (13,16) (Fig. 3-9). Invasion of the pulmonary veins usually occurs around the left atrium and results in a clinical syndrome that closely mimics mitral valve stenosis with pulmonary hypertension (12,41). This complication is usually fatal. Secondary thrombosis of the pul-

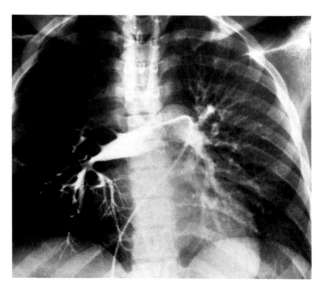

FIG. 3–10. Sclerosing mediastinitis. Right pulmonary angiogram showing almost complete occlusion of the right upper lobe artery and circumferential narrowing of other vessels. (Courtesy of Dr. Jack Rabinowitz, New York.)

monary veins may be associated with pulmonary infarcts (23). Pulmonary artery involvement has also been described (Fig. 3-10) (21,38,39). Histologically, the arteries have infiltration of their media and adventitia by fibrous tissue and intimal proliferation that results in thrombosis secondary to irregular blood flow.

Thrombosis of the pulmonary arteries can also result in pulmonary infarcts. Bronchial and tracheal obstruction is a rare complication in patients with sclerosing mediastinitis, since the airway cartilage usually acts as a barrier against fibrous tissue invasion (Fig. 3-11) (24). When invasion occurs, it is usually accompanied by a secondary ectasia of veins and lymphatic vessels in the airway lamina propria, which in turn leads to hemoptysis, dyspnea, and markedly abnormal pulmonary function tests. This complication is usually fatal. The esophagus is rarely compressed in sclerosing mediastinitis, since it is a freely movable structure that can be displaced by the fibrous mass without being infiltrated by it. However, in patients with severe

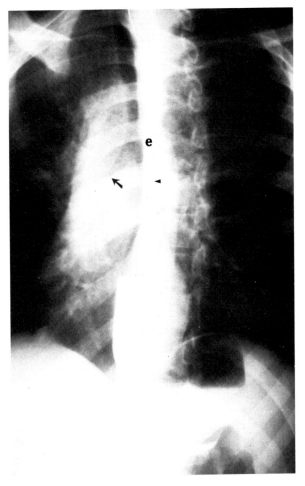

FIG. 3–11. Sclerosing mediastinitis. Esophagram taken at a right anterior oblique position showing marked narrowing of the esophagus (*arrowhead*) and main bronchus (*arrow*). Proximal esophagus is mildly dilated (*e*). (Courtesy of Dr. Jack Rabinowitz, New York.)

forms of the disease in which the entire mediastinum is encased by the fibrosing process, esophageal obstruction does occur (25,52).

Rarely, mediastinal fibrosis is complicated by a syndrome of left vocal cord paresis as a result of involvement of the recurrent laryngeal nerve and esophageal diverticulum formation (26).

The lung may exhibit pathologic changes secondary to pulmonary venous or arterial obstruction in patients with sclerosing mediastinitis (22). They include medial hypertrophy and intimal proliferation of pulmonary medium and small arteries and arterioles and intraalveolar accumulations of hemosiderin-laden macrophages, as seen in patients with pulmonary hypertension secondary to mitral stenosis. Secondary thrombosis can ensue in these small vessels and contribute to a more severe degree of pulmonary hypertension (52). Rare instances of pulmonary infarcts following arterial or venous thrombosis have also been reported (23). A more frequent complication in patients with sclerosing mediastinitis is pulmonary interstitial fibrosis, which can follow a clinical and pathologic course similar to that in patients with usual interstitial pneumonitis (UIP) (59).

In isolated instances, sclerosing mediastinitis may be associated with a similar fibrotic process in the retroperitoneum, thyroid, and other organs (53).

Prognosis and Treatment

In most patients with sclerosing mediastinitis, the disease follows a slow, self-limiting clinical course (12). For example, only one of 31 patients studied at the Mayo Clinic with this syndrome died of cardiorespiratory failure 26 years after the initial diagnosis (12). It is controversial whether the evolution of the disease can be altered by corticosteroid therapy. Few patients with presumed histoplasmosis have received amphotericin B therapy, but most cases have no evidence of active infection, and it is not known whether antifungal therapy has a useful role in the treatment of this syndrome (12,59). Surgery is indicated in most patients, and thoracotomy and biopsy are frequently needed to establish the diagnosis. In approximately 25% of patients with localized granulomas, complete excision of the lesion can be achieved. It appears that in at least some cases excision of local granulomas prevented the development of subsequent progressive fibrosis. In a few patients, reconstructive surgery is necessary to alleviate vascular, esophageal, or airway obstruction. It is, however, advised only in advanced cases (12,13,18,24,25).

MEDIASTINAL HEMORRHAGE

Patients with massive mediastinal hemorrhage that can simulate a mass or a cyst on chest roentgenograms have been described (60–64). Mediastinal hemorrhage can develop spontaneously or following trauma, extracorporeal membrane oxygenation, and intravenous drug abuse. Indeed, one of our surgical residents presented with an enlarging mediastinal cyst that simulated a malignant neoplasm and consisted of a large, spontaneous, anterior mediastinal cystic hematoma present in the thymic area (Color fig. 3).

REFERENCES

1. Payne WS, Larson RH: Acute mediastinitis. *Surg Clin North Am* 1969;49:999–1009.
2. Cogan MIC: Necrotizing mediastinitis secondary to descending cervical cellulitis. *Oral Surg* 1973;36:307–320.
3. Benezra C, Spurgeon L, Light RW: Mediastinal abscess secondary to vertebral osteomyelitis. *Postgrad Med* 1982;71:220–223.
4. North J, Emanuel B: Mediastinitis in a child caused by perforation of pharynx. *Am J Dis Child* 1975;129:962–963.
5. Weinstein RA, Jones EL, Schwarzmann SW, et al: Sternal osteomyelitis and mediastinitis after open-heart operation: pathogenesis and prevention. *Ann Thorac Surg* 1976;21:442–444.
6. Howell HS, Prinz RA, Pickleman JR: Anaerobic mediastinitis. *Surg Gynecol Obstet* 1976; 143:353–359.
7. Moncada R, Warpeha R, Pickleman J, et al: Mediastinitis from odontogenic and deep cervical infection. Anatomic pathways of propagation. *Chest* 1978;73:497–500.
8. Mensah GA, Gold JP, Schreiber T, Isom OW: Acute purulent mediastinitis and sternal osteomyelitis after closed chest cardiopulmonary resuscitation: a case report and review of the literature. *Ann Thorac Surg* 1988;46:353–355.
9. Zachariades N, Mezitis M, Stavrinidis P, et al: Mediastinitis, thoracic empyema, and pericarditis as complications of a dental abscess: report of a case. *J Oral Maxillofac Surg* 1988;46:493–495.
10. Komatsu ES, Costa F, Marchese LT, et al: Abscess of the mediastinum: a case report. *J Pediatr Surg* 1989;24:1125.
11. Levine TM, Wurster CF, Krespi YP: Mediastinitis occurring as a complication of odontogenic infections. *Laryngoscope* 1986;96:747–750.
12. Dines DE, Payne WS, Bernatz PE, et al: Mediastinal granuloma and fibrosing mediastinitis. *Chest* 1979;75:320–324.
13. Ferguson TB, Burford TH: Mediastinal granuloma. A 15-year experience. *Ann Thorac Surg* 1965;1:125–141.
14. Goodwin RA, Nickell JA, Des Prez RM: Mediastinal fibrosis complicating healed primary histoplasmosis and tuberculosis. *Medicine* 1972;51:227–246.
15. Kunkel WM Jr, Clagett OT, McDonald JR: Mediastinal granulomas. *J Thorac Surg* 1954;27:565–574.
16. Salyer JM, Harrison HN, Winn DF Jr, et al: Chronic fibrous mediastinitis and superior vena caval obstruction due to histoplasmosis. *Dis Chest* 1959;35:364–377.
17. Schowengerdt CG, Suyemoto R, Main FB: Granulomatous and fibrous mediastinitis. A review and analysis of 180 cases. *J Thorac Cardiovasc Surg* 1969;57:365–379.
18. Strimlan CV, Dines DE, Payne WS: Mediastinal granuloma. *Mayo Clin Proc* 1975;50:702–705.
19. Zeanah CH, Zusman J: Mediastinal and cervical histoplasmosis simulating malignancy. *Am J Dis Child* 1979;133:47–49.
20. Prager RL, Burney P, Waterhouse G, et al: Pulmonary, mediastinal and cardiac presentations of histoplasmosis. *Ann Thorac Surg* 1980;30:385–390.
21. Wieder S, White TJ, Salazar J, et al: Pulmonary artery occlusion due to histoplasmosis. *Am J Roentgenol* 1982;138:243–251.
22. Light AM: Idiopathic fibrosis of mediastinum: a discussion of three cases and review of the literature. *J Clin Pathol* 1978;31:78–88.
23. Katzenstein AL, Mazur MT: Pulmonary infarct: an unusual manifestation of fibrosing mediastinitis. *Chest* 1980;77:521–524.
24. James EC, Harris SS, Dillenburg CJ: Tracheal stenosis: an unusual presenting complication of idiopathic fibrosing mediastinitis. *J Thorac Cardiovasc Surg* 1980;80:410–413.
25. Albrechtsen D, Nygaard K: Idiopathic mediastinal fibrosis. A case of oesophageal obstruction treated by partial oesophagolysis. *Acta Chir Scand* 1981;147:219–222.
26. Lerner MA, Katz R: A new syndrome of left vocal cord paresis and esophageal diverticulum due to mediastinal fibrosis. *Am J Roentgenol Radium Ther Nucl Med* 1975;125:193–197.
27. Morad N, Strongwater SL, Eypper S, et al: Idiopathic retroperitoneal and mediastinal fibrosis mimicking connective tissue disease. *Am J Med* 1987;82:363–366.
28. Berry DF, Buccigrossi D, Peabody J, et al: Pulmonary vascular occlusion and fibrosing mediastinities. *Chest* 1986;89:296–301.
29. Kountz PD, Molina PL, Sagel SS: Fibrosing mediastinitis in the posterior thorax. *Am J Roentgenol* 1989;153:489–490.
30. Mitchell IM, Saunders NR, Maher O, et al: Surgical treatment of idiopathic mediastinal fibrosis: report of five cases. *Thorax* 1968;41:210–214.
31. Westhoff M: Riedel's struma and fibrous mediastinitis. Positive therapeutic responsiveness to corticoids. *Dtsch Med Wochenschr* 1988;113:337–341.

32. Loyd JE, Tillman BF, Atkinson JB, et al: Mediastinal fibrosis complicating histoplasmosis. *Medicine* 1988;67:295–310.
33. Oulmont N: *Des Obliterations de la Veine Cave Superieure*. Paris, JB Baillère, 1855.
34. Osler W: On obliteration of the superior vena cava. *Bull Johns Hopkins Hosp* 1903;14:169–182.
35. Knox LB: Chronic mediastinitis. *Am J Med Sci* 1925;169:807–820.
36. Puri S, Factor SM, Farmer P: Sclerosing mediastinitis. Presumed to be due to primary aspergillosis. *NY State J Med* 1977;77;1774–1777.
37. Ahmad M, Weinstein AJ, Hughes JA, et al: Granulomatous mediastinitis due to *Aspergillus flavus* in a nonimmunosuppressed patient. *Am J Med* 1981;70:887–890.
38. Arnett EN, Bacos JM, Macher AM, et al: Fibrosing mediastinitis causing pulmonary arterial hypertension without pulmonary venous hypertension. Clinical and necropsy observations. *Am J Med* 1977;63:634–643.
39. Zorn SK, Schachter N, Smith GJW, et al: Pulmonary artery obstruction with fibrosing mediastinitis. *Lung* 1978;155:91–100.
40. Spinola SM, Bell A, Henderson FW: Actinomycosis. A cause of pulmonary and mediastinal mass lesions in children. *Am J Dis Child* 1981;135:336–339.
41. Dye TE, Saab SB, Almond CH, et al: Sclerosing mediastinitis with occlusion of pulmonary veins. Manifestations and management. *J Thorac Cardiovasc Surg* 1977;74:137–141.
42. Sinha P, Naik KG, Bhagwat GP: Mediastinal cryptococcoma. *Thorax* 1978;33:657–659.
43. Leong ASY: Granulomatous mediastinitis due to Rhizopus species. *Am J Clin Pathol* 1978;70:103–107.
44. Jauregui L, Arbulu A, Wilson F: Osteomyelitis, pericarditis, mediastinitis and vasculitis due to *Mycobacterium chelonei*. *Am Rev Respir Dis* 1977;115:699–703.
45. Hache L, Woolner LB, Bernatz PE: Idiopathic fibrous mediastinitis. *Dis Chest* 1962;41:9–25.
46. Graham JR, Suby HI, Le Compte PR, et al: Fibrotic disorders associated with methysergide therapy for headache. *N Engl J Med* 1966;274:359–368.
47. Owen GE, Scherr SN, Segre EJ: Histoplasmosis involving the heart and great vessels. *Am J Med* 1962;32:552–559.
48. Que GS, Mandema E: A case of idiopathic retroperitoneal fibrosis presenting as a systemic collagen disease. *Am J Med* 1964;36:320–329.
49. Yacoub MH, Thompson VC: Chronic idiopathic pulmonary hilar fibrosis: a clinicopathologic entity. *Thorax* 1971;26:365–375.
50. Iversen BM, Johannessen JW, Nordahl E, et al: Retroperitoneal fibrosis during treatment with methyldopa. *Lancet* 1975;2:302–304.
51. Friedman JL, Baum GL, Schwarz J: Primary pulmonary histoplasmosis: associated pericardial and mediastinal manifestations. *Am J Dis Child* 1965;109:298–303.
52. Sobrinho-Simões MA, Saleiro JV, Wagenvoort CA: Mediastinal and hilar fibrosis. *Histopathology* 1981;5:53–60.
53. Comings DE, Skubi KB, Van Eyes J, et al: Familial multifocal fibrosclerosis. Findings suggesting that retroperitoneal fibrosis, mediastinal fibrosis, sclerosing cholangitis, Riedel's thyroiditis and pseudotumor of the orbit may be different manifestations of a single disease. *Ann Intern Med* 1967;66:884–892.
54. Bates M, Cruickshank G: Thoracic actinomycosis. *Thorax* 1957;12:99–124.
55. Weese WC, Smith IM: A study of 57 cases of Actinomycosis over a 36-year period. A diagnostic "failure" with good prognosis after treatment. *Arch Intern Med* 1975;135:1562–1568.
56. Rankin RS, Westcott JL: Superior vena-cava syndrome caused by *Nocardia* mediastinitis. *Am Rev Respir Dis* 1973;108:361–363.
57. Mathisen W, Holta AL: Idiopathic retroperitoneal fibrosis. *Surg Gynecol Obstet* 1966;122:1278–1282.
58. Baum GL, Green RA, Schwartz J: Enlarging pulmonary histoplasmoma. *Am Rev Respir Dis* 1960;82:721–726.
59. Wieder S, Rabinowitz JG: Fibrous mediastinitis: a late manifestation of mediastinal histoplasmosis. *Radiology* 1977;125:305–312.
60. Marquette CH, L'Her P, Cosnard G, et al: Spontaneous hematome of the mediastinum. *Rev Mal Respir* 1989;6:381–384.
61. Weiss RG, Ball WS Jr, Warner BW, et al: Mediastinal hemorrhage during extracorporeal membrane oxygenation. *J Pediatr Surg* 1989;24:1115–1117.
62. Ramani Rao MV, Snyder TC, Tybak B, et al: Mediastinal hematoma in an intravenous drug abuser. *Mt Sinai J Med (NY)* 1986;53:157–159.
63. Suddes KP, Thomas RD: Mediastinal haemorrhage: a complication of thrombolytic treatment. *Br Med J* 1988;297:527.
64. Vergnon JM, Cuilleret J, Fournel P, et al: Difficult diagnosis of a rapidly developing post-traumatic tumor of the thymus region. Encysted hematoma or intracystic hemorrhage? *Rev Pneumol Clin* 1986;42:199–203.

4

The Thymus Gland

The thymus gland is a very important organ of the immune system and is located in the anterior mediastinum. It is an essential structure for the development of cell-mediated immunity, and it can be the site of origin of numerous pathologic conditions including tumors, cysts, and developmental abnormalities (1,2).

ANATOMY

The thymus is a pyramid-shaped organ composed of two closely apposed lobes and located in front of the great vessels at the base of the pericardium and the heart (Fig. 4-1) (3–6). Each lobe is completely covered by a fibrous capsule that extends into the parenchyma in the form of connective tissue septa. These septa divide the thymic tissue into the many lobules that constitute the basic structural units of the thymus; these vary in size from 0.5 to 2 mm.

HISTOLOGY

The lobules are composed of two areas that can be distinctly recognized in histologic sections: cortex and medulla (Fig. 4-2). Each thymic lobule is incompletely surrounded by fibrous septa, and the medullary areas extend continuously from one lobule into others, giving the organ a characteristic "branching" configuration when viewed by low-power microscopy (1,2).

Thymic Cortex

The thymic cortex is the peripheral portion of a thymic lobule and appears darker than the medulla under low-power microscopy (7–15). It has two antigenically distinct types of epithelial cells: the subcapsular and the inner cortical cells admixed with large lymphoid cells (lymphoblasts) and smaller lymphocytes (16–24). Thymic lymphocytes have also been denominated as thymocytes, but the term is now restricted to immature thymic T lymphocytes (16).

The cortical and the medullary epithelial cells of the thymus share several features such as the presence of tonofilaments and desmosomes under electron microscopy and reactivity with antibodies to keratin and monoclonal antibodies such as anti-KiM3 (25).

The subcapsular epithelial cells form an almost continuous row at the periphery of the thymic cortex (25). They have a stellate cytoplasm with a large round to oval

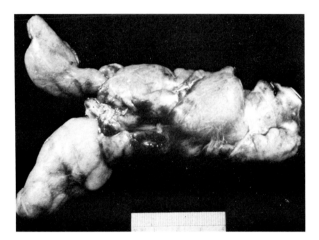

FIG. 4–1. Thymus, showing its typical bilobate pyramidal shape.

nucleus exhibiting a clear chromatin pattern and a medium to large central nucleolus (Fig. 4-3). Ultrastructurally, thymic cortical cells have scanty, peripheral organelles, intermediate filaments, and long cytoplasmic projections covered by basal lamina material (16,26). Subcapsular epithelial cells express strong immunoreactivity with antibodies to class I (A,B,C) and II (DR) HLA antigens, Leu7, and other antigens listed in Table 1 (16). An interesting feature of these cells is their capacity to secrete

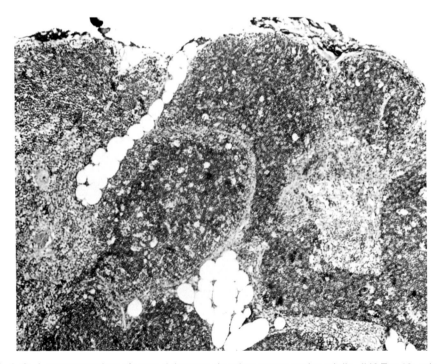

FIG. 4–2. Low-power view of normal thymus showing cortex and medulla. (H&E × 40, original)

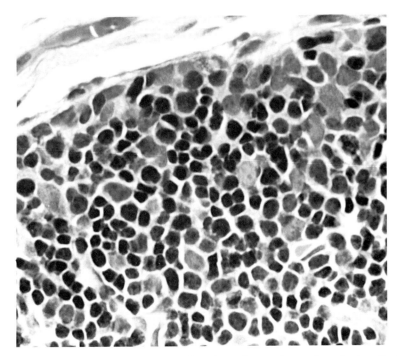

FIG. 4–3. Cortex of a normal thymus showing the subcapsular and cortical epithelial cells admixed with large lymphoid cells. (H&E × 400, original)

TABLE 1. *Epithelial cells of the thymus: antigenic characteristics*

| Antigen | Secretory ("endocrine")* epithelium | | Nonsecretory epithelium | |
	Subcapsular cortical cells	Medullary cells	Inner cortical cells	Hassall's corpuscles
Polyclonal keratin	+	+	+	+ +**
Keratin AE-1	+	−	+	−
Keratin AE-2	−	−	−	+
Keratin AE-3	+	+	+	−
A2B5	+	+	−	−
TE-4	+	+	−	−
Anti-p19	+	+	−	−
HLA Class I	+	+	+	−
HLA-DR	+	−	+	−
TE-3	−	−	+	−
Leu-7	+	−	−	−
PE-35	−	+	−	−

*Immunocytochemical studies have demonstrated intracytoplasmic thymulin, thymosin α-1, thymosin β-3, and thymopoietin in these cells.

A2B5: Monoclonal antibody against complex ganglioside present in neuroendocrine cells and neurons.

TE-4: Monoclonal antibody to thymic epithelial cells.

Anti-p19: Antibody to core protein of the human T cell lymphoma virus (HTLV).

TE-3: Monoclonal antibody to thymic stroma.

Leu-7: Differentiation antigen present also in neuroendocrine cells and human null/killer lymphoid cells.

**Hassall's corpuscles react strongly with antibodies to high molecular weight keratin (AE-2), a finding characteristic of mature epithelial cells.

PE-35: Monoclonal antibody to medullary epithelium.

hormones such as thymosin α-1, thymosin β-3, and thymopoietin, which are able to induce TdT positivity in TdT-prothymocytes derived from the bone marrow (24).

Some large subcapsular cortical epithelial cells of the thymus enclose numerous immature thymocytes with active mitotic activity and are thought to represent the thymic "nurse" cells (24). These cells exhibit immunoreactivity with antibodies to neuropeptides (27).

The inner cortical epithelial cells of the thymus have morphologic features similar to the other cortical cells but exhibit distinct antigenic determinants such as a Leu-7–phenotype and strong immunoreactivity to the monoclonal antibody TE-3 (Fig. 4-4) (Table 1). They lack secretory characteristics (16).

The thymic cortex has medium- or large lymphoblasts with a round nucleus and a narrow cytoplasmic rim that are in close contact with epithelial cells. The nucleus of these thymocytes has an open chromatin structure without a prominent nucleolus (Fig. 4-4). Mitoses are frequent. Thymic lymphoblasts represent up to 5% of thymocytes and exhibit the antigenic characteristics listed in Table 2. The thymic cortex also has smaller, more mature thymocytes with the phenotypic features listed in Table 2. An interesting feature of thymic lymphocytes is the presence of simultaneous T4 and T8 reactivity. Cortical thymocytes comprise the majority (60% to 80%) of thymic lymphoid cells (16).

The thymic cortex has numerous degenerating thymocytes that undergo lympholysis and phagocytosis by cortical macrophages that stain strongly with reagents to α-naphtyl acetate esterase and acid phosphate (16). The presence of phagocytosis

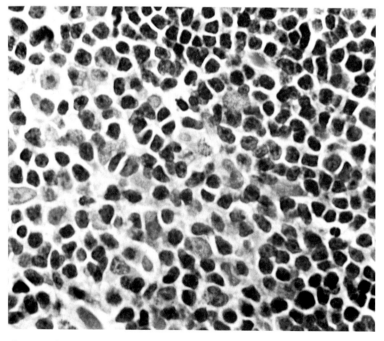

FIG. 4–4. Cortex of a normal thymus showing cortical epithelial cells, lymphoblasts, and smaller lymphocytes. (H&E × 400, original)

TABLE 2. *Antigenic characteristics of thymocytes*

Antigen	Subcapsular thymocytes (0.5–5%)	Cortical thymocytes (60–80%)	Medullary thymocytes (15–20%)
TdT	+	+	−
CD1 (Leu-6)	+	+	−
CD2 (Leu-5)	+	+	+
CD3 (Leu-4)	+	+	+
CD4 (Leu-3a)	+	+	−
CD5 (Leu-1)	+	+	+
CD7 (Leu-9)	+	+	+
CD8 (Leu-2c)	+	+	−
CD14 (Leu-M3)	−	+	−
CD38 (OKT-10)	−	−	+
T200	+	+	+

(From ref. 16.)

becomes prominent in patients with acute thymic involution resulting in a "starry-sky" pattern (see Chapter 5).

Thymic Medulla

The medulla is the central portion of a thymic lobule and appears lighter than the cortex on histologic sections, reflecting the presence of smaller densities of lymphoid cells. It contains characteristic epithelial structures known as Hassall's corpuscles (Fig. 4-5) (7,8). These are complex tubular structures composed of masses of mature

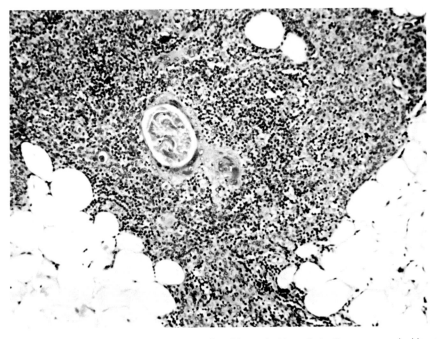

FIG. 4–5. Thymic medulla. Hassall's corpuscle with central keratinization surrounded by reticular epithelial cells admixed with thymocytes. (H&E × 100, original)

epithelial cells forming concentric layers. Hassall's corpuscles exhibit varying degrees of central keratinization and/or calcification and occasionally may become cystic. Cystic corpuscles have a central space containing proteinaceous material and degenerated lymphocytes and eosinophils. The epithelium of Hassall's corpuscles secretes a sulfated acid mucopolysaccharide and is continuous with the medullary reticular cells. Ultrastructurally, the epithelial cells of Hassall's corpuscles have features similar to those of the "reticular" cells present in the cortex and medulla of the thymus, and they exhibit complex interdigitating cell processes bound by prominent desmosomes (Fig. 4-6).

Hassall's corpuscles stain strongly with antibodies to keratin, particularly with a monoclonal antibody to high-molecular keratin (AE-2) that is considered a marker of mature epithelial cells (16,25,27). Immunoglobulins have been described in Hassall's corpuscles (28,29).

The epithelial cells of the thymic medulla have a fusiform shape with an oval or spindle nucleus. The nuclear chromatin is slightly more hyperchromatic than that of cortical epithelial cells (Fig. 4-7). The cytoplasm has numerous tonofilaments, prominent desmosomes, and shorter cytoplasmic projections (16) (Fig. 4-6). Medullary epithelial cells are HLA-DR$^-$, TE-4$^+$, and A2B5$^+$ and exhibit other phenotypic

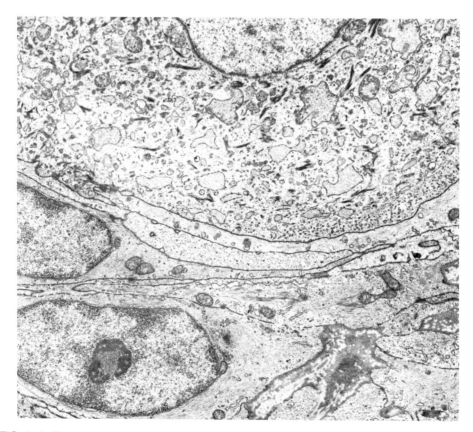

FIG. 4–6. Electron micrograph of Hassall's corpuscle showing thymic medullary epithelial cells with abundant tonofilaments, cytoplasmic processes, and desmosomes. (Courtesy of Dr. H. Sobel, New Jersey.)

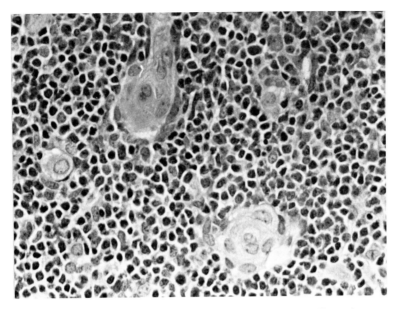

FIG. 4–7. Medulla of a normal thymus showing medullary epithelial cells and mature lymphocytes. (H&E × 200, original)

characteristics listed in Table 1. They also secrete thymosin α-1, thymopoietin, and other thymic hormones (24). Medullary lymphocytes are more mature as expressed by TdT negativity and other phenotypic features listed in Table 2. They represent 15% to 20% of thymic lymphocytes (16).

B Lymphocytes in the Thymus

Although the large majority of thymic lymphoid cells have phenotypic features of T cells, B lymphocytes have been described in the thymus (25,28–30). They are present in germinal centers and as individual B cells. Thymic B lymphocytes are present primarily in the fibrous septa and in the so-called extraparenchymal compartment composed of perivascular spaces, although they have been described within the medulla (16). Intramedullary B cells are particularly prominent in the thymus glands of fetuses, newborns, and children and tend to cluster around Hassall's corpuscles (31).

Immunocytochemical studies have also demonstrated the presence of immunoglobulins in Hassall's corpuscles and in other thymic areas (16). Henry and Anderson (28) demonstrated the presence of IgG, IgA, and IgM in the fetal and adult thymus. In the fetal thymus, IgM cells predominate, while IgG positive cells are more frequent in the adult thymus.

Rare plasma cells can be seen in the connective tissue septa of the thymus and occasionally within the medulla.

The thymic perivascular spaces are difficult to recognize in sections of the normal gland but become prominent in thymomas. They are separated from the thymic parenchyma, comprising the cortex and the medulla, by a basal lamina that can be demonstrated ultrastructurally and by immunocytochemistry with antibodies to laminin and collagen IV (1,8,32,33).

Other Cell Types in the Thymus

In addition to the cell types already described, the thymus has interdigitating reticulum cells, mast cells, eosinophils, neuroendocrine cells, and myoid or striated cells (34–42).

Eosinophils are present in the normal thymus of infants and children but are infrequent in adults (2).

Myoid or striated cells are of great interest because of their potential role in the pathogenesis of myasthenia gravis (13–15,41). They are found in small groups adjacent to Hassall's corpuscles and are more frequent in newborns. They are prominent in the thymus of birds and reptiles but are infrequent in the human thymus. They are more readily identified in the thymus of infants, and they increase in frequency in patients with myasthenia gravis and true thymic hyperplasia (16).

Myoid cells are characterized by an acidophilic cytoplasm that contains cross striations identical to those seen in skeletal muscle. These striations cross react with antisera to actin and myosin, troponin, and acetylcholine receptor (AChR) (41) and have characteristic ultrastructural features (15,41). They exhibit thick actin and myosin myofilaments arranged in a haphazard fashion with focal dense Z-band formation as seen in immature skeletal muscle (8). These striations have, however, no organized sarcomere formation. Myoid cells have no cell-to-cell attachments to reticular epithelial cells.

Several studies have shown that the thymus gland has neuroendocrine functions and is influenced by several hormones (42–47). For example, Geenen and associates (46) have demonstrated the presence in thymic extracts of oxytocin and neurophysin.

Neuroendocrine cells can be readily identified in birds, reptiles, and other animals and have been described in the human thymus (9,16). They may be related embryologically to the C cells of the thyroid gland (16). Cells in the medulla, in the subcapsular epithelium, and, less often, in the cortex exhibit immunoreactivity with antibodies to oxytocin, vasopressin, neurophysin, and other neuropeptides (27,29).

The vasculature of the thymus derives from branches of the internal mammary, inferior thyroid, and pericardiophrenic arteries (48,49). Detailed ultrastructural studies with electron-opaque tracers have demonstrated the presence of a blood–thymus barrier (50).

The thymic innervation derives from the vagus nerve and cervical sympathetic nerves (47).

EMBRYOLOGY

The thymus probably derives from cells of all three germ layers. It arises as paired structures from the endoderm of the third and, to a lesser and inconstant degree, fourth branchial pouches during the sixth intrauterine week (2–5). It is controversial whether the ectoderm of the third branchial clefts also contributes to its origin. The mesoderm contributes its vascular stroma and mesenchymal cells.

The thymus shares a common embryologic origin with the lower pair of parathyroid glands.

From each side of the neck, the embryonal thymic anlagen migrate downward and medially into the anterosuperior mediastinum as epithelial tubules or cords, while the inferior parathyroid glands remain in contact with the lower poles of the thyroid. Only the upper pole of each thymic lobe remains in the neck. The thymic epithelial elements proliferate in the mediastinum, and by the eighth intrauterine week, they lose contact with the branchial clefts.

It is controversial how the primitive epithelial structures of the thymus develop. Hammar (3) maintained that the thymic epithelial cells increase in size and number in an onion-layer fashion and form solid thymic corpuscles that by the 13th to 14th week of intrauterine life become Hassall's corpuscles. Schambacher (4) had a different view. Based on the examination of lymphocyte-depleted thymus glands, he suggested that Hassall's corpuscles derive from a system of discontinuous epithelial tubules whose epithelium proliferates in concentric layers. A study by Shier (5) supports Schambacher's view.

The thymus is an epithelial organ during the second month of intrauterine life, but by the end of this month, the proliferating epithelial tubules and cords become infiltrated by lymphocytes and mesenchymal elements (5).

The origin of thymic lymphocytes has also been the subject of controversy (51). It is now accepted that they derive from migrating bone marrow cells that differentiate and rapidly proliferate in the environment provided by the developing thymic epithelium (51–53). Most thymic lymphocytes have a very short life span and die *in situ*. A few others, however, have a long life span and are seeded into peripheral lymphoid tissues during late fetal and early postnatal life (52).

The origin of thymic myoid cells is unknown. They may be derived from the mesenchyme surrounding the thymic epithelium, or they may arise directly from the epithelial reticular cells (8,15).

The thymus grows rapidly in embryonic life. By the ninth to tenth week of intrauterine life, the two lobes become apposed, and the gland increases in size to reach a mean weight of 15 g at birth (1,54,55). In the neonatal period, the thymus reaches its largest relative size. It continues to grow until puberty to reach a mean weight of 30 to 40 g and then begins a gradual process of involution (54,55).

ECTOPIC THYMIC TISSUE

Small islands of thymic tissue can be found outside the capsule of the gland in the neck, tympanic cavity, different areas of the mediastinum (posterior and anterior compartments and hilum), and the lung (56–58). These islands most likely represent remnants of thymic tissue incorporated in ectopic locations during embryologic development at the time when the thymic anlagen migrate from the branchial clefts into the mediastinum (2).

In rare instances, these islands of ectopic thymic tissue become clinically important since they can become hyperplastic, cystic, or neoplastic (56).

FUNCTIONAL ASPECTS

The role of the thymus as an important part of the immune system has been recognized only in the last three decades after experiments by Miller and associates (58–60) and other investigators demonstrated in the 1960s that the removal of the gland from neonatal mice rendered the animals severely immune deficient and prone to infections. Neonatal thymectomy also resulted in lymphopenia in blood and thoracic duct lymph and in marked lymphoid depletion in the paracortical areas of lymph nodes (60). Additional experiments with thymectomy preceded by sublethal irradiation demonstrated similar defects in adult mice. Moreover, the immune defects produced by these experimental conditions could be restored by grafts of thymic epithelial anlage or of thymic tissue enclosed in cell-impermeable Millipore® diffusion chambers, by infusion of thymic lymphocytes, and by the injection of thymic extracts (60,61).

These experimental data were also supported by the report by Di George and associates (62) in 1967 of patients with congenital absence of the thymus and immunologic abnormalities such as a marked impairment in their capacity to develop delayed hypersensitivity reactions and ability to reject allografts.

Currently, the thymus is viewed as one of the two primary or central lymphoid organs. As such, it is not primarily involved in antibody production, and its development does not appear to be dependent on antigenic stimulation (61).

The thymic epithelial cells create a microenvironment that plays a key role in T-cell maturation (61,63–68). They induce the proliferation and differentiation of lymphoid precursor cells into postthymic T cells through direct contact and through the secretion of thymic hormones (19). In turn, the thymocytes induce thymic epithelial cell proliferation through the secretion of interleukin-1 (IL-1) and other cytokines in tissue culture models (69). As part of this interaction between thymic epithelial cells and thymocytes, there is a process of adhesion of both cell types, mediated through adhesion molecules such as ICAM-1 and LFA-1 that are expressed on the surface of the epithelial cells (70).

The gland appears to function in two phases. During the first phase, undifferentiated lymphoid cells migrating from the bone marrow reach the thymus and establish close contact with the thymic epithelium and its microenvironment (61,71–88). During this phase, lymphoid cells acquire characteristics of T cells such as the capacity to form rosettes with sheep erythrocytes. During the second phase, these T cells migrate to peripheral lymphoid organs, where they are relatively short lived unless exposed to thymic hormones produced by the thymic epithelium. These hormones are a necessary requirement for the differentiation and survival of these postthymic populations of T cells (78,79).

THYMIC HORMONES

The thymus gland produces several polypeptide hormones that are thought to regulate specific immunological roles of lymphoid cells and induce lymphocyte differentiation *in vivo* and *in vitro* (61,81,89–91). A few of these polypeptides have been characterized chemically, and at least three of them have been synthesized (81). The best-known thymic hormones are thymosin fraction V, thymosin α-1, thymopoietin II, thymic humoral factor (THF), thymulin, and serum thymic factor (FTS) (61,44).

The secretion of these peptides is thought to be modulated by the neuroendocrine network, comprising the thyroid, hypophisis, adrenals, gonads, and other glands (44,91–93).

These hormones exert their physiologic effects on so-called postthymic lymphoid precursor cells found in the neonatal spleen and on mature T cells through cellular processes that involve binding to specific membrane receptors, interaction with adenylate cyclase, and an increase in GMP levels (81).

A. Goldstein and associates (91) isolated from calf thymus the first thymic hormone, thymosin, in 1966. This protein fraction has lymphopoietic activity. In 1972, thymosin was further purified and characterized, and one of its active components was isolated: thymosin fraction V (61,81,93). This component of thymosin is a family of 20 or more heat-stable polypeptides with molecular weights ranging from 1,000 to 5,000 that are divided into three regions according to their isoelectric point (pI): α region (pI below 5.5), β (pI 5.5–7), and γ (pI above 7). Thymosin α-1 consists of 28 amino acid residues, has a molecular weight of 3,108, and has been synthesized in the laboratory. It has 10 to 100 times more biologic activity than thymosin fraction V (61).

Thymosin can induce multiple functional changes in lymphocytes, such as production of macrophage migratory inhibitory factor (MIF), increased formation of antibody-forming cells, development of functional suppressor T cells, and induction of TdT formation by immature lymphoid cells (81). Thymosin is also capable of restoring certain immune functions in thymus-deprived or immunodeficient patients or animals (61,81). For example, it increases cytotoxic–suppressor T-cell numbers and stimulates the development of delayed hypersensitivity reactions in immunosuppressed children and cancer patients (94,95).

Thymopoietin was isolated by G. Goldstein and associates (88) as a polypeptide fraction present in calf thymus that interfered with neuromuscular transmission. It is a polypeptide composed of 49 amino acids and is present in two forms: thymopoietin I and II. These two forms differ by only two amino acids (61).

Thymopoietin has been synthesized chemically and is known to be capable of inducing the production of various T-cell antigens *in vitro* and restoring immunological functions of aged mice (81). Its probable role in the pathogenesis of myasthenia gravis is discussed in Chapter 5.

Thymic humoral factor (THF) was isolated by Trainin and associates and is a small peptide with a molecular weight of 3,230 and 31 amino acid residues (81). It is capable of restoring the immunocompetence of lymphoid cells from neonatal athymic mice and of inducing these cells in culture to participate in mixed lymphocyte reactions, develop inducer activities, and acquire graft-versus-host capabilities. Thymic humoral factor also restores cellular immunocompetence to patients suffering from primary or secondary immunodeficiencies and has been used experimentally in the treatment of immune disorders (61).

Serum thymic factor (FTS) was isolated by Bach (81). It is a nonapeptide with a molecular weight of 857. It is capable of inducing lymphoblasts to form T-cell antigens such as θ, Ly 1-2-3, and TL (81). It also retards the growth of Moloney sarcoma virus-induced tumors *in vivo* and enhances T-cell-mediated cytotoxicity in thymectomized mice (81).

Thymic hormones have been under intense investigation during the last decade. Indeed, several hormones such as thymosin and FTS have been localized to the thymic epithelium in immunocytochemical studies (96,97). In addition, thymosin, FTS, and THF have been utilized in clinical trials for the treatment of patients with immunodeficiency, malignancy, viral and fungal infections, and autoimmune disorders (61). Results from these trials are encouraging but difficult to evaluate, given the small number of patients treated with hormonal therapy and the complex nature of their clinical problems.

THE THYMUS IN THE AGING INDIVIDUAL

The thymus undergoes marked morphologic and physiologic changes with aging (55,98,99). The size of the gland increases from birth until puberty and decreases later in life until the age of 50 (55). Histologically, the involuting thymus exhibits a marked decrease in lymphocyte and Hassall's corpuscle numbers, epithelial elements become clumped, cystic changes appear, secretory granules are depleted, and tissues are replaced by lipid-laden macrophages and adipose cells (Fig. 4-8) (2).

However, the widespread belief that the thymus disappears in adult life is no longer accepted, and several anatomic studies have shown that the gland, although atrophic, persists throughout life (Fig. 4-9) (53).

Approximate thymic weights at different ages are 12 to 15 g at birth, 30 to 40 g at puberty, and 10 to 15 g at age 60 (55). The thymic size varies a great deal in different individuals, and at any given age a patient may have a gland that is either larger or smaller than expected from published tables.

A detailed anatomic study of human thymus glands at necropsy by Kendall and associates (55) has demonstrated a gradual age-related decrease in thymus wet weight after puberty and a significant increase in extractable lipid up to the age of 50, supporting the notion of replacement of thymic elements by adipose tissue. This study reported significantly lower wet and lipid thymic weights in patients with chronic stressful conditions. By contrast, individuals dying from cardiovascular disease or asphyxia had higher weights than those found in the normal population.

The thymus retrogresses functionally with increasing age, and these changes are paralleled by a decline of normal immune functions in older individuals (61).

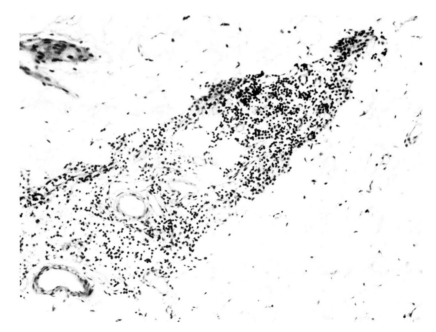

FIG. 4–8. Involuting thymus in adult patient. Thymus shows marked decrease in lymphoepithelial elements and increased adipose tissue. (H&E × 40, original)

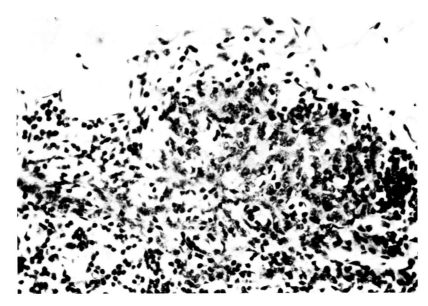

FIG. 4–9. Involuting thymus in adult patient. Persistent reticular epithelial cells admixed with scanty lymphocytes. (H&E × 100, original)

Tissue culture studies by Oosterom and Kater (98,99) have demonstrated changes in the secretory activities of thymic epithelial cells with age. Cells from individuals older than 30 years appear to have lower hormone secretory capabilities than thymic epithelial cells from younger patients. Other studies have shown declines in the serum levels of thymopoietin and FTS with aging. These hormones become nondetectable in normal serum by age 50 (81).

REFERENCES

1. Rosai J, Levine GD: Tumors of the thymus, in: *Atlas of Tumor Pathology*, Ser 2, Fasc 13. Washington, Armed Forces Institute of Pathology, 1976.
2. Henry K: The thymus gland, in Symmers WSTC (ed): *Systemic Pathology*, ed 2, vol 2. Edinburgh, Churchill Livingstone, 1978, pp 894–924.
3. Hammar JA: Zur Histogenese und Involution der Thymus-druse. *Anat Anz* 1905;37:23–31; 1906;39:41–89.
4. Schambacher A: Uber die Persistenz vom DrusenKanalen in der Thymus in ihre Beziehung zur Entstehung der Hassallschen Korperchen. *Virchows Arch [Pathol Anat]* 1903;172:368–394.
5. Shier KJ: The thymus according to Schambacher: medullary ducts and reticular epithelium of thymus and thymomas. *Cancer* 1981;48:1183–1199.
6. Shier KJ: The morphology of the epithelial thymus. Observations on lymphocyte-depleted and fetal thymus. *Lab Invest* 1963;12:316–326.
7. Bearman RM, Levine GD, Bensch KG: The ultrastructure of the normal human thymus. A study of 36 cases. *Anat Rec* 1978;190:755–761.
8. Bloodworth JMB Jr, Hiratsuka H, Hickey RC, et al: Ultrastructure of the human thymus, thymic tumors and myasthenia gravis. *Pathol Ann* 1975;10:329–391.
9. Hackanson R, Larsson LI, Sundler F: Peptide and amine producing endocrine-like cells in the chicken thymus. A chemical, histochemical and electron microscopic study. *Histochemistry* 1974;39:25–34.
10. Hoshino T, Kukita A, Sato S: Cells containing Birbeck granules (Langerhans' cells granules) in the human thymus. *J Electron Microsc* 1970;19:271–276.
11. Vetters JM, Macadam RF: Fine structural evidence for hormone secretion by the human thymus. *J Clin Pathol* 1973;26:194–197.

12. Haar JL: Light and electron microscopy of the human fetal thymus. *Anat Rec* 1974;179:463–476.
13. Hayward AR: Myoid cells in the human foetal thymus. *J Pathol* 1972;106:45–48.
14. Van de Velde RL, Friedman NB: Thymic myoid cells and myasthenia gravis. *Am J Pathol* 1970;59:347–367.
15. Drenckhahn D, von Gaudecker B, Müller-Hermelink HK, et al: Myosin and actin containing cells in the human postnatal thymus. Ultrastructural and immuno histochemical findings in normal thymus and in myasthenia gravis. *Virchows Arch [Cell Pathol]* 1979;32:33–45.
16. Suster S, Rosai J: Histology of the human thymus. *Am J Surg Pathol* 1990;14:284–303.
17. Izon DJ, Boyd RL: The cytoarchitecture of the human thymus detected by monoclonal antibodies. *Hum Immunol* 1990;27:16–32.
18. Kampinga J, Berges S, Boyd RL, et al: Thymic epithelial antibodies: immunohistological analysis and introduction of nomenclature. *Thymus* 1989;13:165–173.
19. Laster AJ, Itoh T, Palker TJ, et al: The human thymic microenvironment: thymic epithelium contains specific keratins associated with early and late stages of epidermal keratinocyte maturation. *Differentiation* 1986;31:67–77.
20. Savino W, Dardenne M: Immunohistochemical studies on a human thymic epithelial cell subset defined by the anti-cytokeratin 18 monoclonal antibody. *Cell Tissue Res* 1988;254:225–231.
21. Timens W, Boes A, Rozeboom-Uiterwijk T, et al: Immuno-architecture of human fetal lymphoid tissues. *Virchows Arch [Cell Pathol]* 1988;413:563–571.
22. von Gaudecker B: The development of the human thymus microenvironment. *Curr Top Pathol* 1986;1–37.
23. von Gaudecker B, Larche M, Schuurman HJ, et al: Analysis of the fine distribution of thymic epithelial microenvironmental molecules by immuno-electron microscopy. *Thymus* 1989;13:187–194.
24. Janossy G, Bofill M, Trejdosiewicz LK, et al: Cellular differentiation of lymphoid subpopulations and their microenvironments in the human thymus. *Curr Top Pathol* 1986;89–124.
25. Henry K: The thymus—what's new? *Histopathology* 1989;14:537–548.
26. Cohen-Kaminsky S, Berrih-Aknin S, Savino W, et al: Immunodetection of the thymic epithelial P19 antigen in cultures of normal and pathological human thymic epithelium. *Thymus* 1987;9:225–238.
27. Geenen V, Robert F, Degresne MP, et al: Neuroendocrinology of the thymus. *Horm Res* 1989;31:81–84.
28. Henry L, Anderson G: Immunoglobulins in Hassall's corpuscles of the human thymus. *J Anat* 1990;168:185–197.
29. Hofmann WJ, Momburg F, Moller P: Thymic medullary cells expressing B lymphocyte antigens. *Hum Pathol* 1988;19:1280–1287.
30. Wirt DP, Grogan TM, Nagle RB, et al: A comprehensive immunotopographic map of human thymus. *J Histochem Cytochem* 1988;36:1–12.
31. Isaacson PG, Norton AJ, Addis BJ: The human thymus contains a novel population of B lymphocytes. *Lancet* 1987;2:1488–1491.
32. Kendall MD: The morphology of perivascular spaces in the thymus. *Thymus* 1989;13:157–164.
33. Karttunen T: Basement membrane proteins and reticulin in a normal thymus and the thymus in myasthenia gravis. *Virchows Arch [Cell Pathol]* 1987;411:245–252.
34. Jung LK, Haynes BF, Nakamura S, et al: Expression of early activation antigen (CD69) during human thymic development. *Clin Exp Immunol* 1990;81:466–474.
35. Landry D, Lafontaine M, Cossette M, et al: Human thymic dendritic cells. Characterization, isolation and functional assays. *Immunology* 1988;65:135–142.
36. Lobach DF, Haynes BF: Ontogeny of the human thymus during fetal development. *J Clin Immunol* 1987;7:81–97.
37. Milan J, Barbijeri M, Kovacevic D, et al: Identification of neuroendocrine oxytocic activity of the human fetal thymus. *Thymus* 1990;15:181–185.
38. Miller JF: The thymus and its role in immunity. *Chem Immunol* 1990;49:51–68.
39. Moll UM, Lane BL, Robert F, et al: The neuroendocrine thymus. Abundant occurrence of oxytocin-vasopressin, and neurophysin-like peptides in epithelial cells. *Histochemistry* 1988;89:385–390.
40. Ruco LP, Rosati S, Monardo F, et al: Macrophages and interdigitating reticulum cells in normal thymus and in thymoma: an immunohistochemical study. *Histopathology* 1989;14:37–45.
41. Sato T, Tamaoki N: Myoid cells in the human thymus and thymoma revealed by three different immunohistochemical markers for striated muscle. *Acta Pathol Jpn* 1989;39:509–519.
42. Savino W, Gagnerault MC, Bach JF, et al: Neuroendocrine control of thymic hormonal production. II. Stimulatory effects of endogenous opioids on thymulin production by cultured human and murine thymic epithelial cells. *Life Sci* 1990;46:1687–1697.
43. Aubray J, Cohen-Kaminsky S, Berrih-Aknin S: Differential expression of carcinoembryonic antigens and non-cross-reacting antigens in the human thymus. Analysis on frozen sections and cultured epithelial cells using monoclonal antibodies. *Thymus* 1990;15:107–123.

44. Dardenne M, Savino W, Gagnerault MC, et al: Neuroendocrine control of thymic hormonal production. I. Prolactin stimulates *in vivo* and *in vitro* the production of thymulin by human and murine thymic epithelial cells. *Endocrinology* 1989;125:3–12.

45. Fukayama M, Hayashi Y, Shiozawa Y, et al: Human chorionic gonadotropin in the thymus. An immunocytochemical study on discordant expression of subunits. *Am J Pathol* 1990;136:123–129.

46. Geenen V, Legros JJ, Franchimont P, et al: The neuroendocrine thymus: coexistence of oxytocin and neurophysin in the human thymus. *Science* 1986;232:508–511.

47. Nilsson B, Ferno M, Von Schoultz B: Estrogen and progesterone receptors in the human thymus. *Gynecol Obstet Invest* 1990;29:289–291.

48. Ghali WM, Abdel-Rahman S, Nagib M, et al: Intrinsic innervation and vasculature of pre- and post-natal human thymus. *Acta Anat (Basel)* 1980;108:115–123.

49. Bearman RM, Bensch KG, Levine GD: The normal human thymic vasculature: an ultrastructural study. *Anat Rec* 1975;183:485–498.

50. Raviola E, Karnovsky MJ: Evidence for a blood–thymus barrier using electron-opaque tracers. *J Exp Med* 1972;136:466–498.

51. Bach JF: B and T lymphocytes, in Bach JF (ed): *Immunology*. New York, John Wiley & Sons, 1978, pp 57–91.

52. Stutman O: Two main features of T cell development: thymus traffic and postthymic maturation, in Stutman O (ed): *Contemporary Topics in Immunobiology*, vol 7. New York: Plenum Press, 1977, pp 1–45.

53. Cantor H, Weissman I: Development and function of subpopulations of thymocytes and T lymphocytes. *Prog Allergy* 1976;20:1–64.

54. Boyd E: The weight of the thymus gland in health and in disease. *Am J Dis Child* 1932;43:1162–1214.

55. Kendall MD, Johnson HRM, Singh J: The weight of the human thymus gland at necropsy. *J Anat* 1980;131:483–497.

56. Masaoka A, Nagaoka Y, Kotake Y: Distribution of thymic tissue at the anterior mediastinum. Current procedures in thymectomy. *J Thorac Cardiovasc Surg* 1975;70:747–754.

57. Barr RJ, Santa Cruz DJ, Pearl RM: Dermal thymus. A light microscopic and immunohistochemical study. *Arch Dermatol* 1989;125:1681–1684.

58. Miller JF: Immunological function of the thymus. *Lancet* 1961;2:748–749.

59. Miller JF, Osoba D: Current concepts of the immunological function of the thymus. *Physiol Rev* 1967;47:437–520.

60. Miller JF: Experimental thymology has come of age. *Thymus* 1979;1:3–25.

61. Pahwa R, Ikehara S, Pahwa SG, et al: Thymic function in man. *Thymus* 1979;1:27–58.

62. Di George AM, Lischner HW, Dacou C, et al: Absence of the thymus. *Lancet* 1967;1:1387.

63. Dezutter-Dambuyant C, Staquet MJ, Schmitt D, et al: The effect of trypsin on CD1a molecule of human thymocytes. *Thymus* 1990;15:213–221.

64. Groh V, Fabbi M, Strominger JL: Maturation or differentiation of human thymocyte precursors *in vitro? Proc Natl Acad Sci USA* 1990;87:5973–5977.

65. Singer KH, Haynes BF: Epithelial-thymocyte interactions in human thymus. *Hum Immunol* 1987;20:127–144.

66. Swerdlow SH, Angermeier PA, Hartman AL: Intrathymic ontogeny of the T cell receptor associated CD3 (T3) antigen. *Lab Invest* 1988;58:421–427.

67. Steinmann GG: Changes in the human thymus during aging. *Curr Top Pathol* 1986;75:43–88.

68. Nakahama M, Mohri N, Mori S, et al: Immunohistochemical and histometrical studies of the human thymus with special emphasis on age-related changes in medullary epithelial and dendritic cells. *Virchows Arch [Cell Pathol]* 1990;58:245–251.

69. Savino W, Dardenne M: Thymic hormone-containing cells. VIII. Effects of colchicine, cytochalasin B, and monensin on secretion of thymulin by cultured human thymic epithelial cells. *J Histochem Cytochem* 1986;34:1719–1723.

70. Galy AH, Hadden EM, Touraine JL, et al: Effects of cytokines on human thymic epithelial cell proliferation and change in morphology. *Cell Immunol* 1989;124:13–27.

71. Gomez-Marquez J, Dosil M, Segade F, et al: Thymosin-beta 4 gene. Preliminary characterization and expression in tissues, thymic cells, and lymphocytes. *J Immunol* 1989;143:2740–2744.

72. Christensson B, Matell G, Biberfeld P: Immunological studies on human thymus. Occurrence and distribution of immunoglobulin and immunological receptors in myasthenia gravis and control patients. *Acta Med Scand* 1980;208:161–168.

73. Pahwa S, Pahwa R, Goldstein G, et al: Immunoregulatory influence of thymic epithelium and thymopoietin on human B-lymphocyte differentiation. *Cell Immunol* 1980;56:40–46.

74. Piantelli M, Musiani P, Lauriola L, et al: Lymphocyte subpopulations in non-neoplastic thymus from myasthenia gravis patients. *Clin Exp Immunol* 1980;41:19–24.

75. Galili U, Polliack A, Okon E, et al: Human prothymocytes. Membrane properties, differentiation patterns, glucocorticoid sensitivity and ultrastructural features. *J Exp Med* 1980;152:796–807.

76. von-Gaudecker B, Müller-Hermelink HK: Ontogeny and organization of the stationary non-lymphoid cells in the human thymus. *Cell Tissue Res* 1980;207:287–306.
77. Haines KA, Siskind GW: Ontogeny of T cell function. I. Acquisition of helper cell activity by the thymus. *J Immunol* 1980;124:1878–1882.
78. Janossy G, Thomas JA, Bollum FJ, et al: The human thymic microenvironment: an immunohistologic study. *J Immunol* 1980;125:202–212.
79. Papiernik M, Bach JF: Postnatal development of T cells. I. Study of the respective contribution of thymic cellular export, thymic humoral function and T cell environment. *J Immunol* 1979;123:2311–2315.
80. Jenkinson EJ, Owen JJT, Aspinall R: Lymphocyte differentiation and major histocompatibility complex antigen expression in the embryonic thymus. *Nature* 1980;284:177–179.
81. Bach J-F: Thymic hormones. *J Immunopharmacol* 1979;1:277–310.
82. Musiani P, Lauriola L, Carbone A, et al: Lymphocyte subsets in human thymus: expression of IgM-Fc receptor by peanut agglutinin positive and negative thymocytes. *Thymus* 1981;2:225–233.
83. Shirai T, Miyata M, Nakase A, et al: Lymphocyte subpopulation in neoplastic and non-neoplastic thymus and in blood of patients with myasthenia gravis. *Clin Exp Immunol* 1976;26:118–123.
84. Haaijman JJ, Micklem HS, Ledbetter JA, et al: T cell ontogeny. Organ location of maturing populations as defined by surface antigen markers is similar in neonates and adults. *J Exp Med* 1981;153:605–614.
85. Wagner H, Hardt C, Bartlett R, et al: Intrathymic differentiation of cytotoxic T lymphocyte (CTL) precursors. I. The CTL immunocompetence of peanut-agglutinin-positive (cortical) and negative (medullary) Lyt 123 thymocytes. *J Immunol* 1980;125:2532–2538.
86. Bhan AK, Reinherz EL, Poppema S, et al: Location of T cell and major histocompatibility complex antigens in the human thymus. *J Exp Med* 1980;152:771–782.
87. Janossy G, Tidman N, Papageorgiou ES, et al: Distribution of T lymphocyte subsets in the human bone marrow and thymus: an analysis with monoclonal antibodies. *J Immunol* 1981;126:1608–1613.
88. Goldstein G, Lau CY: Immunoregulation by thymopoietin. *J Supramol Struct* 1980;14:397–403.
89. Galili U, Schlesinger M: Subpopulations of human thymus cells differing in their capacity to form stable E-rosettes and in their immunologic reactivity. *J Immunol* 1975;115:827–833.
90. Moretta L, Ferrarini M, Cooper MD: Characterization of human T-cell subpopulations as defined by specific receptors for immunoglobulins, in Warner NL, Cooper MD (eds): *Contemporary Topics in Immunobiology*, vol 8. New York, Plenum Press, 1978, pp 19–53.
91. Goldstein AL, Slater FD, White A: Preparation, assay and partial purification of a thymic lymphocytopoietic factor (thymosin). *Proc Natl Acad Sci USA* 1966;56:1010–1017.
92. Fabris N, Mocchegiani E, Mariotti S, et al: Thyroid-thymus interactions during development and aging. *Horm Res* 1989;31:85–89.
93. Goldstein G: Isolation of bovine thymin: a polypeptide hormone of the thymus. *Nature* 1974;274:11–14.
94. Lavastida MT, Goldstein AL, Daniels JC: Thymosin administrators in autoimmune disorders. *Thymus* 1981;2:287–295.
95. Wara DW, Goldstein AL, Doyle W, et al: Thymosin activity in patients with cellular immunodeficiency. *N Engl J Med* 1975;292:70–74.
96. Dalakas MC, Engel WK, McLure JE, et al: Immunocytochemical localization of thymosin-alpha$_1$ in thymic epithelial cells of normal and myasthenia gravis patients and in thymic cultures. *J Neurol Sci* 1981;50:239–247.
97. Schmitt D, Monier JC, Dardenne M, et al: Cytoplasmic localization of FTS *(facteur thymique serique)* in thymic epithelial cells. An immunoelectromicroscopical study. *Thymus* 1980;2:177–186.
98. Oosterom R, Kater L: The thymus in the aging individual. I. Mitogen responsiveness of human thymocytes. *Clin Immunol Immunopathol* 1981;18:187–194.
99. Oosterom R, Kater L: The thymus in the aging individual. II. Thymic epithelial function *in vitro* in aging and in thymus pathology. *Clin Immunol Immunopathol* 1981;18:195–202.

5

Pathology of Nonneoplastic Conditions of the Thymus

THYMIC INVOLUTION

The thymus undergoes a normal process of involution with aging that starts approximately after puberty and is completed by age 40 (1,2). Involution with marked reduction in the weight of the gland can also occur as a response to stress, the so-called accidental, acute, or stress involution of the thymus (3,4). This process is mediated by endogenous corticosteroid secretion, as demonstrated by Selye (3). Acute involution can be followed radiologically and is associated with hyaline membrane disease in newborns, trauma, infection, and/or radiotherapy (4).

Microscopically, the thymus in acute involution shows widespread lympholysis that is more prominent in the cortex. Macrophages become prominent, giving the gland a typical "starry-sky" appearance (Fig. 5-1). Van Baarlen and associates (5,6) have reported that the degree of acute thymic involution in infancy and childhood is a reliable marker for the duration of the acute illness. Immunohistologic studies have demonstrated that in the acutely involuted thymus the epithelial network remains unchanged, while there is a progressive loss of immature proliferating lymphoid cortical cells and medullary interdigitating cells (6).

In situations of chronic stress, the gland undergoes marked involution with complete loss of differentiation between the cortex and the medulla. The thymus remains as two irregular lobes composed mostly of adipose tissue with occasional perivascular spindle epithelial cells, scanty lymphocytes, and focal elongated cystic Hassall's corpuscles lined with squamous epithelium (Fig. 5-2).

Seemayer and Bolande (7) have reported a peculiar form of involution mimicking thymic dysplasia in a premature infant with transfusion-induced graft-versus-host disease.

THYMIC HYPERPLASIA

The concept of thymic hyperplasia has been the subject of controversy since Paltauf proposed his concept of "status thymicolymphaticus" in 1889 (8,9). His theory that diffuse enlargement of lymphoid tissues and the thymus is a predisposing factor in sudden death has been discarded. Hyperplasia of the thymus is currently divided into two types based on morphologic criteria (9):

1. True thymic hyperplasia (TTH) is characterized by an increase in the size and weight of a gland that retains a normal morphology for age. Included in this type

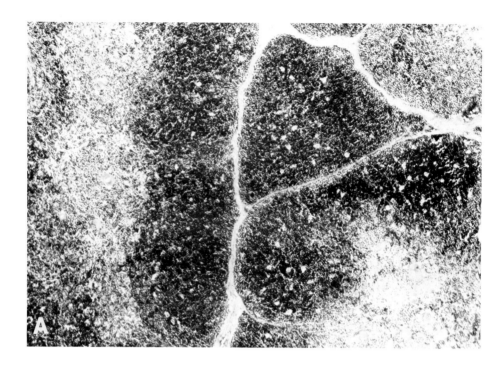

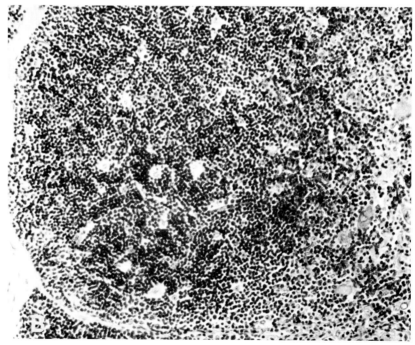

FIG. 5–1. **A:** Acute thymic involution. The gland shows a typical "starry-sky" appearance. (H&E, × 40, original) **B:** Higher magnification showing multiple histiocytes in "starry-sky" areas. (H&E × 100, original)

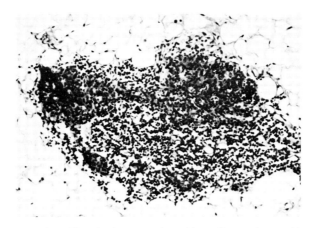

FIG. 5–2. Thymic involution. Thymic tissue replaced by adipose tissue. Hassall's corpuscles are absent. (H&E × 40, original)

are two rare clinicopathologic forms of hyperplasia: (a) thymic hyperplasia with massive enlargement and (b) thymic rebound after treatment of childhood tumors (10–16).

2. Lymphoid hyperplasia (LH), or follicular hyperplasia is defined by the presence of lymphoid follicles with germinal centers in a thymus gland of normal or abnormal size and/or weight. The germinal centers develop in the thymic medulla, and the gland is usually of normal size.

Patients with combined TTH and LH have been described (15,17).

The diagnosis of TTH is difficult to establish unless the size and weight of the gland are compared with tables of thymic weight in relation to age (Table 1) (18). These tables are based, however, on data obtained in autopsy studies in which values from different patients classified as "normal" varied considerably. This variability should be taken into consideration in establishing the diagnosis of TTH in a given patient. For example, a study by Kendall and associates (18) has demonstrated that a large number of thymic weights at any age can be larger or smaller than those expected from the standard data of Young and Turnbull (8) presented in Table 1. Therefore, the thymic weight has to be considered in conjunction with morphometric data regarding the relative proportions of lymphoepithelial, vascular, and adipose

TABLE 1. *Thymic weight and age*

Age group (years)	Thymic mean weights (g)
0–1	24.77
1–6	23.30
6–11	28.70
11–16	33.91
16–21	20.50
21–26	18.38
26–31	14.90
36–46	13.98
56–66	12.65

From Young and Turnbull (8), with permission.

tissues present in the gland. Judd and Welch (15) have proposed to utilize a cutoff value of 2 standard deviation above the mean weight for age as the upper limit of normal thymus.

Thymic Hyperplasia with Massive Enlargement

There are several documented cases in the literature of patients presenting with massive enlargement of the thymus (19–22). Approximately 55% of these patients present with an asymptomatic mediastinal mass, and the other 45% present with respiratory distress, chest pain, and/or other signs secondary to compression of mediastinal structures (14). Patients with massive enlargement of the thymus do not have an associated autoimmune disorder or myasthenia gravis and frequently have peripheral lymphocytosis (14). In these instances, the problem is usually not a determination of whether the gland is hyperplastic or not but whether the patient has a thymoma (19). The glands of some patients with massive hyperplasia grossly exhibit the typical bilobate shape of the thymus; however, in others the lobulation of the gland cannot be readily recognized (14). The thymic glands are markedly enlarged and have varied in size from 120 to 950 g (14). Histologically, the thymic architecture is well preserved, and germinal centers are absent. Judd and associates (15,17) have demonstrated (utilizing antibodies to myoglobin and desmin) the presence of myoid cell in TTH and in LH.

Morphologic criteria that are helpful to distinguish massive hyperplasia from thymomas include the lack of clear distinction between cortical and medullary areas and the paucity of Hassall's corpuscles in thymomas. These tumors also have, in most instances, a characteristic low-power-microscopy pattern of islands of lymphoepithelial tissue separated by thick, irregular fibrous trabecula. In small biopsies, however, this distinction may be difficult.

Another form of thymic hyperplasia recently reported is that occurring in children treated for malignancies such as Hodgkin's disease (23–25). This form of thymic hyperplasia may simulate radiologically a recurrence of the original neoplasm. Shin and Ho (26) suggested that this unusual form of diffuse thymic hyperplasia probably represents an immunologic rebound phenomenon that can be used clinically as a favorable prognostic sign of successful control of the malignant neoplasm.

Rare instances of thymic hyperplasia have also been described in children treated for hypothyroidism, in patients with sarcoidosis, and in infants with Beckwith-Wiedemann syndrome and pulmonary hypoplasia (11,27,28).

Lymphoid Hyperplasia

Lymphoid or follicular hyperplasia is characterized by the presence of germinal centers in the medullary areas of the thymus irrespective of the size and/or weight of the gland (Fig. 5-3) (29,30).

There is controversy regarding the significance of germinal centers in the thymus. Indeed, their incidence in different autopsy series varies from 2% to 51% (31–34). In the normal thymus, however, germinal centers are small and scanty and tend to occur in the fibrous septa of the gland and the medulla (34).

Lymphoid hyperplasia of the thymus has been the subject of numerous studies because of its association with autoimmune diseases such as myasthenia gravis, sys-

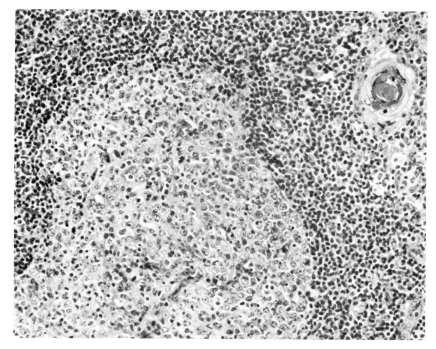

FIG. 5–3. Follicular hyperplasia of the thymus. The thymus has a well-formed germinal center. (H&E × 100, original)

temic lupus erythematosus, scleroderma, and rheumatoid arthritis (2,35–39). It can also be seen in patients with endocrine disorders such as hyperthyroidism, Addison's disease, acromegaly, and in cases of liver disease (40,41). The thymic germinal centers in those conditions are similar to those encountered in lymph nodes. They contain large amounts of immunoglobulins, occur most frequently in the thymic medulla, and are accompanied by its expansion with development of a sharp corticomedullary junction that can be demonstrated with reticulum stains as suggested by Rosai and Levine (2).

The density, size, and configuration of germinal centers in lymphoid hyperplasia of the thymus varies considerably from patient to patient and in different histologic slides from a single individual (42). These parameters can be quantitated utilizing simple morphometric techniques (29).

THE THYMUS IN DISORDERS OF THE IMMUNE SYSTEM

The thymus is one of the primary lymphoid organs and is essential for the development of a normal immune system. Failure in the development of the gland results in or is associated with various immunodeficiency syndromes, which are listed in Table 2 (43–56).

A detailed review of the pathology of immunodeficiency syndromes is beyond the scope of this volume. However, the surgical pathologist needs to become acquainted with the various pathologic changes present in the thymus of patients with immune deficiency, as these individuals may undergo thymic biopsy to characterize the na-

TABLE 2. *Cysts of the thymus*

Congenital
Inflammatory
  Syphilis (Dubois abscess)
  Tuberculosis
  Hydatidosis
Neoplastic
  Cystic thymoma
  Cystic teratoma
  Lymphangioma

ture of their immunologic defect, and determine whether they will respond to immunologic reconstitution or other therapeutic modalities (43).

Indeed, Borzy and associates (44) have demonstrated that thymic biopsy through an extrapleural cervical approach is a valuable procedure in the evaluation of patients with severe immune deficiency.

The Thymus in Congenital Immune Deficiencies

The pathologic changes in the thymus of patients with congenital immune deficiencies vary from complete absence or severe hypoplasia of the gland to syndromes in which the gland is smaller than expected for age but has a normal microscopic morphology (43–45). A small thymus may also exhibit abnormal histologic features and be dysplastic.

Thymic dysplasia is characterized by the presence of a small, rudimentary gland containing only epithelial elements, scant or absent Hassall's corpuscles, and no thymocytes.

Clinicopathologic Forms of Immunodeficiency

Reticular dysgenesis is the most severe form of immune deficiency. This rare condition results from a failure of development of bone marrow stem cells and is characterized by the presence of a vestigial thymus, lymphopenia, granulocytopenia, and death of the patient *in utero* or in the newborn period (43).

Hypogammaglobulinemia of the Swiss type (Glanzmann–Riniker disease) is a rare autosomal recessive disease presenting with severe thymic hypoplasia or dysplasia (36,47,48). Infants with this disorder exhibit total absence of lymphocytes and Hassall's corpuscles in the thymus and die, usually within a few years after birth, with severe bacterial, viral, fungal, and/or protozoal infections. This disease is attributed to a failure in the development of lymphoid stem cells with the resulting lack of thymic lymphocytes and marked hypoplasia of peripheral lymphoid tissues (43). Studies have demonstrated the failure of the thymic anlage to descend from the neck into the superoanterior mediastinum in patients with hypogammaglobulinemia of the Swiss type (43,44).

Infants with this disorder present clinically with manifestations of a severe combined (T and B cell) immunodeficiency (SCID) syndrome. T-cell defects result from thymic dysplasia or severe hypoplasia, whereas B-cell defects are thought to be secondary to the lack of inducer T lymphocytes (44).

In addition to Glanzmann–Riniker disease, there are two other forms of hypogamma globulinemia that are not accompanied by aplasia or severe hypoplasia of the thymus: *Bruton's X-linked type of hypogammaglobulinemia* and *acquired hypogammaglobulinemia*. In both syndromes, the thymus is normal and exhibits only changes of stress involution secondary to repeated infections.

Di George's syndrome is another rare condition that results from a failure in the development of the third and fourth branchial pouches with the resulting total or partial absence of the thymus and absence or hypoplasia of the parathyroid glands (46,47). In cases in which a small amount of thymic tissue is present (partial Di George's syndrome), the gland exhibits a normal microscopic morphology. Patients with Di George's syndrome usually have associated congenital cardiovascular defects such as truncus arteriosus (47). Peripheral lymphoid tissues of patients with Di George's syndrome have severe depletion of T-cell areas (45).

The prognosis of this condition is guarded, although some patients who have survived the clinical manifestations of hypoparathyroidism and the severe recurrent infections that are so frequent in patients with Di George's syndrome have been treated successfully by thymic transplants (45,57).

Nezelof's syndrome is a rare immune disorder characterized by immunologic abnormalities similar to those seen in Di George's syndrome. Individuals with Nezelof's syndrome, however, exhibit normal parathyroids (52).

Wiscott–Aldrich syndrome is a sex-linked, recessive hereditary disease characterized by the triad of severe immune deficiency, eczema, and thrombocytopenia (55,56). Patients with this disorder usually have a hypoplastic thymus that is either normal histologically or exhibits changes of acute involution (43). They also exhibit marked depletion of parafollicular thymus-dependent areas in peripheral lymphoid tissues. Patients with Wiscott–Aldrich syndrome have a shortened life span and die of infection or malignancy (malignant lymphoma) (55,56).

Thymic Dysplasia

Thymic dysplasia is characterized by the absence of lymphoid tissue in an epithelial thymus. Hassall's corpuscles are also absent or very scanty. Thymic dysplasia may exhibit nine morphologic patterns, described in detail by Landing and associates (43), including the pinealoid pattern, the dark spindle-celled pattern, the epithelial "stem-only" pattern, and others.

The classical form of thymic dysplasia is the pinealoid pattern, shown in Fig. 5-4, in which the gland has only solid nests of round epithelial cells surrounded by fibrovascular septa. A second variant of dysplasia is the dark spindle-celled epithelial pattern characterized by irregular nests of hyperchromatic spindle epithelial cells. Tissue clefts ("stem cystosis") may be prominent in this morphologic type of dysplasia. A third variant of thymic dysplasia is the epithelial "stem-only" pattern, characterized by large aggregates of round epithelial cells surrounded by a pale myxoid stroma.

The distinction among these morphologic variants of thymic dysplasia has clinical relevance. For example, patients with SCID or Nezelof's syndrome who have thymic dysplasia with the pinealoid pattern exhibit a less severe immune deficiency and respond better to immunologic reconstitution than patients with epithelial "stem-only" features. Patients with the thymic epithelial "stem-only" pattern usu-

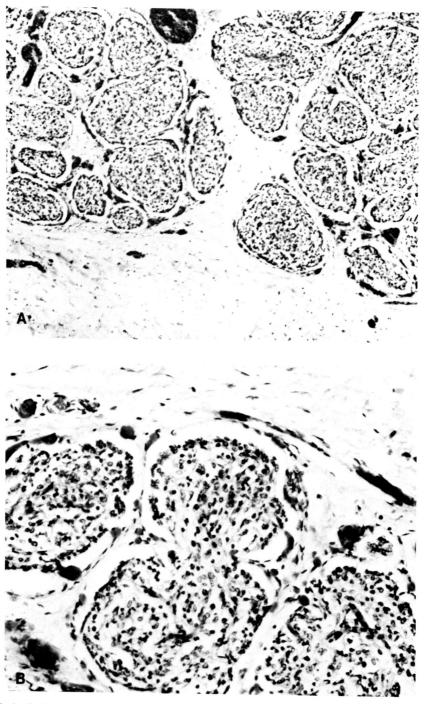

FIG. 5–4. A: Thymic dysplasia with pinealoid pattern. The gland has solid nests of epithelial cells. Note absence of thymocytes and Hassall's corpuscles. (H&E × 40, original) **B:** Higher magnification showing round to oval epithelial cells. (H&E × 100, original)

ally have SCID syndrome with severe immunologic deficits and associated deficiency of the enzyme adenosine deaminase (ADA) in lymphoid cells. Patients with the small dark spindle-celled pattern usually exhibit pure T-lymphocyte deficiency (so-called thymic alymphoplasia) and have a relatively better survival rate than those with the SCID syndrome.

The classification of thymic dysplasia proposed by Landing and associates is based on the observation of a small number of patients, and it is not accepted by all authors. For example, Borzy and associates (44) distinguish five morphologic patterns of thymic abnormalities in patients with the SCID syndrome: total dysplasia, partial dysplasia, partial dysplasia with phagocytosis, heterogeneous, and late fetal pattern.

In their view, the thymus in total dysplasia (TDP) is characterized by small lobules that exhibit no clear distinction between cortical and medullary areas and are composed of small spindle-epithelial cells that can form distinct glands (alveolar pattern) or rosettes. There are few if any lymphocytes and no Hassall's corpuscles. The thymus in partial dysplasia (PDP) has similar lobules composed, however, of larger epithelial cells that have abundant eosinophilic cytoplasms. The thymus with a heterogeneous cell population (HCP) is characterized by small distinct lobules composed of epithelial cells admixed with mononuclear cells and scanty lymphocytes. Occasional Hassall's corpuscles and a hint at corticomedullary distinction are also present. The thymus with partial dysplasia with phagocytosis (PDPP) has lobules of thymic tissue larger than those in the previous three forms, composed of epithelial cells, lymphocytes, and large numbers of phagocytic mononuclear cells. Hassall's corpuscles are absent. No corticomedullary demarcation is present. The thymus with the late fetal pattern (LFP) resembles the fetal gland. It has lobules composed of a central area of pale epithelial cells surrounded by a mantle of lymphocytes and monocytes. Focal corticomedullary distinction is present; however, Hassall's corpuscles are absent.

In this study (44) the degree of thymic dysplasia could not be predicted from laboratory studies of immune functions, a fact that underscores the value of thymic biopsy in the evaluation of patients with immune deficiency.

More studies are needed to determine which classification of thymic dysplasia has a better prognostic value.

The Thymus in Other Congenital and Acquired Immune Deficiencies

Patients with congenital diseases such as ataxia–telangiectasia, Zinsser Cole–Engman syndrome (X-linked congenital dyskeratosis with pancytopenia), and acquired conditions such as Hodgkin's disease, histiocytosis X, acquired immune deficiency syndrome (AIDS), and others may develop immunodeficiency associated with thymic abnormalities.

These abnormalities are seldom present at birth and usually develop progressively in a previously normal gland (36–41). For example, patients with biliary atresia develop a progressive loss of thymic epithelium over several months, and those with dysgammaglobulinemia exhibit a small thymus with cystic Hassall's corpuscles, the so-called "central Hassall's corpuscle" pattern. Patients with systemic lupus erythematosus also occasionally have large cystic Hassall's corpuscles (37–40,43).

In addition, serologic studies of patients with SCID or Di George's syndrome or

other forms of immune deficiency can exhibit low serum levels of thymopoietin and
FTS (45). Unfortunately, these abnormal hormonal levels do not correlate well with
the pathologic abnormalities present in the thymus. Serum levels of thymopoietin
and FTS can return to normal values following transplants of fetal thymus to these
patients (45).

The Thymus in the Acquired Immune Deficiency Syndrome (AIDS)

Several thymic abnormalities have been described in thymic biopsies from patients
with AIDS and at autopsy. Patients at autopsy have dysplastic thymuses devoid of
Hassall's corpuscles and lymphocytes (Fig. 5-5) (58–60). It has been postulated that
the epithelial cells may be the primary thymic site to be injured in AIDS, a view that
is supported by immunohistologic studies demonstrating the loss of the epithelial
reticular pattern in thymic samples from patients with the syndrome (61,62).

Joshi and associates (59,60) have described several histopathologic patterns in
thymic biopsies from children with AIDS: precocious involution, involution mimicking dysplasia, and thymitis. Biopsies with precocious involution had an obscured
corticomedullary differentiation, marked decrease in lymphocytes, and microcystic
Hassall's corpuscles. Thymic dysinvolution was characterized by a decrease in
thymic weight, loss of the corticomedullary differentiation, normal blood vessels,
marked lymphocyte depletion, and absence of Hassall's corpuscles. Patients with
thymitis had thymuses with normal location, size, weight, and vascularity; medullary germinal centers; lymphomononuclear or plasmacytic infiltrates that obscured
the corticomedullary differentiation, and medullary giant cells (60).

It is controversial whether these morphologic findings are secondary to injury by
the Human Immunodeficiency Virus 1 (HIV-1) or the result of accelerated involution
in very sick patients. Schuurman and associates (63) compared the thymuses taken
at autopsy from patients who died from AIDS, from congenital immunodeficiency,
or after allogeneic bone marrow transplantation and detected no significant morpho-

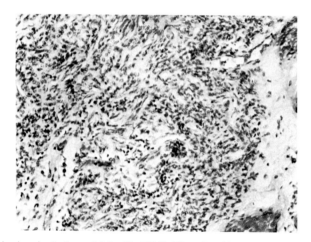

FIG. 5–5. Thymic dysplasia in a child with AIDS. The gland has lost its corticomedullary distinction and Hassall's corpuscles and is composed of small round and spindle epithelial cells.
Lymphocytes are scanty. (H&E × 100, original)

logic differences between the three groups. Furthermore, utilizing immunohisto-chemistry for HIV-1 gag and env proteins and other molecular biology techniques, the authors described only low numbers of positive cells, disputing the theory that the thymic epithelial cells are preferentially injured by the virus. This study also confirmed the presence of epitopes of retroviral antigens in the thymic epithelium (63).

The Thymus in Bone Marrow Allograft Recipients

Several studies have demonstrated that the thymus gland undergoes atrophy or hyperinvolution in bone marrow allograft recipients (64,65). The glands are small and composed of subcapsular and medullary epithelium, small remants of cortical epithelium, and only mature thymocytes (64). It has been postulated that these changes may be secondary to graft-versus-host disease (GVHD), chemotherapy, and lethal total body irradiation (63). Some patients show evidence of partial reconstitution of normal thymic structures or of lymphopoiesis (63).

THE THYMUS IN MYASTHENIA GRAVIS

Myasthenia gravis (MG) is a neurological disease characterized by muscular weakness and fatigability resulting from a postsynaptic defect that impairs neuromuscular transmission (66–78).

There is substantial clinical and experimental evidence indicating the autoimmune pathogenesis of the disease and the role of the thymus gland in its immunobiology, including the frequent association of MG with other autoimmune disorders and the presence in these patients of low serum levels of complement, high levels of circulating antibodies to acetylcholine receptors (AChR), and pathologic abnormalities in the thymus (66–79). Moreover, MG can be produced experimentally by immunizing animals with purified AChR isolated from the electric organs of eels and rays (67).

The role of the thymus in the pathogenesis of MG has been studied in detail (80–88). The autoantigen in MG is the nicotinic AChR encountered at the neuromuscular junction and in the myoid cells of the thymus (85–89). The number of functioning AChRs is reduced in patients with MG, as a result of circulating anti-AChR antibodies that are present in over 90% of patients with the disease (88). These antibodies are thought to be produced in the thymus, peripheral lymphoid organs, and the blood. The secretion of these antibodies may be modulated by AChR-specific helper T cells (88). The anti-AChR autoantibodies are thought to inactivate the receptor sites at the neuromuscular junctions by (a) activation of complement with destruction of the postsynaptic muscle cell membrane, (b) accelerated turnover and loss of the AChR, or (c) pharmacologic block of the receptor with inhibition of acetylcholine binding (66,68,88).

The thymus has myoid cells, described in the human thymus by van de Velde and Friedman in 1966 (89). These cells are more readily found in the medulla of the thymus of patients with MG than in controls (89). Myoid cells express AChR immunoreactivity and probably provide the autoantigen for intrathymic autosensitization (90–95). In the thymus of a patient with MG, there is also an increase in the number of interdigitating cells expressing strong HLA-DR immunoreactivity (96). These cells are in close contact with the myoid cells and may play an important role as antigen-presenting cells in the process of T-cell activation that takes place in the thymus of a patient with MG.

Wekerle and associates (85,97) have proposed a three-stage model of the pathogenesis of MG based on pathological and experimental evidence. In their view, the primary event in MG is the appearance of thymic myogenic cells followed by autosensitization against AChR present in those cells. In a later stage, autosensitized thymocytes interact with thymic B cells to produce anti-AChR antibodies (97). Several other studies support the hypothesis of the thymus as the primary site of autosensitization in MG (98–100). The mechanisms by which the tolerance to normal antigenic epitopes is lost in patients with MG are not well known (90).

Heredity appears to play a significant role in the pathogenesis of MG (68,72,73). For example, Caucasian patients with MG have an increased incidence of the major histocompatibility complex antigens HLA-B8 and DR3, whereas their Japanese counterparts more frequently have HLA-B12. In female patients the DRw15-Dx3-positive haplotype strongly correlates with the presence of a thymoma in association with MG (47).

This association of HLA antigens with MG is potentially interesting because human genes in the D and DR regions are probably involved in the control of immune recognition and the generation of helper and suppressor T-cell responses (68).

Congenital Myasthenia Syndromes

There are several unusual forms of myasthenia that have a different pathogenesis than MG (74). These syndromes are usually congenital or familial and are associated with a normal thymus. They include myasthenic syndromes caused by either endplate acetylcholinesterase deficiency or a putative abnormality of the acetylcholine-induced ion channel or a postulated defect of acetylcholine resynthesis or mobilization (74).

Thymic Pathology in Myasthenia Gravis

Myasthenia gravis is frequently associated with several thymic abnormalities including lymphoid hyperplasia (60–90% of patients), increased densities of B lymphocytes, T-helper cells, epithelial cells containing detectable intracytoplasmic thymosin, and myoid cells, and decreased numbers of T lymphocytes (101–107). In 10% to 20% of the cases, the disease is associated with a thymoma (2).

The hyperplastic follicles encountered in the thymus of a patient with MG are located both in the interlobular/perivascular spaces and within the thymic medulla. They are associated with a remodeled thymic architecture resulting from an expanded medulla, a compressed cortex, and a partial destruction of the normal network of thymic medullary epithelial cells (108). The medulla also has a prominent increase in individual B lymphocytes, supporting the theory of autoimmune activation of thymic B cells in MG (87–89).

Thymic Lymphoid Hyperplasia in Myasthenia Gravis

The thymus is normal in 10% to 25% of MG patients who do not have thymomas and hyperplastic in the other 60% to 90% (109–118). Hyperplastic thymic glands have germinal centers composed of B lymphocytes with intracytoplasmic immuno-globulins (lymphoid hyperplasia) (Fig. 5-3). These thymocytes may also have de-tectable anti-AChR antibodies in their cytoplasm (45).

The presence of lymphoid hyperplasia in the thymus of a patient with MG has been the subject of controversy, and there have been several studies that have quan-titated morphometrically the degree of thymic lymphoid hyperplasia in MG (111–119). Slightly different methods have been utilized to determine (a) the presence and density of germinal centers in thymic sections (0, absent; 1 +, equivocal, rare; 2 +, present; 3 +, frequent; 4 +, numerous), (b) the degree of lymphoid cell loss and fat replacement as a measure of involution (none, less than expected, partial, complete), and (c) the number of epithelial elements present (42,109–122). Penn and associates (117) also quantitated the number of myoid cells detected in thymic sections with labeled bungarotoxin.

These parameters, in particular the number of germinal centers, have been cor-related with the age and sex of MG patients, duration of symptoms prior to thymec-tomy, and response to therapy to determine their prognostic value (120). Results have been conflicting. Most studies report large numbers of germinal centers in the thymuses of MG patients and indicate that their presence is, indeed, significant (118). Middleton (33), however, reported germinal centers in the thymuses of 71% of sudden death patients. The density and size of thymic follicles present in their cases appear to be significantly smaller than those in MG (33).

Alpert and associates (42) reviewed the experience with nonthymomatous thymic glands of MG patients at The Mount Sinai Hospital, New York, and indicated that the presence of a gland of normal or involuted size with few germinal centers cor-related well with a favorable response to surgery and a rapid remission rate of the disease. Other investigators, however, have had different experience. For example, Mackay and associates (109) detected a significant association between thymic ger-minal centers and MG but no correlation between their number and prognosis.

In a recent study utilizing computerized interactive morphometric analysis, Moran and associates (29) evaluated the germinal centers of the thymuses of patients with nonthymomatous MG and demonstrated a correlation between the size of germinal centers and clinical improvement following thymectomy. Patients with germinal cen-ters with a cross-sectional area of 0.02 mm^2, perimeter of 0.58 mm, and diameter of 0.17 mm had better clinical outcomes than those with larger follicles. There was no correlation between the number of germinal centers and the clinical outcome.

THYMIC CYST

Cysts of the thymus, thymogenous cysts, are uncommon lesions that can be found at any location along the embryologic course of the thymus gland, including the mediastinum and the lateral neck (123–134). Their nature is controversial, and sev-eral pathologic classifications have been proposed. Krech and associates (126) di-vided thymic cysts into three groups: inflammatory, congenital, and neoplastic (Ta-ble 2). Inflammatory cysts of the thymus are very unusual. They were described at autopsy during the 19th century in children with congenital syphilis as multiple small cysts (Dubois abscesses) (123). Krech and associates argue that tuberculosis may also have played a role in their pathogenesis. Giraud and associates (135) reported exceptional cases of hydatid cysts of the thymus. Jaramillo and associates (136) re-ported the development of thymic cysts in patients with a previous history of thoracotomy and postulated that 15% of the thymic cysts observed in their institution were related to surgical trauma. Epidermoid cysts of the thymus have been described in patients with Gardner's syndrome (137).

Most thymic cysts are probably congenital in origin and derive from an anomaly of the third pharyngeal pouches with persistence of small tubular remnants of thymic anlage that became distended as a result of fluid accumulation or hemorrhage (125). They may also be the result of cystic degeneration of Hassall's corpuscles. Indeed, multiple small thymic cysts can be induced experimentally in rats by injecting estrogens. In this experimental model, they probably originate in Hassall's corpuscles (126).

Clinical Findings

Mediastinal cysts are found in children or adults of both sexes and are usually asymptomatic. They represent approximately 1% of mediastinal masses (2). Rarely, they may be symptomatic and present with pain, fullness in the chest, dyspnea and acute respiratory distress because of tracheal compression, dysphagia, Horner's syndrome, vocal cord paralysis, or loculated pneumomediastinum (2). Radiologically, mediastinal thymic cysts appear as smooth, round anterior and superior mediastinal lesions that can exhibit partial calcification. Occasionally, they may be confused with cardiomegaly on routine chest roentgenograms. Computed tomographic scans are useful to determine their cystic nature (130).

Cervical cysts are unusual. Fewer than 40 cases have been reported (131). They are usually found in children under the age of 10, although they have been reported in a 74-year-old patient and are more frequent in males (male/female ratio = 2:1), where they present as a slowly growing, painless lateral neck mass (131–133). They are usually present for several years before surgery. Rarely, they can simulate a thyroid tumor (131).

Thymic cysts in both locations are usually excised with no recurrences. Their prognosis is also excellent without treatment. Malignant transformation of a thymic cyst is very unusual. Leong and Brown (138) reported a patient who developed a well-differentiated papillary squamous cell carcinoma in a pre-existent thymic cyst.

Pathology

Thymic cysts are round or ovoid in the mediastinum and tubular and elongated in the neck (Fig. 5-6). Their shape in the neck presumably arises from compression by adjacent structures. They are usually multiloculated and, less frequently, uniloculated and are lined by a thin, smooth, fibrous wall, which can become focally calcified. They contain clear to straw-colored fluid or chocolate-colored material composed of degenerated blood and cellular debris. They can reach a giant size (Fig. 5-7).

The inner aspect of the cyst wall is lined by flattened, columnar, cuboidal, ciliated columnar, or stratified squamous epithelium (Fig. 5-8). The cyst wall has focal islands of thymic tissue. Not infrequently, the epithelial lining of a thymic cyst is destroyed by infection or pressure necrosis, and only a fibrous wall with chronic inflammation, cholesterol granulomas, hemorrhage, and focal calcifications remain. The identification of islands of thymic tissue is crucial to determine the true thymic

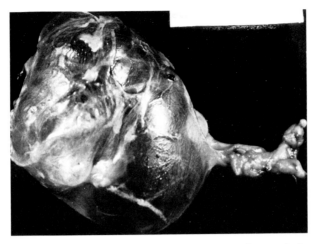

FIG. 5–6. Thymic cyst with attached remnant of normal gland.

nature of the cyst in these situations. These diagnostic areas, however, can be present very sparsely, and the surgical pathologist may have to sample the cyst wall extensively to establish the correct diagnosis.

The wall of an inflamed thymic cyst can have foci of epithelial proliferation with cytologic atypia that may be misdiagnosed as areas of malignant transformation. They are similar to foci of pseudoepitheliomatous hyperplasia observed in the skin and other epithelia following severe inflammation.

Differential Diagnosis—Neoplastic Cysts

Neoplastic cysts of the thymus include teratomas, cystic thymomas, and lymphangiomas. Dermoid cysts (teratomas) may have the same location and radiologic

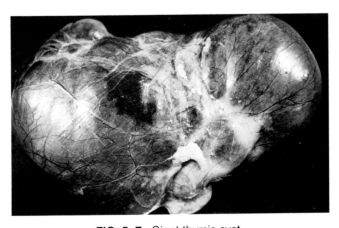

FIG. 5–7. Giant thymic cyst.

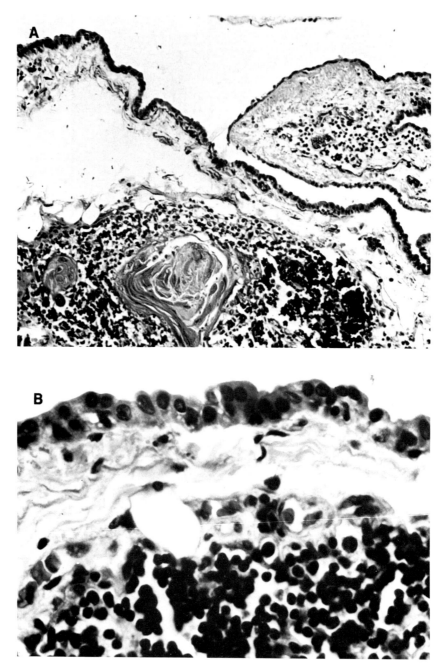

FIG. 5–8. A: Thymic cyst lined by single cuboidal epithelium. Note presence of thymic tissue within the cyst wall. (H&E × 100, original) **B:** Higher magnification showing simple cuboidal epithelium and thymic tissue. (H&E × 400, original)

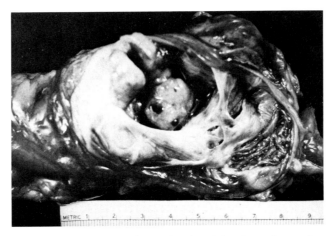

FIG. 5–9. Cystic thymoma. The cyst has a focal nodule of gray tumor tissue in its wall.

appearance as thymic cysts and can pose diagnostic problems to radiologists. However, they are simple to distinguish pathologically from thymic lesions (2).

Cystic thymomas may pose difficult diagnostic problems (19). Indeed, their cystic degeneration can be so extensive that only focal areas of thymoma can be identified (139). These islands of tumor appear grossly as small, irregular, white nodules located within the cystic wall and should be sampled histologically to establish the correct diagnosis (Fig. 5-9). Histologically, these focal areas of thymoma are composed of solid nests of epithelial and lymphoid cells without Hassall's corpuscles and with no corticomedullary organization as seen in the normal thymus.

Basaloid carcinomas of the thymus are also frequently cystic and may be difficult to distinguish from inflamed cysts that exhibit pseudoepitheliomatous hyperplasia.

Less frequently, cystic germ cell tumors or Hodgkin's disease of the thymus with cystic degeneration pose similar diagnostic problems (2). The differential diagnosis of thymic cysts also includes mesothelial, enteric, and bronchogenic cysts, which are discussed in Chapter 10.

Inflammatory Pseudotumor of the Thymus

Harpaz and associates (140) reported a patient with a markedly enlarged thymic gland that radiologically and grossly simulated a malignant thymoma (Color fig. 4).*
The thymic gland exhibited severe chronic inflammation with fibrosis and foci of epithelial hyperplasia (Color fig. 5).

REFERENCES

1. Boyd E: The weight of the thymus gland in health and in disease. *Am J Dis Child* 1932;43:1162–1214.
2. Rosai J, Levine GD: Tumors of the thymus, in: *Atlas of Tumor Pathology*, Fasc 13. Washington, Armed Forces Institute of Pathology, 1976.

*Color figures 4 and 5 appear following page 64.

3. Selye H: Thymus and adrenals in the response of the organism to injuries and intoxications. *Br J Exp Pathol* 1936;17:234–248.

4. Gewolb IH, Lebowitz RL, Taeusch HW Jr: Thymus size and its relationship to the respiratory distress syndrome. *J Pediatr* 1979;95:108–111.

5. van Baarlen J, Schuurman HJ, Huber J: Acute thymus involution in infancy and childhood: a reliable marker for duration of acute illness. *Hum Pathol* 1988;19:1155–1160.

6. van Baarlen J, Schuurman HJ, Reitsma R, et al: Acute thymus involution during infancy and childhood: immunohistology of the thymus and peripheral lymphoid tissues after acute illness. *Pediatr Pathol* 1989;9:261–275.

7. Seemayer TA, Bolande RP: Thymic involution mimicking thymic dysplasia. A consequence of transfusion-induced graft versus host disease in a premature infant. *Arch Pathol Lab Med* 1980;104:141–144.

8. Young M, Turnbull HM: An analysis of the data collected by the Status Lymphaticus Investigation Committee. *J Pathol* 1931;34:213–258.

9. Levine GD, Rosai J: Thymic hyperplasia and neoplasia: a review of current concepts. *Hum Pathol* 1978;9:495–515.

10. Arliss J, Scholes J, Dickson PR, et al: Massive thymic hyperplasia in an adolescent. *Ann Thorac Surg* 1988;45:220–222.

11. Balcom RJ, Hakanson DO, Werner A, et al: Massive thymic hyperplasia in an infant with Beckwith-Wiedemann syndrome. *Arch Pathol Lab Med* 1985;109:153–155.

12. Hendrichx P, Dohring W: Thymic atrophy and rebound enlargement following chemotherapy for testicular cancer. *Acta Radiol* 1989;30:263–267.

13. Nezelof C, Normand C: Tumor-like massive thymic hyperplasia in childhood: a possible defect of T-cell maturation, histological and cytoenzymatic studies of three cases. *Thymus* 1986;8:177–186.

14. Ricci C, Pescarmona E, Rendina EA, et al: True thymic hyperplasia: a clinicopathological study. *Ann Thorac Surg* 1989;47:741–745.

15. Judd RL, Welch SL: Myoid cell differentiation in true thymic hyperplasia and lymphoid hyperplasia. *Arch Pathol Lab Med* 1988;112:1140–1144.

16. Carmosino L, DiBenedetto A, Feffer S: Thymic hyperplasia following successful chemotherapy. A report of two cases and review of the literature. *Cancer* 1985;56:1526–1528.

17. Judd RL: Massive thymic hyperplasia with myoid cell differentiation. *Hum Pathol* 1987;18:1180–1183.

18. Kendall MD, Johnson HRM, Singh J: The weight of the human thymus gland at necropsy. *J Anat* 1980;131:485–499.

19. Lack EE: Thymic hyperplasia with massive enlargement. Report of two cases with review of diagnostic criteria. *J Thorac Cardiovasc Surg* 1981;81:741–746.

20. Katz SM, Chatten J, Bishop HC, et al: Massive thymic enlargement. Report of a case of gross thymic hyperplasia in a child. *Am J Clin Pathol* 1977;68:786–790.

21. O'Shea PA, Pansatiankul B, Farnes P: Giant thymic hyperplasia in infancy: immunologic, histologic and ultrastructural observations. *Lab Invest* 1978;38:391.

22. Lee Y, Moallem S, Clauss RH: Massive hyperplastic thymus in a 22 month old infant. *Ann Thorac Surg* 1979;27:356–358.

23. Durkin W, Durant J: Benign mass lesions after therapy for Hodgkin's disease. *Arch Intern Med* 1979;139:333–336.

24. Cohen M, Hill CA, Cangir A, et al: Thymic rebound after treatment of childhood tumors. *Am J Roentgenol* 1980;135:151–156.

25. Due W, Dieckmann KP: Stein H: Thymic hyperplasia following chemotherapy of a testicular germ cell tumor. Immunohistological evidence for a simple rebound phenomenon. *Cancer* 1989;63:446–449.

26. Shin MS, Ho KJ: Diffuse thymic hyperplasia following chemotherapy for nodular sclerosing Hodgkin's disease. *Cancer* 1983;51:30–33.

27. Yulish BS, Owens RP: Thymic enlargement in a child during therapy for primary hypothyroidism. *Am J Roentgenol* 1980;135:157–158.

28. Pardo-Mindan FJ, Crisci CD. Serrano M, et al: Immunological aspects of sarcoidosis associated with true thymic hyperplasia. *Allergol Immunopathol* 1980;8:91–96.

29. Moran CS, Suster S, Gil J, et al: Morphometric analysis of germinal centers in nonthymomatous patients with myasthenia gravis. *Arch Pathol* 1990;114:689–691.

30. Grody WW, Jobst S, Keesey J, et al: Pathologic evaluation of thymic hyperplasia in myasthenia gravis and Lambert-Eaton myasthenic syndrome. *Arch Pathol Lab Med* 1986;110:843–846.

31. Castleman B, Norris EH: The pathology of the thymus in myasthenia gravis. A study of 35 cases. *Medicine* 1949;28:27–58.

32. Goldstein G, Mackay IR: The thymus in systemic lupus erythematosus: a quantitative histopathological analysis and comparison with stress involution. *Br Med J* 1967;2:475–478.

33. Middleton G: The incidence of follicular structures in the human thymus at autopsy. *Aust J Exp Biol Med Sci* 1967;45:189–199.
34. Vetters JM, Barclay RS: The incidence of germinal centers in thymus glands of patients with congenital heart disease. *J Clin Pathol* 1973;26:583–591.
35. Gunn A, Michie W: Biopsy of the thymus. *Br J Surg* 1965;52:957–963.
36. Biggart JD, Nevin NC: Hyperplasia of the thymus in progressive systemic sclerosis. *J Pathol* 1967;93:334–337.
37. Mackay IR, de Gail P: Thymic "germinal centers" and plasma cells in systemic lupus erythematosus. *Lancet* 1963;2:667.
38. Goldstein G, Abbot A, Mackay IR: An electron microscopic study of the human thymus: normal appearances and findings in myasthenia gravis and systemic lupus erythematosus. *J Pathol* 1968;95:211–215.
39. Burnet FM, Mackay IR: Lymphoepithelial structures and autoimmune diseases. *Lancet* 1962;2:1030–1033.
40. Corridan M: The thymus in hepatic cirrhosis. *J Clin Pathol* 1963;16:445–447.
41. Kamegaya K, Tsuchiya M, Sambe K: Thymic abnormalities and the chronicity of liver disease—report of 10 cases and follow-up study. *Keio J Med* 1971;20:77–90.
42. Alpert LI, Papatestas A, Kark A, et al: A histologic reappraisal of the thymus in myasthenia gravis. A correlative study of thymic pathology and response to thymectomy. *Arch Pathol* 1971;91:55–61.
43. Landing BH, Yutuc IL, Swanson VL: Clinicopathologic correlations in immunologic deficiency diseases of children, with emphasis on thymic histologic patterns, in: *Proceedings of the International Symposium on Immunodeficiency.* Tokyo, Tokyo University Press, 1976, pp. 3–33.
44. Borzy MS, Schult-Wissermann H, Gilbert E, et al: Thymic morphology in immunodeficiency diseases: results of thymic biopsies. *Clin Immunol Immunopathol* 1979;12:31–51.
45. Pahwa R, Ikehara S, Pahwa SG, et al: Thymic function in man. *Thymus* 1979;1:27–58.
46. DiGeorge AM, Lischner HW, Dacou C, et al: Absence of the thymus. *Lancet* 1967;1:1387.
47. Pahwa RN, Pahwa SG, Good RA: T-lymphocyte differentiation in severe combined immunodeficiency: defects of the thymus. *Clin Immunol Immunopathol* 1978;11:437–444.
48. Pahwa RN, Pahwa SG, O'Reilly RJ, et al: Stem cell defects in severe combined immunodeficiency. *Pediatr Res* 1978;12:484.
49. Aiuti F, Businco C, Gatti RA: Reconstitution of T-cell disorders following thymus transplantation. *Birth Defects* 1975;11:370–376.
50. Ammann AJ, Wara DW, Salmon S, et al: Thymus transplantation. Permanent reconstitution of cellular immunity in a patient with sex-linked combined immunodeficiency. *N Engl J Med* 1973;289:5–9.
51. Astaldi A, Astaldi GCB, Wijermans P, et al: Experience with thymosin in primary immunodeficiency disease. *Cancer Treat Rep* 1978;62:1779–1785.
52. Smith SD, Lindsley CB, Abdou NI: Suppressor-cell-mediated leukopenia and T-cell dysfunction in Nezelof's syndrome. *Clin Immunol Immunopathol* 1980;17:406–414.
53. Webster AD: Combined immunodeficiency and thymic abnormalities. *J Clin Pathol [Suppl]* 1979;13:10–14.
54. Barret DJ, Wara DW, Ammann AJ, et al: Thymosin therapy in the DiGeorge's syndrome. *J Pediatr* 1980;97:66–71.
55. Shapiro RS, Perry GS, Krivit W, et al: Wiscott-Aldrich syndrome: detection of carrier state by metabolic stress of platelets. *Lancet* 1978;1:121–123.
56. Parkman R, Rappeport J, Geha R, et al: Complete correction of the Wiscott-Aldrich syndrome by allogeneic bone marrow transplantation. *N Engl J Med* 1978;298:921–927.
57. Mayumi M, Kimata H, Suehiro Y, et al: DiGeorge syndrome with hypogammaglobulinemia: a patient with excess suppressor T cell activity treated with fetal thymus transplantation. *Eur J Pediatr* 1989;148:518–522.
58. Elie R, Laroche AC, Arnoux E, et al: Thymic dysplasia in acquired immunodeficiency syndrome. *N Engl J Med* 1983;308:841–842.
59. Joshi VV, Oleske JM, Saad S, et al: Thymus biopsy in children with acquired immunodeficiency syndrome. *Arch Pathol Lab Med* 1986;110:837–842.
60. Joshi VV, Oleske JM: Pathologic appraisal of the thymus gland in acquired immunodeficiency syndrome in children. *Arch Pathol Lab Med* 1985;109:142–146.
61. Linder J: The thymus gland in secondary immunodeficiency. *Arch Pathol Lab Med* 1987;111:1118–1122.
62. Savino W, Dardenne M, Marche C, et al: Thymic epithelium in AIDS. An immunohistologic study. *Am J Pathol* 1986;122:302–307.
63. Schuurman HJ, Krone WJ, Broekhuizen R, et al: The thymus in acquired immune deficiency syndrome. Comparison with other types of immunodeficiency diseases, and presence of components of human immunodeficiency virus type 1. *Am J Pathol* 1989;134:1329–1338.

64. Thomas JA, Sloane JP, Imrie SF, et al: Immunohistology of the thymus in bone marrow transplant recipients. *Am J Pathol* 1986;122:531–540.

65. Muller-Hermelink HK, Sale GE, Borisch B, et al: Pathology of the thymus after allogeneic bone marrow transplantation in man. A histologic immunohistochemical study of 36 patients. *Am J Pathol* 1987;129:242–256.

66. Drachman DB, Adams RN, Josifek LF, et al: Antibody-mediated mechanisms of ACh receptor loss in myasthenia gravis: clinical relevance. *Ann NY Acad Sci* 1981;377:175–187.

67. Niemi WD, Nastuk WL, Chang HW: Factors in the production of experimental autoimmune myasthenia gravis in acetylcholine receptor immunized rabbits. *Ann NY Acad Sci* 1981;377:222–236.

68. Christadoss P, Lennon VA, Krco CJ, et al: Genetic control of autoimmunity to acetylcholine receptors: role of Ia molecules. *Ann NY Acad Sci* 1981;377:258–276.

69. Tindall RSA: Humoral immunity in myasthenia gravis: clinical correlations of anti-receptor antibody avidity and titer. *Ann NY Acad Sci* 1981;377:316–329.

70. Kelley RE, Keesey JC, Goymerac V, et al: Immunoregulation of total IgG synthesis in myasthenia gravis. *Ann NY Acad Sci* 1981;377:403–410.

71. Levine GD: Pathology of the thymus in myasthenia gravis: current concepts, in Dau PC (ed): *Plasmapheresis and the Immunobiology of Myasthenia Gravis.* Boston, Houghton-Mifflin Professional Publishers, 1978, pp 113–123.

72. Feltkamp TW, Van den Berg-Loonen PM, Nijenhuis LE, et al: Myasthenia gravis, autoantibodies and HLA antigens. *Br Med J* 1974;1:131–133.

73. Compston DAS, Vincent A, Newsom-Davis J, et al: Clinical, pathological, HLA antigen and immunological evidence for disease heterogeneity in myasthenia gravis. *Brain* 1980;103:579–601.

74. Engel AG, Lambert EH, Mulder DM, et al: Recently recognized congenital myasthenia syndromes: (A) Endplate acetylcholine (ACh) esterase deficiency, (B) putative abnormality of the ACh induced ion channel, (C) putative defect of ACh resynthesis or mobilization—clinical features, ultrastructure and cytochemistry. *Ann NY Acad Sci* 1981;377:614–637.

75. Dalakas MC, Engel WK, McClure JE, et al: Identification of human thymic epithelial cells with antibodies to thymosin alpha₁ in myasthenia gravis. *Ann NY Acad Sci* 1981;377:477–484.

76. Sambrook MA, Reid H, Mohr PD, et al: Myasthenia gravis: clinical and histological features in relation to thymectomy. *J Neurol Neurosurg Psychiatry* 1976;39:38–43.

77. Dalakas MC, Engel WK, McClure JE, et al: Immunocytochemical localization of thymosin alpha₁ in thymic epithelial cells of normal and myasthenia gravis patients and in thymic cultures. *J Neurol Sci* 1981;50:239–247.

78. Castleman B: The pathology of the thymus gland in myasthenia gravis. *Ann NY Acad Sci* 1966;135:496–505.

79. Zbieranowski I, Kahn HJ, Hanna W: Epithelial proliferation in thymic hyperplasia. *Arch Pathol Lab Med* 1989;113:385–389.

80. Kirchner T, Tzartos S, Hoppe F, et al: Pathogenesis of myasthenia gravis. Acetylcholine receptor-related antigenic determinants in tumor-free thymuses and thymic epithelial tumors. *Am J Pathol* 1988;130:268–280.

81. Marchiori PE, dos Reis M, Quevedo ME, et al: Acetylcholine receptor antibody in myasthenia gravis. *Acta Neurol Scand* 1989;80:387–389.

82. Marx A, Kirchner T, Hoppe F, et al: Proteins with epitopes of the acetylcholine receptor in epithelial cell cultures of thymomas in myasthenia gravis. *Am J Pathol* 1989;134:865–877.

83. Matsui M, Fukuyama H, Akiguchi I, et al: Circulating CD4 + CD8 + cells in myasthenia gravis: supplementary immunological parameter for long-term prognosis. *J Neurol* 1989;236:329–335.

84. Tesch H, Hohlfeld R, Toyka KV: Analysis of immunoglobulin and T cell receptor gene rearrangements in the thymus of myasthenia gravis patients. *J Neuroimmunol* 1989;21:169–176.

85. Wekerle H, Muller-Hermelink HK: The thymus in myasthenia gravis. *Curr Top Pathol* 1986;75:179–206.

86. Cohen-Kaminsky S, Levasseur P, Binet JP, et al: Evidence of enhanced recombinant interleukin-2 sensitivity in thymic lymphocytes from patients with myasthenia gravis: possible role in auto-immune pathogenesis. *J Neuroimmunol* 1989;24:75–87.

87. Hofmann WJ, Momburg F, Moller P, et al: Intra- and extrathymic B cells in physiologic and pathologic conditions. Immunohistochemical study on normal thymus and lymphofollicular hyperplasia of the thymus. *Virchows Arch [Cell Pathol]* 1988;412:431–432.

88. Hohlfeld R: Myasthenia gravis and thymoma: paraneoplastic failure of neuromuscular transmission. *Lab Invest* 1990;62:241–243.

89. van de Velde RL, Friedman NB: The thymic "myoidzellen" and myasthenia gravis. *JAMA* 1966;198:287–288.

90. Engel WK, Trotter JL, McFarlin DE, et al: Thymic epithelial cell contains acetylcholine receptor. *Lancet* 1977;1:1310–1311.

91. Scadding GK, Vincent A, Newsom-Davis J, et al: Acetylcholine receptor antibody synthesis by thymic lymphocytes: correlation with thymic histology. *Neurology* (NY) 1981;31:935–943.

92. Goldstein AL, Thurman GB, Low TLK, et al: Hormonal influences on the reticuloendothelial system—current status of the role of thymosin in the regulation and modulation of immunity. *J Reticuloendothel Sci* 1978;23:253–266.
93. Kao I, Drachman DB: Thymic muscle cells bear acetylcholine receptors: possible relation to myasthenia gravis. *Science* 1977;195:74–75.
94. Mittag T, Kornfeld P, Tormay A, et al: Detection of antiacetylcholine receptor factors in serum and thymus from patients with myasthenia gravis. *N Engl J Med* 1976;294:691–694.
95. Wekerle H, Ketelsen UP, Zurn AD, et al: Intrathymic pathogenesis of myasthenia gravis: transient expression of acetylcholine receptors on thymus derived myogenic cells. *Eur J Immunol* 1978;8:579–582.
96. Kirchner T, Hoppe F, Schalke B, et al: Microenvironment of thymic myoid cells in myasthenia gravis. *Virchows Arch [Cell Pathol]* 1988;54:295–302.
97. Wekerle H, Hohlfeld R, Ketelsen U-P, et al: Thymic myogenesis, T-lymphocytes and the pathogenesis of myasthenia gravis. *Ann NY Acad Sci* 1981;377:455–475.
98. Piantelli M, Musiani P, Lauriola L, et al: Lymphocyte subpopulations in non-neoplastic thymus from myasthenia gravis patients. *Clin Exp Immunol* 180;41:19–24.
99. Scadding GK, Thomas HC, Havard CWH: The immunological effects of thymectomy in myasthenia gravis. *Clin Exp Immunol* 1979;36:205–213.
100. Scadding GK, Webster ADB, Ross M, et al: Humoral immunity before and after thymectomy in myasthenia gravis. *Neurology (Minneap)* 1979;29:502–506.
101. Carlsson B, Wallin J, Pirskanen R, et al: Different HLA DR-DQ associations in subgroups of idiopathic myasthenia gravis. *Immunogenetics* 1990;31:285–290.
102. Apostolski S, Gospavic J, Isakovic K, et al: Functional difference between cortical and medullary thymic epithelial cells in patients with myasthenia gravis. *Ann NY Acad Sci* 1987;496:707–710.
103. Apotolski S, Micic M, Popeskovic L, et al: Thymic microenvironment in myasthenia gravis. *J Neuroimmunol* 1989;24:1–8.
104. Chilosi M, Iannucci A, Fiore-Donati L, et al: Myasthenia gravis: immunohistological heterogeneity in microenvironmental organization of hyperplastic and neoplastic thymuses suggesting different mechanisms of tolerance breakdown. *J Neuroimmunol* 1986;11:191–204.
105. Savino W, Emonard H, Grimaud JA: Thymic extracellular matrix in myasthenia gravis. II. Immunohistochemical evidence for increased type I collagen degradation. *J Neuroimmunol* 1988;18:223–230.
106. Savino W, Takacs L, Monostori E, et al: Phenotypic changes of the subseptal thymic epithelium in myasthenia gravis. *Thymus* 1988;89:111–116.
107. Kirchner T, Schalke B, Melms A, et al: Immunohistological patterns of non-neoplastic changes in the thymus in myasthenia gravis. *Virchows Arch [Cell Pathol]* 1986;52:237–257.
108. Christensson B, Biberfeld P, Matell G: B-cell compartment in the thymus of patients with myasthenia gravis and control subjects. *Ann NY Acad Sci* 1988;540:293–297.
109. Mackay IR, Whittingham S, Goldstein G, et al: Myasthenia gravis: clinical, serological and histological studies in relation to thymectomy. *Aust Ann Med* 1968;17:1–11.
110. Vetters JM, Simpson JA: Comparison of thymic histology with response to thymectomy in myasthenia gravis. *J Neurol Neurosurg Psychiatry* 1974;37:1139–1145.
111. Goldstein G: Thymic germinal centers in myasthenia gravis: a correlative study. *Clin Exp Immunol* 1967;2:103–107.
112. Osserman KE, Genkins G: Studies in myasthenia gravis: review of a twenty-year experience in over 1200 patients. *Mt Sinai J Med* 1971;38:497–537.
113. Papatestas AE, Alpert LI, Osserman K, et al: Studies in myasthenia gravis: effects of thymectomy. Results on 185 patients with non-thymomatous and thymomatous myasthenia gravis, 1941–1969. *Am J Med* 1971;50:465–474.
114. Genkins G, Papatestas AE, Horowitz SH, et al: Studies in myasthenia gravis: early thymectomy. Electrophysiological and pathologic correlations. *Am J Med* 1975;58:517–524.
115. Papatestas AE, Genkins G, Kornfeld P: Comparison of the results of the transcervical and transsternal thymectomy in myasthenia gravis. *Ann NY Acad Sci* 1981;377:766–778.
116. Leong ASY, Vignaendra V, Ghee LT: A reappraisal of the significance of thymic germinal centers in myasthenia gravis. *Eur Neurol* 1976;14:53–59.
117. Penn AS, Jaretzki A III, Wolff M, et al: Thymic abnormalities: antigen or antibody? Response to thymectomy in myasthenia gravis. *Ann NY Acad Sci* 1981;377:786–803.
118. Zeldowicz LR, Saxton GD: Myasthenia gravis; comparative evaluation of medical and surgical treatment. *Can Med Assoc J* 1969;101:609–614.
119. Seybold ME, Howard FM, Duane DD, et al: Thymectomy in juvenile myasthenia gravis. *Arch Neurol* 1971;25:385–392.
120. Maggi G, Casadio C, Cavallo A, et al: Thymectomy in myasthenia gravis. Results of 662 cases operated upon in 15 years. *Eur J Cardiothorac Surg* 1989;31:504–509.
121. Molnar J, Szobor A: Myasthenia gravis: effect of thymectomy in 425 patients. A 15-year experience. *Eur J Cardiothorac Surg* 1990;4:8–14.

122. Papatestas AE, Genkins G, Kornfeld P, et al: Effects of thymectomy in myasthenia gravis. *Ann Surg* 1987;206:79–88.
123. Bieger RE, McAdams AJ: Thymic cysts. *Arch Pathol* 1966;82:535–541.
124. Rastegar H, Arger P, Harken AH: Evaluation and therapy of mediastinal thymic cyst. *Am Surg* 1980;46:236–238.
125. Indeglia RA, Shea MA, Grage TB: Congenital cysts of the thymus gland. *Arch Surg* 1967;94:149–152.
126. Krech WG, Storey CF, Umiker WC: Thymic cysts: a review of the literature and report of two cases. *J Thorac Cardiovasc Surg* 1954;27:477–493.
127. Cuasay RS, Fernandez J, Spagna P, et al: Mediastinal thymic cyst after open heart surgery. *Chest* 1976;70:296–298.
128. Fahmy S: Cervical thymic cysts: their pathogenesis and relationship to branchial cysts. *J Laryngol Otol* 1974;88:47–60.
129. Gouliamos A, Striggaris K, Lolas C, et al: Thymic cysts. *J Comput Assist Tomogr* 1982;6:172–174.
130. Benveniste GL, Holoyda A, Hamilton DW: Cervical thymic cyst: report of an unusual presentation of a rare lesion. *Aust NZ J Surg* 1980;50:309–310.
131. Singh RP, Zamora I, Pia F, et al: Congenital thymic cyst in the neck. *Int Surg* 1979;64:37–41.
132. Mikal S: Cervical thymic cyst. Case report and review of the literature. *Arch Surg* 1974;109:558–562.
133. Fielding JF, Farmer AW, Lindsay WK, et al: Cystic degeneration in persistent cervical thymus. A report of four cases in children. *Can J Surg* 1963;6:178–186.
134. Davis JW, Florendo FT: Symptomatic mediastinal thymic cysts. *Ann Thorac Surg* 1988;46:693–694.
135. Giraud G, Negre E, Thevenet A, et al: Kyste hydatique du thymus. *Presse Med* 1963;71:1375–1376.
136. Jaramillo D, Perez-Atayde A, Griscom NT: Apparent association between thymic cysts and prior thoracotomy. *Radiology* 1989;172:207–209.
137. Delamarre J, Dupas JL, Muir JF, et al: Gardner's syndrome and epidermoid cyst of the thymus. *Gastroenterol Clin Biol* 1987;11:421–423.
138. Leong ASY, Brown JH: Malignant transformation in a thymic cyst. *Am J Surg Pathol* 1984;8:471–475.
139. Dyer NH: Cystic thymomas and thymic cysts. A review. *Thorax* 1967;22:408–421.
140. Harpaz N, Gribetz AR, Krellenstein DJ, et al: Inflammatory pseudotumor of the thymus. *Ann Thorac Surg* 1986;42:331–333.

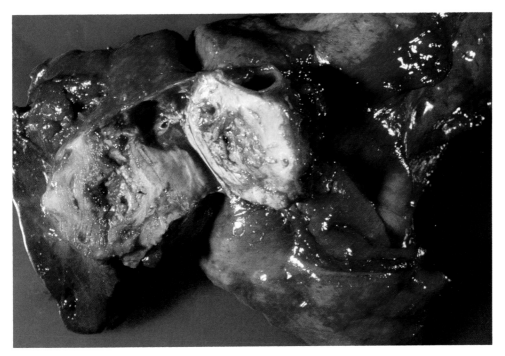

COLOR FIG. 1. Sclerosing mediastinitis presenting as a large peribronchial mass.

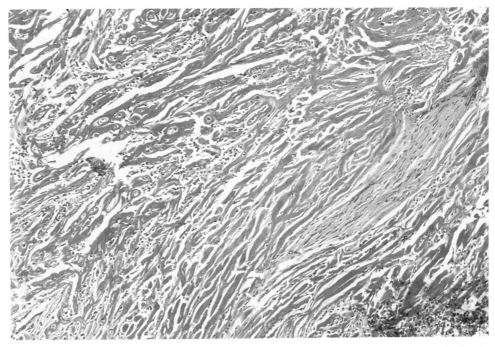

COLOR FIG. 2. Sclerosing mediastinitis composed of dense connective tissue with thick collagenous bands (Hematoxylin and Eosin × 40 original).

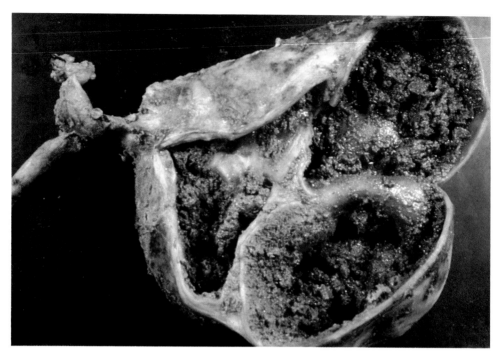

COLOR FIG. 3. Thymic cyst with extensive hemorrhage. The lesion presented clinically as a rapidly growing anterior mediastinal mass that simulated a malignant neoplasm.

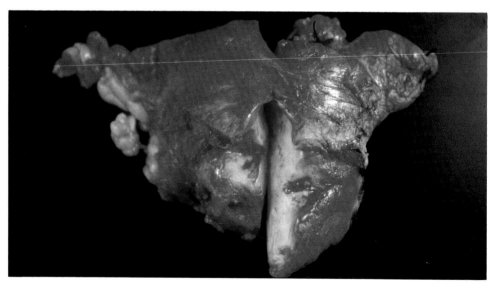

COLOR FIG. 4. Pseudotumor of the thymus. The lesion presented as a large, well encapsulated thymic mass.

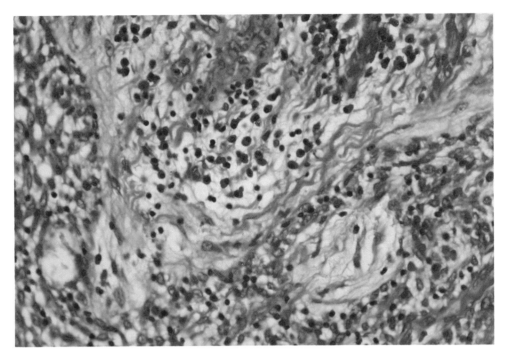

COLOR FIG. 5. Pseudotumor of the thymus composed histologically of inflamed thymic tissue with foci of fibrosis. The thymic epithelium shows foci of proliferation that simulate a neoplasm (Hematoxylin and Eosin × 100 original).

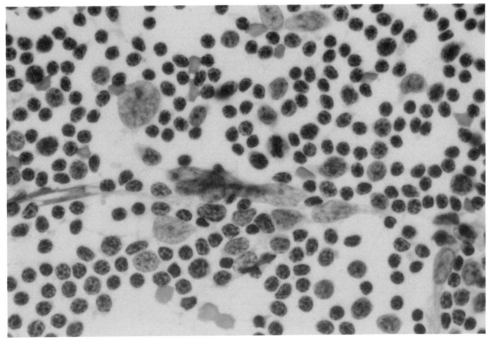

COLOR FIG. 6. Fine needle aspirate biopsy of a thymoma showing lymphoid cells and scanty, larger epithelial cells (Diff-Quick stain, 400× original)

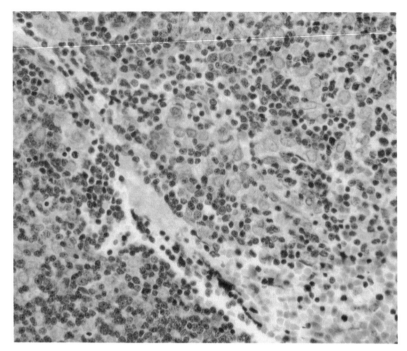

COLOR FIG. 7. Lymphoepithelial thymoma. The epithelial cells exhibit strong keratin immune-reactivity (PAP stain, 200 × original).

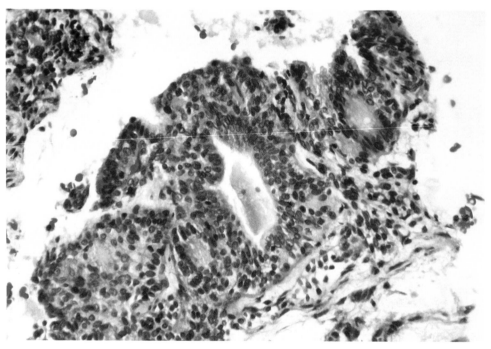

COLOR FIG. 8. Mixed tumor (pleomorphic adenoma) of the mediastinum composed of epithelial cells forming acini, myoepithelial cells and a myxoid stroma (Hematoxylin and eosin, 200 × original).

6

Tumors of the Thymus: Thymomas

The thymus gland can be the site of origin of a large variety of benign and malignant neoplasms (1). Although these tumors are relatively uncommon in the general population, they have been the subject of a great deal of interest in the medical literature because of their protean clinical and pathologic manifestations and their association with myasthenia gravis, red cell aplasia, and other diseases (2–17).

CLASSIFICATION OF THYMIC NEOPLASMS

There have been several classifications of thymic tumors. The most widely used is that proposed by Rosai and Levine (1,18). Their classification is used throughout this volume with several modifications.

Thymic neoplasms are classified according to their morphologic features and presumed histogenesis and include tumors arising from the thymic epithelium, neuroendocrine cells, germ cells, lymphoid tissue, and adipose tissue. These neoplasms are listed in Table 1. The thymus can also be the site of metastases, especially in patients with lung, breast, and thyroid cancer.

TUMORS OF THE THYMIC EPITHELIUM

Thymomas

The term thymoma has been applied in the literature to indicate any type of tumor that originates in the thymus. However, in accordance with the concepts of Rosai, Levine, and others, we have restricted the term to tumors originating from thymic epithelium (1,4,18). Thymoma is one of the most frequent mediastinal tumors and the most common neoplasm in the anterosuperior compartment (19–21).

Epidemiology

Thymomas have no predilection for any particular age group, sex, race, or geographic area (1). Although this tumor can affect patients of all ages, most cases are encountered in patients older than 40 years of age. Indeed, as many as 70% of patients with this neoplasm are in the fifth and sixth decades of life (1,21). Thymomas are unusual in children. Although it is unusual, patients with familial thymoma rarely associated with autoimmune myasthenia gravis have been reported (22).

TABLE 1. *Classification of tumors of the thymus*

Tumors of the thymic epithelium
  Benign
    Encapsulated thymoma
      Epithelial
      Lymphocytic
      Mixed lymphocytic and epithelial
  Malignant
    Invasive thymoma
      Epithelial
      Lymphocytic
      Mixed lymphocytic and epithelial
    Thymic carcinoma
      Squamous cell carcinoma
      Lymphoepithelioma-like carcinoma
      Basaloid carcinoma
      Mucoepidermoid carcinoma
      Sarcomatoid carcinoma
      Adenocarcinoma
      Adenosquamous carcinoma
      Mixed small-cell–undifferentiated-squamous cell carcinoma
      Clear-cell carcinoma
      Undifferentiated carcinoma
Tumors of neuroendocrine cell origin
  Carcinoid
  Oat-cell carcinoma
  Melanocytic neuroendocrine carcinoma
Tumors of germ cell origin
  Seminoma
  Embryonal carcinoma
  Endodermal sinus tumor
  Teratoma
    Benign cystic teratoma
    Immature teratoma
    Malignant teratoma
  Choriocarcinoma
  Combined germ cell tumors
Tumors of lymphoid origin
  Malignant lymphoma
    Hodgkin's disease
    Non-Hodgkin's lymphomas (lymphoblastic, others)
Tumors of adipose tissue
  Thymolipoma
Metastatic tumors to the thymus

Location

Approximately 95% of thymomas occur in the anterosuperior compartment of the mediastinum (Fig. 6-1). Less frequently, they can occur at any site in which thymic tissue can be normally found and have been described in the neck, middle mediastinum, pulmonary hilus, supradiaphragmatic area, and posterior mediastinum (1,23–28). Thymomas have rarely been found as intrapulmonary tumors (29–31). A particularly unusual presentation of thymoma was as an intratracheal polypoidal mass (32,33).

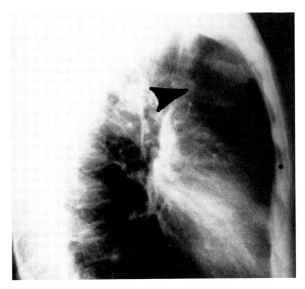

FIG. 6–1. Thymoma. Chest roentgenogram shows a round anterior mediastinal mass (*arrowhead*).

Clinical Features

Patients with thymomas present with varied clinical and radiologic manifestations. In approximately 50% of instances, the tumor is found incidentally in chest roentgenograms of asymptomatic patients (2–20). Twenty-five to 30% of patients present with local signs or symptoms from compression or invasion of adjacent structures. These may be cough, chest pain, dysphagia, dyspnea, hoarseness, and/or respiratory infections (34–39). Thymomas can also present as a neck mass with manifestations of the superior vena cava syndrome or with bronchial obstruction from polypoid endobronchial extension of an invasive mediastinal tumor (25,36,40). Infrequently, sudden death may follow compression of the right atrium. Thymomas can also simulate clinically and radiologically other conditions such as Hodgkin's disease, pulmonary stenosis, and constrictive pericarditis (41–44). As many as a third of patients have myasthenia gravis or one of the systemic disorders listed in Table 2 (45–101).

Thymoma and Myasthenia Gravis

The association between myasthenia gravis (MG) and thymic neoplasms was first established by Weigert in 1901 (45). It is estimated that 8% to 15% of patients with MG have a thymoma, and approximately 30% of thymomas are accompanied by MG (1–3). In some clinical studies, however, the incidence of MG in patients with thymomas has been reported to be as high as 60% (3,52). These high estimates derive, however, from selected groups of patients evaluated at MG clinics.

Myasthenia gravis usually becomes clinically evident prior to the discovery of the thymic tumor, but it can occur after the recognition of a mediastinal mass on chest

---

TABLE 2. *Clinical disorders associated with thymomas*

Neuromuscular syndromes
  Myasthenia gravis
  Myotonic dystrophy
  Eaton–Lambert syndrome
  Myositis
  Subacute motor neuronopathy
  Progressive systemic sclerosis
  Limbic encephalitis
Hematologic syndromes
  Red cell hypoplasia
  Erythrocytosis
  Pancytopenia
  Megakaryocytopenia
  T-cell lymphocytosis
  Acute leukemia
  Multiple myeloma
  Others
Immune deficiency syndromes
  Hypogammaglobulinemia
  T-cell deficiency syndrome
  Epstein–Barr virus infections
Collagen diseases and autoimmune disorders
  Systemic lupus erythematosus
  Rheumatoid arthritis
  Polymyositis
  Myocarditis
  Sjögren's syndrome
  Scleroderma
Dermatologic diseases
  Pemphigus (vulgaris, erythematosus)
  Chronic mucocutaneous candidiasis
Endocrine disorders
  Hyperparathyroidism
  Hashimoto's thyroiditis
  Addison's disease
  Chemodectoma
Renal diseases
  Nephrotic syndrome
  Minimal-change nephropathy
Bone disorders
  Hypertrophic osteoarthropathy
Malignancy
  Malignant lymphoma (Hodgkin's disease, non-Hodgkin's lymphomas)
  Carcinomas (lung, colon, others)
  Kaposi's sarcoma

---

roentgenograms taken from an asymptomatic patient (3). Myasthenia gravis can also develop after thymectomy for removal of a thymoma (46).

Patients with synchronous or metachronous thymomas, MG, and other associated conditions such as aplastic anemia, stiff-man syndrome, multiple schwannomas, gammopathies, relapsing polychondritis, and demyelinating neuropathy have also been described (104–108).

Patients with MG are more likely to be found to have a thymoma in the fourth to sixth decades of life (1). Yet, thymomas associated with MG are detected in younger patients, more so than those not associated with MG. This may be related to the presence of smaller thymic tumors in patients with MG and may reflect the fact that the neoplasms are more likely to be found earlier in symptomatic patients (1,3).

Controversy persists about the possibility that MG is associated more frequently with invasive thymoma than with encapsulated lesions. Studies by Slater and associates (52), Wilkins and Castleman (3), and Rosai and Levine (1) indicate that thymomas are invasive in 29% to 50% of patients with MG. These figures are higher than the overall proportion of invasiveness in all thymomas, suggesting that an individual with the invasive form of the tumor does have a greater likelihood of developing MG.

The prognostic significance of the presence of thymomas in patients with MG has also been the subject of controversy. Severe clinical studies have addressed this question to determine if the presence of the thymic neoplasm in patients with MG is a good prognostic indicator and if the neuromuscular disease can be cured by thymectomy (3). Wilkins and Castleman (3) report beneficial clinical effects with remission of the neuromuscular symptoms in about 25% of patients with MG undergoing thymectomy for removal of a thymoma. The improvement of symptoms, however, can be delayed for periods of up to 2 years following surgery.

In contrast, it has been accepted for many years that the presence of MG is a bad prognostic sign in a patient with a thymoma (1). Wilkins and Castleman (3) indicated that the two principal factors leading to adverse results in the treatment of patients with thymomas were local invasion of tissues by the tumor and the presence of MG. Recent improvements in the clinical management of MG, however, have lessened the importance of the neuromuscular disease as a prognostic sign in patients with thymic neoplasms. Indeed, in more recent studies several investigators have reported that the presence of MG has no effect on the long-term survival of patients with thymomas (3,109–111). Indeed, Monden and associates (103) reported better survival rates in patients with thymoma and myasthenia gravis, as these neoplasms were detected at an earlier stage.

It is less apparent whether surgical pathologists can find specific morphologic findings in the thymomas or in adjacent nonneoplastic thymic tissues in patients with MG (1). There is no agreement as to the possibility of accurately predicting by histologic examination of thymic tissues that patients with thymomas are at a high risk of developing MG. Indeed, as Rosai and associates (1) have shown, although a number of features have a significant association with the neuromuscular disease, there is no morphologic feature of a thymoma that is specifically associated with MG.

Thymomas in myasthenic patients are more likely to have germinal centers and Hassall's corpuscles within the tumor. Thymomas in nonmyasthenic patients are more likely to exhibit rosettes, a spindle cell morphology, and pseudogland formation.

However, the most significant pathologic finding associated with MG can be detected in the nonneoplastic thymic tissue adjacent to a thymoma (1). Alpert and associates (101) in an analysis of thymomas from one of our institutions, reported that 53% of patients with both thymoma and MG had germinal centers in the nontumoral thymic tissue, whereas none of the nonmyasthenic patients with thymoma exhibited that finding. Others have described similar results but, in addition, have documented the occasional occurrence of germinal centers in the nonneoplastic thymic tissue of patients who have no clinical evidence of MG (1).

Thymomas and Other Neurologic Disorders

Thymoma has been encountered in patients with myotonic dystrophy, Eaton–Lambert syndrome, myositis, subacute motor neuronopathy, progressive systemic sclerosis, limbic encephalitis, and myasthenia gravis–Lambert-Eaton syndrome (55–57,112–115). The role played by the thymic neoplasm in the pathogenesis of these disorders is unknown (116).

Thymoma and Hematologic Disorders

Red cell aplasia is a rare hematologic disorder characterized by the almost total absence of bone marrow erythroblasts and blood reticulocytes (58–72). Thymomas have been described in 50% of these patients. However, only 5% of patients with thymoma exhibit this hematologic disorder. Pure red cell aplasia also has been described in association with other thymic neoplasms such as thymolipomas and Hodgkin's disease. Patients with thymomas can present with pure red cell aplasia, myasthenia gravis, and hypogammaglobulinemia (117). They can also have positive Coombs and antinuclear antibody tests (117).

Pure red cell aplasia is mainly associated with epithelial thymomas that are noninvasive and are of the spindle cell type (70% of cases) (58). Anemia is usually diagnosed when the mediastinal mass is being clinically evaluated, but occasionally the tumor is unexpectedly encountered in a patient being studied for the hematologic disorder (68). There are also a few instances of pure red cell aplasia developing after thymectomy for a thymoma (58–69).

The role of either the thymus gland or thymomas in the pathogenesis of red cell aplasia is unclear. Several autoantibodies have been described in patients with pure red cell aplasia including antierythroblast antibody, antierythropoietin antibody, and antiprogenitor antibody (117). They can also exhibit an altered cellular immune system with increase of suppressor T cells against the erythrocyte maturation cycle, increase of gamma interferon, and decrease in interleukin-3 (117).

Masaoka and associates (117) reported that the nonneoplastic thymus adjacent to thymomas associated with pure red cell aplasia is involuted with no germinal centers present. They suggested that thymomas may produce suppressor T cells that inhibit erythrocyte maturation. Approximately a third of patients have remission of their symptoms following thymectomy (117).

Thymomas have also been described with other hematologic disorders including leukopenia, thrombocytopenia, pancytopenia, T-cell lymphocytosis, megakaryocytopenia, lymphocytic leukemias, multiple myeloma, bone marrow eosinophilia, agranulocytosis, chronic lymphocytic leukemia, pure white blood cell aplasia, pernicious anemia, and polycythemia vera (118–126).

Thymoma and Immune Deficiency Syndromes

Thymoma has been described in association with a form of hypogammaglobulinemia affecting mostly elderly people (Good's syndrome), although it has been recently reported in a child (82,127). Patients present with repeated episodes of severe bacterial infections and opportunistic viral infections by cytomegalovirus, herpes virus, and/or mucocutaneous candidiasis (82–85). Hypogammaglobulinemia is usually apparent when the mediastinal neoplasm is discovered, but it may develop following thymectomy for removal of a thymoma. In most instances, the removal of the thymic neoplasm does not have a beneficial effect on the immunoglobulins (82).

A few of these patients have been shown to lack surface immunoglobulin-bearing cells in their peripheral blood. Waldmann and associates (82) also demonstrated a population of suppressor T cells inhibiting immunoglobulin synthesis in two of three patients with thymoma and hypogammaglobulinemia. However, most patients with the syndrome have normal numbers of circulating T cells, normal *in vitro* immunologic tests (mitogenic responsiveness, antigen-stimulated lymphocyte transformation), and normal skin reactivity to common antigens (82–85).

A few patients with thymomas have had severe opportunistic skin infections such as herpes simplex and mucocutaneous candidiasis with increased numbers of T suppressor lymphocytes and decreased numbers of circulating B cells (82–85,128).

Epstein–Barr Virus Infection and Thymoma

The incidence of thymoma associated with MG appears to be considerably higher in patients from China, where the incidence of Epstein–Barr virus (EBV) is more prevalent than in Western countries (129–132). Antibodies of EBV have been detected in patients with thymic tumors, and the viral genome has been demonstrated by Southern blot hybridization analysis in thymomas studied in Hong Kong. Western thymomas studied with Southern blot hybridization and polymerase chain reaction for EBV genome have been negative (130).

Thymomas Associated with Skin Diseases and Other Autoimmune Disorders

Pemphigus vulgaris and pemphigus erythematosus have been described in patients with thymoma (86–88). These autoimmune bullous diseases are usually present at the time of diagnosis of a mediastinal mass but may develop after thymectomy for removal of a thymoma. Patients with these diseases have elevated serum levels of antibodies to striated muscle, skin, and DNA antigens. Gibson and Muller (133) reported cutaneous fungal diseases, lichen planus, pemphigus, myositis, and lupus-like disease in a review of 172 patients with thymoma.

Thymomas have also been described in patients with other autoimmune diseases such as systemic lupus erythematosus, rheumatoid arthritis, polymyositis, scleroderma, Sjögren's syndrome, and Hashimoto's thyroiditis (89,90,134–136).

The role of the thymic neoplasm in the pathogenesis of these diseases is unclear, but it has been postulated that the autoimmune disorder may be the result of a lack of immunologic surveillance by thymic T cells (85). Thymus-derived lymphocytes are thought to prevent autoimmunity in normal individuals, and their derangement could be "permissive," resulting in the formation of clones of lymphocytes that produce autoantibodies. Excess numbers of helper T cells also could result in increased production of autoantibodies.

Thymoma and Renal Disorders

Nephrotic syndrome related to membranous glomerulonephritis or minimal-change "lipoid" nephropathy has been described in a few patients with thymomas and is a well-recognized systemic manifestation of other neoplasms such as Hodgkin's disease (91,92). It may be related to the formation of antigen–antibody complexes that cross react with the patients' neoplasm and glomeruli.

Glomerular injury in minimal-change nephropathy may also represent a T-cell-mediated abnormality secondary to the production of abnormal lymphokines by thymocytes or to the abnormal production of a normal lymphokine by T lymphocytes (91,92).

Thymoma and Other Neoplasms

Thymomas have been reported in association with extrathymic malignancies including non-Hodgkin's lymphomas, Hodgkin's disease, carcinomas of the gastrointestinal tract, genitourinary system, lung, breast, and thyroid, brain tumors, leukemia, multiple myeloma, and Kaposi's sarcoma (93–98,137). Souadjian and associates (95) encountered second neoplasms in 21% of 146 patients with thymomas. These second malignancies may develop as a consequence of defective immunologic surveillance mechanisms in these patients with immune deficiency (94). A similar increased incidence of lymphoreticular and other neoplasms has been reported in immunosuppressed renal transplant recipients and in patients with congenital or acquired immunodeficiency syndromes involving T-cell defects in particular (94).

Thymoma and Bone Disorders

Hypertrophic osteoarthropathy has been reported in two patients with malignant thymomas (99). In one patient reported by Lesser and associates (99), the subjective and objective findings of the osteoarticular disease disappeared following the surgical resection and postoperative radiotherapy of the thymoma.

Thymoma and Endocrine Disorders

Palmer and Sawyers (100) and Byrne and associates (138) reported patients with thymoma and hyperparathyroidism. There is no evidence of a causal relationship. Hashimoto's thyroiditis and Addison's disease also have been associated with thymomas (1).

Diagnosis of Thymomas Using Imaging Techniques

Thymomas can be detected with different imaging techniques and appear as round or oval well-circumscribed, coarsely lobulated masses in the anterior and superior mediastinum or in any of the other locations discussed previously (Fig. 6-2) (139–143). In 6% to 20% of instances, the tumors have coarse, dense, irregular or ringlike calcifications that may be confused with those seen in mediastinal teratomas or aortic aneurysms. Cystic degeneration is seen in a small number of thymomas.

Thymic neoplasms are not always visible on routine posteroanterior or lateral roentgenograms of the chest because they are smaller than 1.5 to 2.0 cm or because their margins overlay the heart and/or pulmonary hilus shadows. These tumors can be detected, however, with more selective roentgenologic procedures such as oblique views guided by fluoroscopy, plain-film tomography, lateral tomograms, pneumomediastinography, selective thymic venography, CT scan, and MRI (Fig. 6-3). In a study from the Mayo Clinic (141), approximately 23% of tumors could only

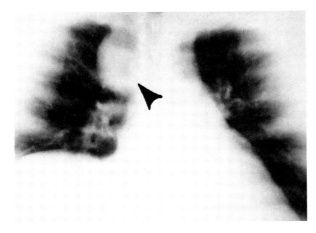

FIG. 6–2. Thymoma. Tomogram of the chest shows an oval, well-circumscribed mass (*arrowhead*).

be detected with these selective procedures. The CT scan is the single most sensitive method for detecting thymomas, but it is no more sensitive than a combination of other techniques (142–150). The CT scan is excellent for revealing the tumor site, size, and extent but does not demonstrate conclusively the presence of tumor invasiveness and malignancy. For example, Brown and associates (139) demonstrated that only 8 of 16 tumors predicted to be malignant by the demonstration of poorly marginated tumor margins on CT scan proved to be truly malignant after morphologic study. Frija and associates (147) reported that the CT scan offered 80% efficacy for the diagnosis of tumors of the mediastinum and a 59% sensitivity for the detection of malignancy. Rendina and associates (148) reported that the procedure was associated with overall positive and negative predictive values of 78% and 58% in the identification of resectability.

When the thymoma is metastatic to the pleura, lungs, or thoracic wall, radio-

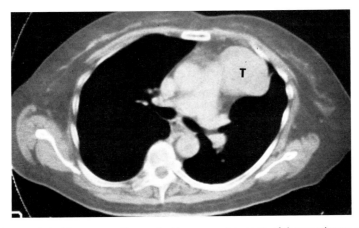

FIG. 6–3. Encapsulated thymoma. Computed tomographic scan of thorax shows a large, well-circumscribed anterior mediastinal mass (*T*).

graphic techniques can predict the presence of malignancy with greater specificity (Fig. 6-4).

Detection of Thymomas with Radionuclide Scans

Thymomas can be detected with ^{99m}Tc-pertechnetate or gallium scans (151,152). Radioiodinated tracers also are useful to differentiate thymic from thyroid mediastinal lesions (153).

Serological Detection of Thymoma

Small thymomas can occasionally remain undetected after examination of the mediastinum with various imaging techniques, and there is a need for ancillary tests for the detection of these occult neoplasms.

Van der Geld and associates (154) as well as other authors (155–163) have demonstrated that most patients with MG and thymoma have elevated serum levels of antibodies to skeletal muscle (so-called antistriational antibodies). These antibodies can be demonstrated by immunofluorescence, complement fixation, indirect hemagglutination, or other immunologic techniques. About 30% of MG patients lacking a thymic neoplasm and 24% of individuals with thymomas and lacking the neuromuscular disease have elevated serum levels of these antibodies. Antistriational antibodies are not, therefore, totally specific for the detection of thymomas in MG patients (158). However, their absence in the sera of these patients is a strong indication against the presence of a thymic epithelial neoplasm. Utilizing a new enzyme immunoassay (EIA) for striational autoantibodies (StrAb), Cikes and associates (164) reported that 53% of patients with MG and thymoma had a positive serum test. The test was also positive in patients with thymoma without MG.

Aarli and associates (157) have developed an indirect hemagglutination test for the detection of thymomas in patients with MG utilizing sheep red blood cells coated with a purified citric acid extract of skeletal muscle (CAE). In a study of 64 sera of

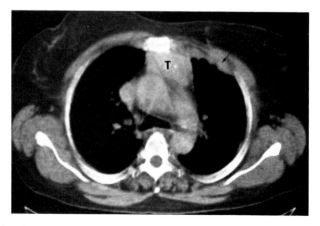

FIG. 6–4. Invasive thymoma. CT scan of the thorax shows an anterior mediastinal mass (*T*) with focal calcification. Adjacent irregular pleural change (*arrow*) represents tumor invasion.

patients with MG, they found five instances in which the CAE test was positive (158). One of these patients had a small thymoma on chest roentgenograms. The other four individuals were found only at surgery to have small thymomas. These authors also studied the sera of patients with MG and thymic hyperplasia and found no elevation of CAE antibodies.

More recently Aarli and associates (165) reported that 85% of patients with thymoma exhibited serologic evidence of CAE antibodies. Ohta and associates (166) recently reported the presence of antiskeletal (SM) antibodies in the sera from myasthenic patients with thymoma. The high serum antibody titers in thymoma patients were characterized by radioimmunoassay (RIA) and Western blotting analysis and were shown to be related to antimyosin and antiactomyosin antibodies. Patients with thymomas and GM also have different immunoglobulin allotypes than controls (167).

Needle Biopsy of Thymomas

Most patients with thymomas undergo thoracotomy after the clinical and radiologic diagnosis of an anterior mediastinal mass is established. The clinical diagnosis of thymoma is almost certain in a patient with MG and an anterosuperior mediastinal mass. However, in some instances, the tumor is biopsied preoperatively in order to confirm the clinical impression (168–174). Biopsies of the thymus can be done at the time of mediastinoscopy or by large-needle biopsy under radioscopic guidance or ultrasonic guidance (175,176). Examination of these relatively large samples of tissue enables the surgical pathologist to distinguish thymomas from other mediastinal neoplasms such as malignant lymphomas, germ cell tumors, metastatic lesions (i.e., small-cell carcinoma of the lung), and others. It is more difficult, however, to establish the benign or malignant nature of the neoplasm on a small tissue sample. Except for unusual instances of thymic carcinomas, described later in this chapter, most encapsulated, benign thymomas have identical histologic and cytologic features to invasive, malignant thymomas.

It may be a diagnostic problem to distinguish between a thymoma and a malignant lymphoma. In small tissue samples, thymic epithelial cells closely resemble large ("histiocytic") lymphoid cells. This type of problem can be resolved, however, with the use of electron microscopy or by utilizing immunocytochemical techniques for the detection of keratin and other antigens in tumor cells. Keratin can be demonstrated in tumor cells by indirect immunofluorescent staining of frozen tissue samples or peroxidase–antiperoxidase (PAP) staining of paraffin sections of a thymic neoplasm, confirming the epithelial nature of thymoma cells (177). It can also be helpful to distinguish spindle cell epithelial thymomas from other spindle cell mesenchymal neoplasms such as neurogenic tumors (177).

Keratins are a group of water-insoluble proteins isolated from epidermis that can be demonstrated with immunopathologic techniques in Hassall's corpuscles, epithelial reticular cells of the thymus, and epithelial thymomas (177).

Immunocytochemical stains for leukocyte common antigen and other lymphoid markers discussed in Chapter 4 are very helpful for the differential diagnosis between malignant lymphoma and thymoma. Stains for the detection of placental alkaline phosphate, AFP, CEA, and HCG can be helpful for the differential diagnosis between thymomas and seminomatous and nonseminomatous germ cell tumors of the mediastinum (178). Nabarra and associates (178) reported the use of monoclonal antibodies to thymulin to confirm the diagnosis of thymoma. Stains for the detection of neuron-specific enolase, chromogranin, synaptophysin, and other neuroendocrine markers can be helpful for the differential diagnosis between thymomas and thymic carcinoid tumors.

Ultrastructural studies of thymic tumors reveal epithelial tumor cells with bundles of tonofilaments, cell processes, and desmosomes (179–187). In contrast, large ("histiocytic") lymphoid cells lack these features but can exhibit instead the presence of intracytoplasmic immunoglobulins. True histiocytes have intracytoplasmic alpha-1-antitrypsin, lysozyme (muramidase), or esterases (188–190).

Fine-Needle Aspiration Cytology

Fine-needle aspiration (FNA) cytology of mediastinal lesions is being increasingly used for the accurate preoperative diagnosis of anterior mediastinal lesions (168–174,191–197). Fine needles (22–23 gauge) are placed in the mediastinum under ultrasound, television fluoroscopy, or CT guidance. Samples of the tumors are aspirated and examined with standard cytologic techniques. The study of these samples enables the pathologist to distinguish thymomas from lymphomas and other malignant lesions in most instances. Often, surgery can be avoided. For example, the cytologic diagnosis of a metastatic carcinoma such as small-cell carcinoma of the lung in the anterior mediastinum precludes the surgical resection of the tumor.

In a recent review of their experience, van Sonnenberg and associates (191) reported that 90.3% of their 31 patients with mediastinal lesions were diagnosed by CT-guided fine-needle biopsies. Linder and associates (192) reported that in 55% of their 29 patients with mediastinal lesions a thoracotomy was avoided by a positive FNA diagnosis.

Smears from thymomas usually exhibit thick, multilayered, cohesive fragments of tissues composed of lymphoid and epithelial cells with separate free lymphoid cells. Lymphocytes are small and uniform with no nuclear atypia but occasional mitotic figures. Epithelial cells appear as oval or spindle cells with scanty cytoplasm and a slightly irregular, folded pale nucleus containing a small nucleolus (Color fig. 6*). Occasionally, the tumor cells form rosette-like clusters.

Thymomas may be difficult to distinguish from thymic hyperplasia on smears of aspirated material, but their cytologic features are distinct from those seen in other mediastinal lesions. For example, metastatic small-cell carcinomas of the lung exhibit dispersed small round, ovoid, or spindle cells with scanty cytoplasm and hyperchromatic nuclei. Lymphomas usually exhibit large, irregular lymphoid cells with obvious cytologic atypia. Lymphoblastic lymphomas, frequent in the mediastinum, show convoluted lymphoid cells. Well-differentiated lymphocytic lymphomas, however, may pose diagnostic problems. They exhibit small, round lymphocytes with minimal nuclear atypia, as seen in thymomas. They lack, however, the presence of clusters of epithelial cells seen in thymic neoplasms. Other mediastinal lesions such as teratomas exhibit cytologic features that are distinct from those seen in thymomas.

The materials obtained by FNA of a mediastinal lesion can be studied with elec-

---

*Color figures 6 and 7 appear following page 64.

tron microscopy and immunocytochemical methods, increasing the sensitivity and specificity of the procedure (194–197).

Classification of Thymomas

The most widely used classification of thymomas in the United States divides the neoplasms into encapsulated thymomas, invasive thymomas, and thymic carcinomas (Table 1) (1,18). Encapsulated and invasive thymomas are classified on the basis of their histopathological features into epithelial, lymphocytic, and mixed lymphocytic and epithelial. Spindle cell thymoma has been recognized as a particular subtype of epithelial thymoma with particular clinicopathologic features including a benign clinical course in most patients, low incidence of associated MG, and high incidence of pure red cell aplasia and hypogammaglobulinemia (198).

Other classifications of thymomas based on the morphologic features of the epithelial cells have also been proposed (199,200).

Marino and Müller-Hermelink (198,201) have developed a conceptually attractive classification of thymomas that takes into account the morphologic, immunohistochemical, and cytochemical features and the histogenesis of the neoplastic epithelial cells. Thymomas are divided into cortical, medullary, and mixed types (Table 3). Several recent publications have shown that this classification has prognostic significance (148,202–207), a view that has been disputed by Kornstein and associates (208).

Pathologic Features of Encapsulated Thymomas

Gross Pathology

As many as 90% of thymomas are well encapsulated and easily excised from the mediastinum (1–10). They are round or oval and may be minute or huge; one of the largest recorded was $34 \times 18 \times 16$ cm and weighed 5,700 g (13) (Fig. 6-5). Thymomas can also be multiple, raising the possibilities of intrathymic metastasis or multicentric development (209). Thymomas usually have a bosselated outer surface. They occasionally appear as flattened masses adherent to the chest wall, simulating a fibrotic plaque.

The parenchyma of thymomas is characteristic and consists of a soft, tan or gray–pink "fishflesh" tissue with macroscopic resemblance to lymphoid tissue and clear separation into visible lobules by generally uniform white–gray fibrous tissue septa (Fig. 6-6). In most instances, the tumor is contiguous with a portion of visible thymic tissue (Fig. 6-5). Although other tumors may occasionally simulate a thymoma, these

TABLE 3. *Histological classification of thymomas*

Cortical
Mixed
Common
With cortical predominance
With medullary predominance
Medullary

From Marino and Müller-Hermelink (198, 201).

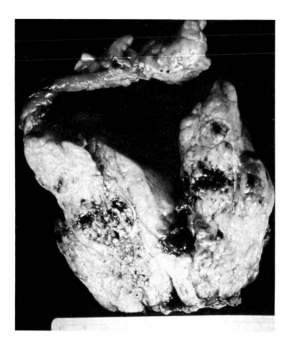

FIG. 6–5. Encapsulated thymoma. The tumor is oval, well-encapsulated, tan, with multiple fibrous septa. Note the presence of adjacent normal thymic tissue.

features in a mediastinal mass are almost pathognomonic of a thymoma. For example, the nodular sclerosis variant of Hodgkin's disease can present as a lobulated lymphoid mass of the thymus but is usually firmer, less well circumscribed, and composed of smaller nodules than a thymoma, with considerable irregularity of the fibrous tissue component (Fig. 6-7). Other thymic lymphomas as well as seminoma with abundant lymphoid stroma may also have a soft, tan, "fishflesh" appearance. These tumors, however, are usually not lobulated.

Thymomas may show varying degrees of cystic change in up to 40% of instances

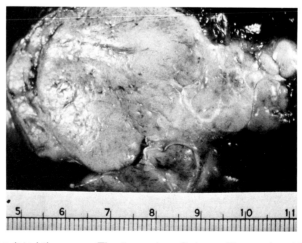

FIG. 6–6. Encapsulated thymoma. The tumor is soft, tan, with prominent lobules separated by white–gray fibrous septa. Note resemblance of the tumor surface to lymphoid tissue.

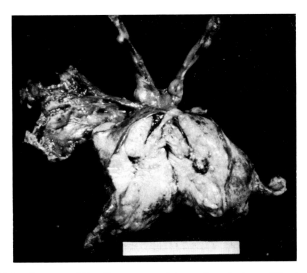

FIG. 6–7. Hodgkin's disease of the thymus, nodular sclerosis type. The lesion has nodules that are smaller and more irregular than those of thymomas. The tumor is firm and not encapsulated.

and frequently exhibit areas of calcification of the capsule or the tumor stroma (Fig. 6-8) (1,2). Foci of hemorrhage and necrosis are not infrequent and may be seen in a third of cases (Fig. 6-9). Rarely, the tumor becomes almost completely cystic, and multiple histologic sections taken from focal solid areas in the cyst wall are necessary to distinguish this lesion from a thymic cyst (Fig. 5-8) (11).

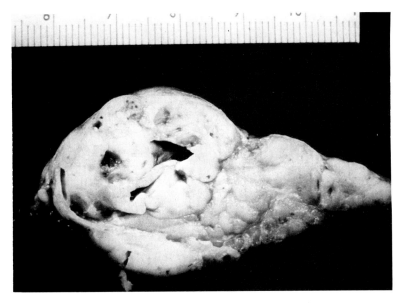

FIG. 6–8. Encapsulated thymoma with cystic change.

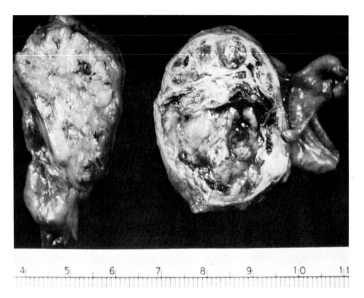

FIG. 6–9. Encapsulated thymoma with foci of hemorrhage and necrosis.

Lymphocytic, Epithelial, and Mixed Lymphocytic-Epithelial Thymomas

Microscopically encapsulated thymomas exhibit varied morphologic features that may pose diagnostic problems and have caused the development of a number of classifications of the tumor (1).

The lobulation observed macroscopically is apparent at low magnification and characteristically consists of irregularly shaped lobules with angulated borders enclosed by thick fibrous bands that are continuous with the tumor capsule (Fig. 6-10). These fibrous bands and the tumor capsule frequently have foci of calcification.

The tumor lobules are composed of variable proportions of two types of cells: lymphocytes and epithelial cells (Figs. 6-11 and 6-12). These cells are usually intermingled with each other, although they can, in rare instances, be in separate portions of the neoplasm (Fig. 6-13). Classification is based on the relative proportions of lymphocytes and epithelial cells. Thymomas may be predominantly lymphocytic, predominantly epithelial, and mixed lymphocytic and epithelial (Figs. 6-14, 6-15, and 6-16). Fisher (210) utilizes the term mixed lymphocytoid and epithelial synonymously with lymphoepithelioma. The latter diagnosis is best reserved, however, for the malignant tumors whose features are similar to those seen in anaplastic nasopharyngeal carcinomas (211,212).

Most thymomas have mixed lymphocytic and epithelial components. Masaoka and associates (213) determined the ratio of lymphocytes to epithelial cells (L/E ratio) in 22 thymomas; L/E ratios ranged from 0.27 to 4.10. In three recurrent lesions, the L/E ratios were lower than those of the original tumors, suggesting that the epithelial elements of thymomas increase in proportion to the progression of the tumor. Indeed, the epithelial component is considered the neoplastic element of the tumor, and it is not agreed whether the lymphocytic infiltrates are inflammatory or neoplastic in nature (1–10).

In most thymomas, lymphocytes are small and mature appearing, although they

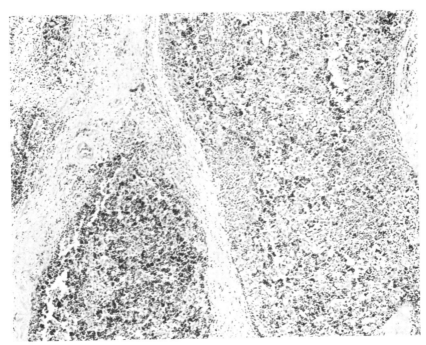

FIG. 6–10. Encapsulated thymoma at low-power microscopy showing typical "lobules" separated by fibrous septa. (H&E × 40, original)

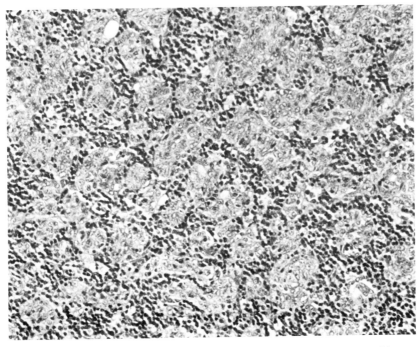

FIG. 6–11. Lymphoepithelial thymoma showing lymphocytes closely admixed with small clusters of larger epithelial cells. (H&E × 100, original)

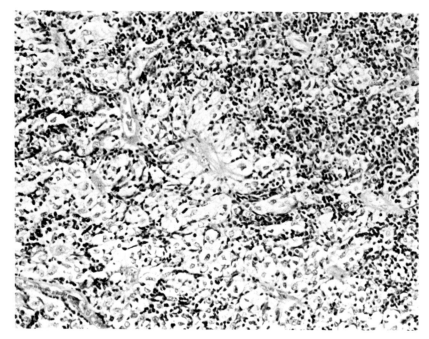

FIG. 6–12. Lymphoepithelial thymoma. Epithelial cells have a clear cytoplasm. (H&E × 100, original)

can be large and have a vesicular nucleus with open chromatin and a small nucleolus. Lymphocytes form diffuse infiltrates in which epithelial cells are admixed. In as many as 24% of thymomas, lymphoid cells aggregate to form ill-defined "nodules" that simulate germinal centers or a nodular malignant lymphoma at low-magnification microscopy. Rosai and Levine (1) designated this as "medullary differentiation" and emphasized features that differentiate it from the nodules of malignant lymphomas. The latter generally consist of large, pleomorphic, atypical lymphoid cells differing cytologically from the small, mature lymphocytes found in thymomas.

True germinal centers are seen in fewer than 10% of thymomas (1). They are heterogeneous and composed of different lymphoid cells and histiocytes with tingible intracytoplasmic bodies (1,2).

The epithelial cells of thymomas are round, oval, or spindle-shaped. They are best distinguished from histiocytes and mesenchymal cells by the fact that they tend to be grouped into cell clusters (Fig. 6-17). The nuclei of round or oval epithelial cells are vesicular with small, inconspicuous nucleoli and a pale, eosinophilic or amphophilic cytoplasm with indistinct cell borders. They are usually in the midst of lymphoid infiltrates as isolated cells, cell clusters, or anastomosing cords. They also can form sharply circumscribed lobules composed almost exclusively of round epithelial cells and can simulate a carcinoma. Examination at high magnification, however, fails to demonstrate cytologic evidence of malignancy.

Spindle-shaped epithelial cells may be indistinguishable from fibroblasts (Fig. 6-18) and were considered to be of mesenchymal origin prior to ultrastructural studies confirming their epithelial nature. Spindle cells grow in a number of patterns. They

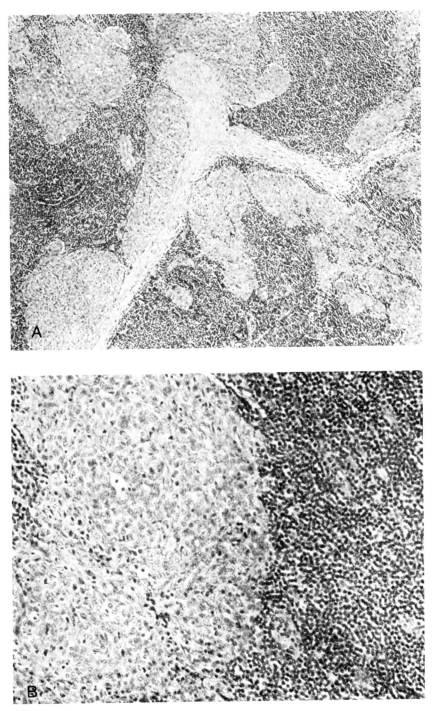

FIG. 6–13. A: Lymphoepithelial thymoma showing clusters of epithelial cells adjacent to lymphocytes. (H&E × 40, original) **B:** Higher power shows sharp separation between epithelial cells and lymphocytes. (H&E × 100, original)

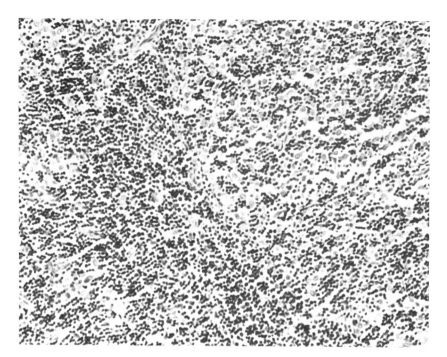

FIG. 6–14. Lymphocytic-predominant thymoma. (H&E × 40, original)

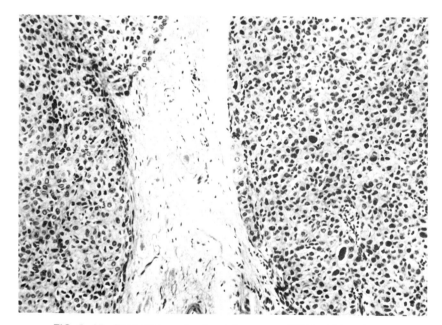

FIG. 6–15. Epithelial-predominant thymoma. (H&E × 100, original)

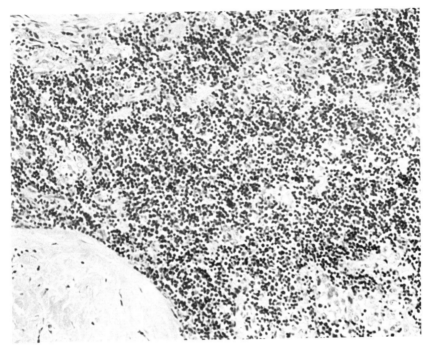

FIG. 6–16. Lymphoepithelial thymoma. (H&E × 40, original)

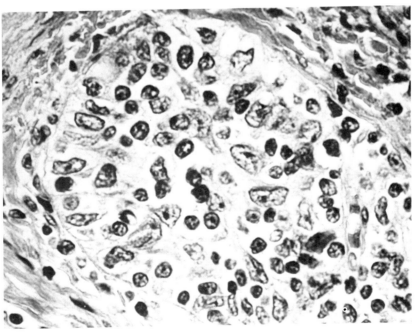

FIG. 6–17. Lymphoepithelial thymoma. Epithelial cells are round to oval and form clusters. Note their resemblance to "histiocytes." (H&E × 400, original)

CHAPTER 6

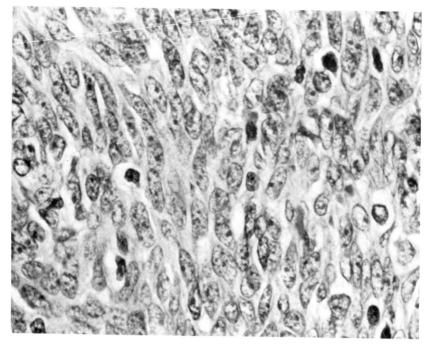

FIG. 6–18. Epithelial thymoma with spindle cells. (H&E × 400, original)

may form whorls, parallel bundles, or even interlacing bundles mimicking the storiform pattern of fibrous histiocytomas (Fig. 6-19) (1,2). This latter feature can be seen in as many as 11% of thymomas that have a spindle cell component. Spindle cells also can follow blood vessels in a hemangiopericytoma-like pattern (17% of instances) (1,2).

Most encapsulated thymomas have only minimal focal cellular atypia and low mitotic activity. Occasionally, however, epithelial cells in benign thymomas become very large and pleomorphic (Fig. 6-20). However, the diagnosis of malignancy should not be considered unless there is marked cytologic atypia with intense nuclear hyperchromasia and pleomorphism, prominent nucleoli, and increased mitotic activity.

Other Microscopic Features in Thymomas

Thymomas may show several other interesting microscopic features, including rosettes, pseudoglands, glands, papillary structures, Hassall's corpuscles, myoid cells, keratinizing squamous epithelium cells, and perivascular spaces.

Rosettes can be found in as many as 20% of thymomas and are formed by elongated epithelial cells arranged radially around a central core of eosinophilic amorphous material (1,2). A true central lumen is not present. Rosettes most frequently occur in predominantly lymphocytic thymomas. They are distinct from the rosettes of neurogenic tumors, which consist of small, dark, round or oval tumor cells, which typically have a "salt and pepper" chromatin pattern and are arranged around a central core of neurofibrils.

Pseudoglands are present in approximately 20% of thymomas (1). These are round

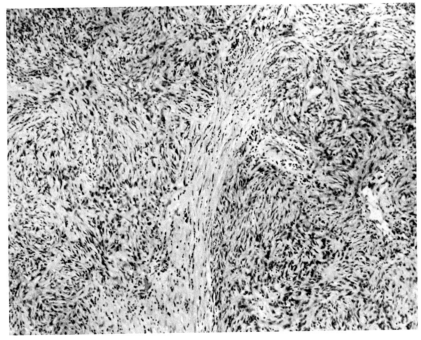

FIG. 6–19. Lymphoepithelial thymoma composed of spindle cells forming whorls and simulating a fibrous histiocytoma. (H&E × 40, original)

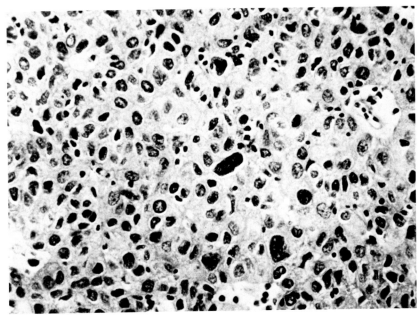

FIG. 6–20. Epithelial-predominant encapsulated thymoma showing focal cellular pleomorphism. This feature alone is not diagnostic of malignancy. (H&E × 400, original)

or elongated spaces of varying sizes lined by cuboidal or flattened spindle cells (Figs. 6-21 and 6-22) (1). These cells closely resemble trapped pleural mesothelial cells but have been shown to have ultrastructural features of thymic epithelium (Fig. 6-22).

True glands, lined by goblet cells or ciliated mucous epithelium, have also been described in thymomas (Fig. 6-23) (1,2).

Papillary structures and Hassall's corpuscles are unusual in thymomas. Hassall's corpuscles are found in 9% of thymomas (Fig. 6-24). They may be in various stages of development: small solid clusters of keratinized cells, cysts lined by squamous cells with intracytoplasmic keratohyaline granules, or variations of these growth patterns (1,2).

Myoid cells having eosinophilic cytoplasm and cross striations of the type seen in striated muscle are distinctly unusual in thymomas (214,215). They are best identified with special stains such as Masson's trichrome or phosphotungstic acid hematoxylin (PTAH) with immunocytochemical methods for the detection of actin, myosin, or other muscle-specific antigens, or with the electron microscope. Rarely, they are a prominent component of malignant spindle cell thymomas.

Shimosato and associates (216) described islands of keratinizing squamous epithelium in thymomas.

Rosai and Levine have emphasized the presence of perivascular spaces in thymomas as a useful morphologic feature for distinguishing these lesions from malignant lymphomas. Perivascular spaces are present in 35% to 56% of thymomas and are characterized by a central capillary or postcapillary venule surrounded by a continuous layer of epithelial cells (Fig. 6-25) (1,2). The intervening space contains pro-

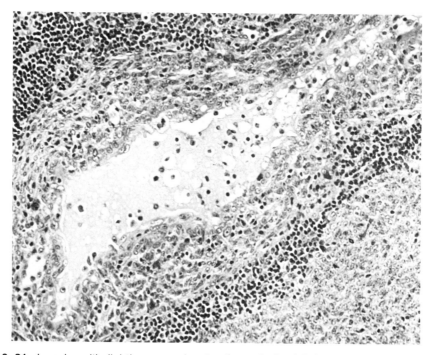

FIG. 6–21. Lymphoepithelial thymoma showing "pseudoglands" lined by flattened epithelial cells. (H&E × 100, original)

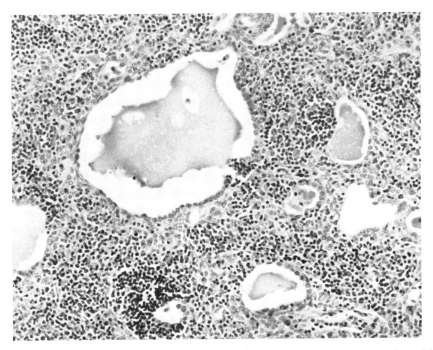

FIG. 6–22. Lymphoepithelial thymoma showing "pseudoglands" lined by cuboidal epithelial cells that resemble mesothelial cells. (H&E × 100, original)

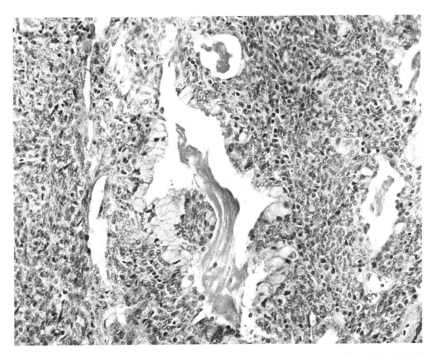

FIG. 6–23. Lymphoepithelial thymoma with true glands lined by goblet cells. (H&E × 100, original)

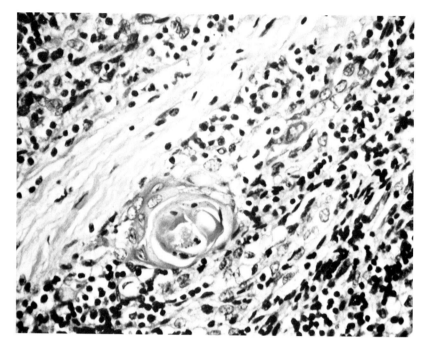

FIG. 6–24. Lymphoepithelial thymoma with Hassall's corpuscle. (H&E × 100, original)

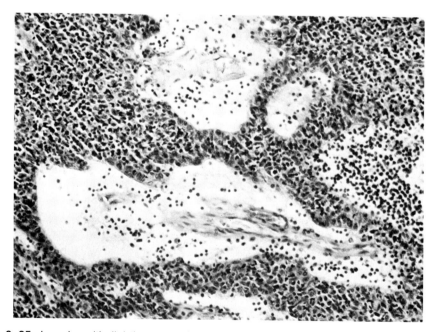

FIG. 6–25. Lymphoepithelial thymoma showing perivascular space with central venule. The space contains lymphocytes and is surrounded by epithelial cells. (H&E × 100, original)

teinaceous material, variable numbers of lymphocytes, plasma cells, and mast cells, erythrocytes, and/or foamy histiocytes. The space may become obliterated by hyalinized fibrous tissue. We have found perivascular spaces to be a useful diagnostic feature. However, in our material, they have been seen only focally and have seldom been present in small biopsies, where the distinction of predominantly lymphocytic thymomas from lymphomas is often difficult.

Degenerative Changes in Thymomas

Thymomas frequently exhibit a variety of microscopic changes that are probably degenerative. They include a "starry-sky" pattern, collections of "foamy histiocytes," microcystic degeneration, areas of old and recent hemorrhage, granulomas, and calcification with occasional formation of "sclerosiderotic nodules" (Figs. 6-26, 6-27, and 6-28) (1,217,218).

The "starry-sky" pattern is characterized by the presence of large numbers of phagocytic histiocytes among the lymphocytic component of thymomas. They may represent a response to cellular destruction (Fig. 6-28). Foamy histiocytes are found in clusters admixed with tumor cells or in perivascular spaces in 15% to 27% of thymomas (1,2).

Microcysts are present in 16% to 41% of thymomas and appear as round, empty holes containing either degenerated or viable cells in their lumina (Fig. 6-29) (1,2). They are found most frequently in lymphoid areas of the tumor and have no cyst lining.

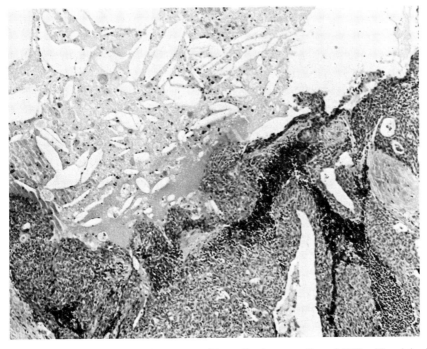

FIG. 6–26. Lymphoepithelial thymoma with cystic degeneration. (H&E × 40, original)

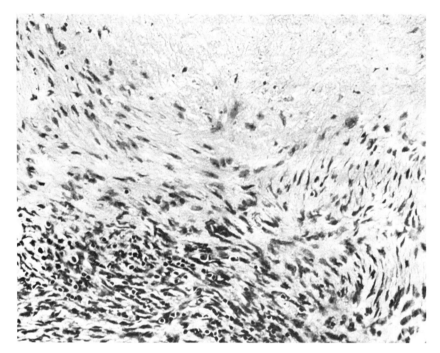

FIG. 6–27. Lymphoepithelial thymoma with spindle cells and focal necrosis. The lesion was well encapsulated and noninvasive. (H&E × 100, original)

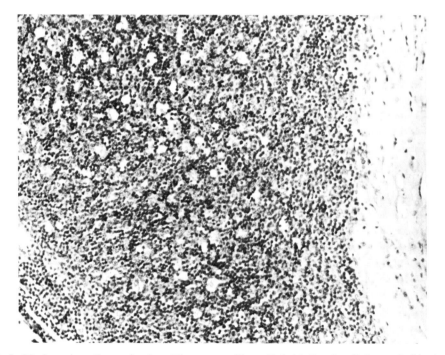

FIG. 6–28. Lymphocytic-predominant thymoma with multiple histiocytes ("starry-sky" feature). (H&E × 100, original)

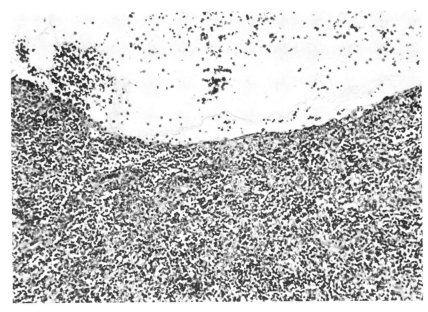

FIG. 6–29. Lymphocytic-predominant thymoma with microcyst formation. Note absence of cyst lining. (H&E × 100, original)

Hemorrhagic foci are not infrequent in thymomas. They may become calcified. Sclerosiderotic nodules similar to Gamna–Gandy nodules can occur (217). Epithelioid granulomas are infrequent in thymomas (Fig. 6-30) (218).

Cystic Thymoma

Grossly visible cysts are seen in as many as 40% of thymomas (Fig. 5-8) (2). The cystic spaces probably follow liquefactive necrosis of tumor cells or fluid accumulation secondary to hemorrhage. Cysts vary in size from a few millimeters to several centimeters in diameter and contain serous, pasty brown, or hemorrhagic material in their lumen.

Cystic degeneration is a feature of larger thymomas and can be seen in encapsulated as well as invasive lesions. Occasionally, the cysts occupy most of the tumor mass, and the neoplastic nature of the lesion can be determined only by study of small areas of tumor tissue in the cyst wall (11). Complete cystic degeneration of an invasive thymoma offers no guarantee of a good prognosis. Effler and McCormack (15) described a cyst from which a definitive histological diagnosis could not be established. The lesion recurred 3 years later; local and pericardial nodules had histologic features of an invasive thymoma. Other cases of invasive, recurrent cystic thymomas have been reported (1).

Cystic thymomas may be quite large and can compress mediastinal structures such as the heart and great vessels (42,43). In these instances, they can clinically simulate syndromes of constrictive pericarditis or pulmonary stenosis.

Cystic change in a thymoma has no particular association with clinical syndromes such as MG, hypogammaglobulinemia, anemia, or others (42).

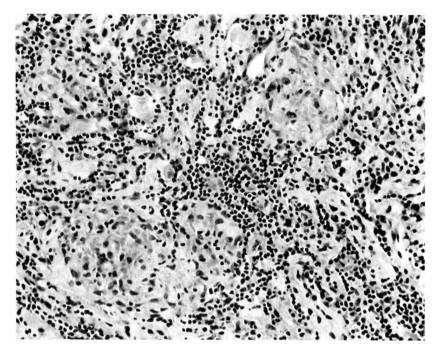

FIG. 6–30. Lymphoepithelial thymoma with epithelioid cell granulomata. (H&E × 100, original)

Giant Thymoma

Rarely, thymomas are so large at the time of diagnosis that they completely fill a hemithorax (6,13). The epithelial thymoma reported by Smith and associates (13) in a 15-year-old boy weighed 5,700 g.

Ectopic Hamartomatous Thymoma

In 1984 Rosai and associates (219) described several adult patients with ectopic thymomas of the lower neck with distinct morphologic features and proposed to classify them as ectopic hamartomatous thymomas. More recently Fetsch and Weiss (220) reported four additional cases. The lesions are located either superficially or deep in the sternoclavicular area and present as well-circumscribed, nonencapsulated tumors that can reach a large size. Their gross surface is solid, gray–white with a fasciculated pattern (220). Histologically the tumors are composed of spindle cell elements that can become very cellular and can be confused with a sarcoma, epithelial cells arranged in solid nests and trabeculae, small glands, cysts lined by squamous epithelium, adipose tissue, and lymphocytes (219). The spindle cells and epithelial cells exhibit keratin and muscle actin immunoreactivity (219). Ectopic hamartomatous thymomas are benign tumors that probably arise from ectopic abnormal thymic tissue derived from the third pharyngeal pouch (220–222).

We have observed a patient with a lymphoepithelial thymoma located adjacent to the thyroid gland (Figs. 6-31 and 6-32).

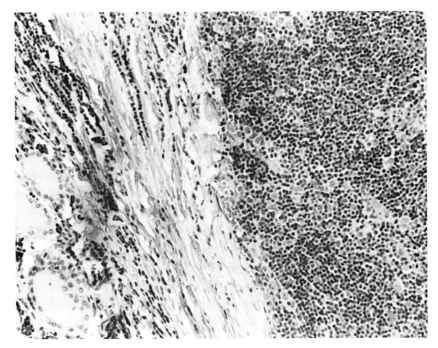

FIG. 6–31. Ectopic thymoma. The lymphoepithelial lesion presented as a neck mass adjacent to the thyroid gland. (H&E × 100, original)

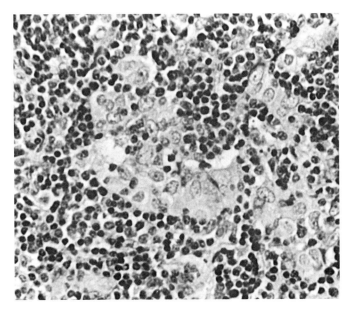

FIG. 6–32. Ectopic thymoma composed of lymphoid cells and solid nests of epithelial cells. (H&E × 400, original)

Cortical, Medullary, and Mixed Thymomas

As discussed in Chapter 3, cortical and medullary epithelial cells of the thymus are thought to have different embryological derivation and exhibit different enzyme histochemical and immunohistological features. At the light microscopic level, cortical epithelial cells are stellate in shape with a medium-sized, oval–round nucleus with thin nuclear membrane, scanty chromatin, and a prominent nucleolus. Medullary epithelial cells are spindle-shaped with indistinct cytoplasmic processes and a small- to medium-sized oval–spindle nucleus with small nucleolus.

Cortical thymomas are composed of neoplastic cortical epithelial cells admixed with small, medium, or large lymphoid cells with morphologic features of lymphoblasts (Fig. 6–33). Small cysts lined by epithelial cells can be present as well as a variable number of "thymic nurse cells" containing lymphocytes within intracytoplasmic vacuoles (198). The tumors usually exhibit a nodular growth pattern with areas of starry-sky appearance exhibiting numerous macrophages (Fig. 6-34). The tumor cells exhibit Leu-7 immunoreactivity (Fig. 6-35). Müller-Hermelink and associates (198) emphasize the presence of conspicuous perivascular palisading as a characteristic finding in cortical thymomas.

Medullary thymomas are composed of proliferating oval or spindle-shaped epithelial cells admixed with small lymphocytes (Fig. 6-36). They also have a prominent number of interdigitating cells (IDC) that exhibit intracytoplasmic S-100 protein immunoreactivity (198).

Mixed thymomas have intermediate features between cortical and medullary thy-

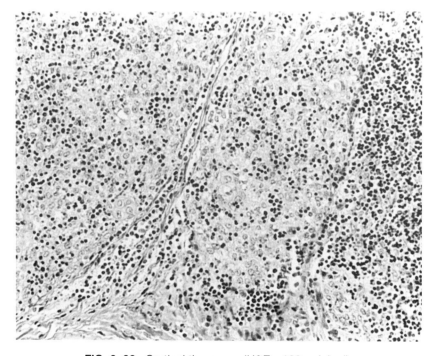

FIG. 6–33. Cortical thymoma. (H&E × 100, original)

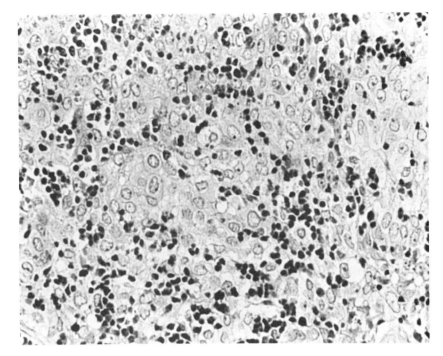

FIG. 6–34. Higher magnification of tumor in Fig. 6-33. The epithelial cells are large and form solid nests admixed with small lymphocytes. The epithelial cells are larger than those of medullary thymomas. (H&E × 200, original)

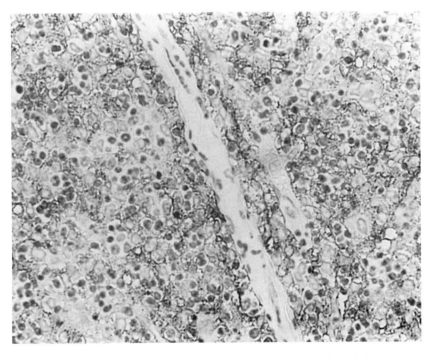

FIG. 6–35. Cortical thymoma. The epithelial cells exhibit Leu-7 cytoplasmic immunoreactivity. (PAP method × 400, original).

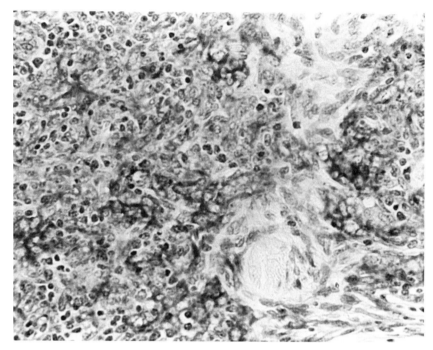

FIG. 6–36. Medullary thymoma. The cells exhibit keratin immunoreactivity. Immunostains for Leu-7 were negative. (PAP method × 400, original)

momas with lymphocyte-rich areas, perivascular spaces, epithelial-rich areas, and other morphologic features described in detail in the previous section.

Invasive (Malignant) Thymomas

The presence of capsular invasion and extension into other mediastinal organs are the most important prognostic features in patients with thymomas. Unfortunately, these features usually cannot be determined with accuracy in biopsy materials or in radiographic studies.

Well-encapsulated thymomas are usually benign and recur locally in fewer than 2% of instances following thymectomy (1). Encapsulated thymomas tend to grow slowly over many years and may remain stationary in size for long periods of time. For example, Rosai and Levine (1) reported a thymoma that was followed radiologically for 15 years without significant progression.

There are, however, exceptional instances of encapsulated thymomas that metastasize as malignant tumors. A case reported by Yoshida and associates (36), for example, was a 49-year-old woman with an encapsulated epithelial thymoma that was not locally invasive yet metastasized to the lungs, spleen, brain, liver, kidney, and ovary.

Thymomas are incompletely encapsulated in 7% to 33% of instances and tend to invade adjacent thoracic structures such as the lungs and pleura (223–243). These locally invasive thymomas tend to recur locally and occasionally metastasize widely in 14% to 15.5% of patients (233).

The infiltrative character of a thymoma is the most significant prognostic factor (Fig. 6-37) (1). Indeed, most authors classify thymomas as benign or malignant solely on the basis of the absence or presence of local invasion (223–242).

The prognostic value of other factors such as the size of lesion, histologic classification of the tumor, and presence of MG has been controversial. It is generally accepted, however, that these parameters are unreliable indicators of the biologic behavior of a thymoma (1). Moreover, the presence of focal cellular atypia and/or increased mitotic activity has no proven prognostic value in these tumors.

Several recent studies have shown that the subclassification of thymomas according to the scheme of Marino and Müller-Hermelink has prognostic significance (198). Cortical thymomas are more frequently invasive and are likely to behave as malignant tumors, while medullary thymomas are benign in most instances. Mixed thymomas have an intermediate prognosis. For example, in a recent study by Elert and associates (203) all epithelial thymomas with cortical differentiation showed a malignant course; however, medullary thymomas did not recur. Ricci and associates (204) reported 100% 20-year actuarial survival in patients with medullary thymoma versus 45% 20-year actuarial survival for patients with cortical thymoma. Patients in this study with mixed thymomas had 65% 20-year actuarial survival. Myasthenia gravis was also more frequent (approximately 33% of the cases) in patients with cortical and mixed thymomas than in patients with medullary thymoma (approximately 11% of the cases).

The macroscopic impression of invasion in a thymoma must be documented histologically for one to consider a lesion malignant. Not infrequently, for example, well-encapsulated benign thymomas are firmly adherent to the lungs, pleura, or thoracic wall because of fibrous adhesions. These lesions should not be diagnosed as malignant unless histologic examination documents the presence of tissue infiltration by the tumor (Fig. 6-38).

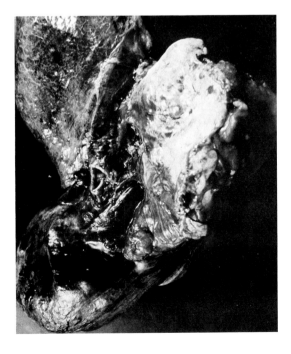

FIG. 6–37. Invasive thymoma infiltrating lung parenchyma.

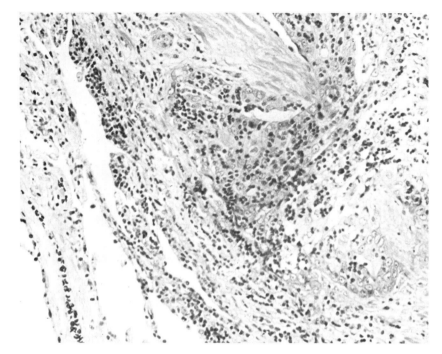

FIG. 6–38. Invasive thymoma extending into lung parenchyma. (H&E × 100, original)

It is also important to document the presence of microscopic capsular invasion in thymomas, as studies have suggested that tumors with this feature have a higher local recurrence rate than noninvasive neoplasms (208).

Invasive thymomas infiltrate adjacent mediastinal structures such as blood vessels, mediastinal and lower cranial nerves, and lymph nodes by direct extension and penetrate into the pleura, lung, pericardium, superior vena cava, and the right atrium of the heart (222, 244). In addition, implants may develop throughout the pleural and pericardial cavities and present as well-circumscribed satellite nodules that have no anatomical connection with the primary lesion (Fig. 6-39).

Invasive thymomas frequently recur within the thoracic cavity but usually do not metastasize widely (245–253).

Clinicopathological Staging of Patients with Thymomas

Several schemes have been developed for the clinicopathological staging of patients with thymomas (Table 4).

Bergh and associates (253) have classified patients with thymomas into three stages: I, intact capsule or growth within the capsule; II, pericapsular growth into the mediastinal fat tissue; and III, invasive growth into the surrounding organs and/or intrathoracic metastases (Figs. 6-40 and 6-41) (Table 4). In their experience, all stage I and II lesions are resectable, whereas only some stage III tumors can be completely removed. Almost 50% of their patients with stage III disease had pleural implants.

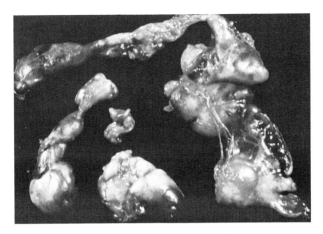

FIG. 6–39. Multiple nodules of invasive thymoma resected from the pleura and pericardium.

Wilkins and Castleman (3) used similar criteria but included pleural or pericardial invasion in stage II (Table 4).

Masaoka and associates developed a four-stage system (Table 4) (254). In their experience with 96 patients with thymoma, the overall 5-year survival was 74.1% and the 10-year survival was 57.1%. Five-year survival rates by clinical stage were 92.6% in stage I, 85.7% in stage II, 69.6% in stage III, and 50% in stage IV.

Treatment and Prognosis of Thymomas

Since the publication of our previous edition there have been numerous reports of the treatment of encapsulated and invasive thymomas with surgery, radiotherapy, and/or chemotherapy (255–275). A detailed review of these studies is beyond the

TABLE 4. *Clinicopathological staging of thymomas*

Stage	Bergh et al. (253)	Wilkins and Castleman (3)	Masaoka et al. (254)
I	Intact capsule or growth within capsule	(Same as in Bergh et al.)	Encapsulated lesion with no macroscopic or microscopic invasion
II	Pericapsular invasion into the mediastinal fat	Pericapsular invasion into the mediastinal fat or adjacent pleura or pericardium	1. Macroscopic invasion surrounding fat or mediastinal pleura or adjacent pleura 2. Microscopic invasion into capsule
III	Invasive growth into the surrounding organs and/ or intrathoracic metastases	(Same as in Bergh et al.)	Macroscopic invasion into adjacent organs (i.e., pericardium, lung)
IVa			Pleural or pericardial dissemination
IVb			Distant metastasis (lymphatic or hematogenous spread)

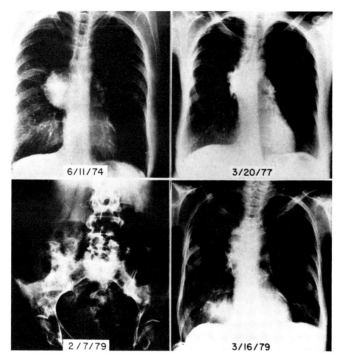

FIG. 6–40. Top left: Chest film showing mediastinal tumor before surgery. **Top right:** After surgical resection and radiotherapy. **Bottom left:** Large, semicircular lytic defect in right ileum. **Bottom right:** Chest film showing right pleural mass as well as a large, well-circumscribed parenchymal mass at the right lung base. (From Chahinian et al, ref. 228, with permission.)

scope of this volume. In general, stage I thymomas are treated with surgical resection with excellent results, except for the few reports discussed above. Most thymectomies are performed through a thoracotomy. Papatestas and associates (270), however, reported high remission rates and low mortality rates in patients with occult thymomas and MG following transcervical thymectomy.

Some patients with thymomas in stage I or stage II due to microscopic invasion of the tumor capsule (according to the Masaoka staging system) recur following complete resection, and it has been suggested that radiotherapy may play a role in their treatment (257). To our knowledge, this topic remains controversial.

Patients with invasive thymomas (stages II and III) benefit from aggressive surgical resection that can include resection of mediastinal veins and replacement by vascular grafts and adjuvant radiotherapy. In a recent report by Nakahara and associates (268), for example, patients with stage III thymomas that underwent complete resection and radiotherapy had survival rates of 100% at 5 years and 94.7% at 15 years. These survival rates were similar to those of stage I patients resected surgically (268). Other authors report lower survival rates for patients with invasive thymoma with overall 5-year survival rates of approximately 40% to 60% (256–275).

Chemotherapy has also been utilized in patients with advanced and/or metastatic thymoma (stages III and IV) (258–261). In a recent review of the experience of a cooperative oncology group trial, Loehrer and associates (266) reported objective

remissions in the majority of patients with thymoma treated with combination chemotherapy of cisplatin, doxorubicin, and cyclophosphamide. Fornasiero and associates (260), utilizing a similar regimen plus vincristine, reported high complete response and overall response rates in patients with stage III and stage IV thymomas.

Radiotherapy and chemotherapy have also been used preoperatively followed by
reoperation for resection of a previously unresectable invasive thymoma (273).

The results of therapy are difficult to assess with accuracy in patients with thymomas as the tumors can recur and/or metastasize many years after the initial treatment. For example, Denayer and associates (255) reported a patient that developed
hepatic metastases and a myasthenic crisis 22 years after apparent cure of an invasive mediastinal thymoma.

Thymic Carcinomas

Thymic carcinomas represent a small group of epithelial neoplasms of the thymus
gland characterized by the presence of marked cytologic and architectural atypia,
increased mitotic activity, and necrosis (276–293).

The incidence of thymic carcinoma varies at different institutions. There is no sex
prevalence, and thymic carcinomas occur in patients of different ages (4 to 81 years
old; mean age 55 years old) (284,285). We have encountered only a few cases of
thymic carcinoma among several hundred thymic epithelial tumors. This may be
related to the fact that many of our patients were referred to The Mount Sinai Hospital for the study of MG. Other medical centers report incidences of thymic carcinomas ranging from 18.3% to 21.3% (201,284,285).

Snover and associates (18) described nine variants of thymic carcinoma based on
the histologic characteristics of the tumors: squamous cell carcinoma, lymphoepithelioma-like carcinoma, undifferentiated carcinoma, small-cell carcinoma (oat-cell
carcinoma), basaloid carcinoma, mucoepidermoid carcinoma, clear-cell carcinoma,
sarcomatoid carcinoma, and mixed small-cell–undifferentiated-squamous cell carcinoma. More recent studies have reported patients with other lesions of the thymus:
adenocarcinoma lymphoepithelial lesions associated with signet-ring cell adenocarcinoma of the anterior mediastinum, adenosquamous carcinoma, melanocytic neuroendocrine carcinoma, and thymic carcinoma with focal neuroblastoma differentiation (282,285,287,291). These pathologic variants probably represent divergent
patterns of differentiation of thymic tumors arising from pluripotential epithelial
stem cells of endodermal origin. Indeed, thymic carcinomas often have different cell
types combined with areas suggestive of a thymoma.

The diagnosis of thymic carcinomas as primary neoplasms is made in the absence
of other possible primary tumors elsewhere. The presence of residual nonneoplastic
thymic tissue at the periphery of the carcinoma also is considered additional evidence of a thymic origin, although it does not rule out the possibility of a metastasis
to the gland.

Clinical Conditions Associated with Thymic Carcinomas

Patients with thymic carcinomas differ from those with thymoma and usually present with no associated clinical syndromes. DiMario and associates (283) reported a

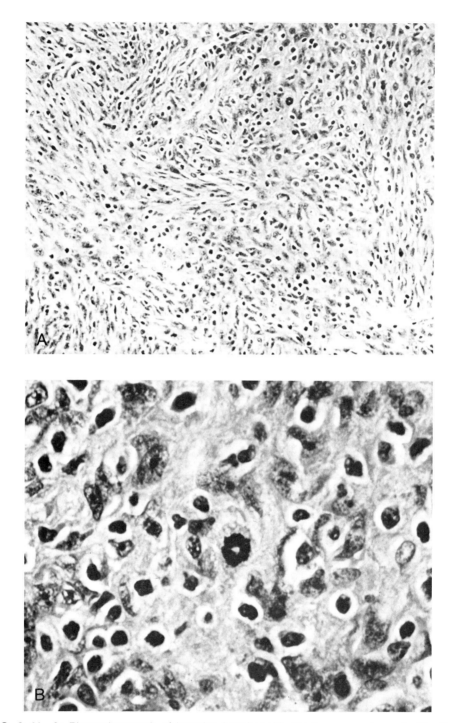

FIG. 6–41. A: Photomicrograph of invasive lymphoepithelial thymoma shown in Fig. 6-40. (H&E × 100, original) **B:** Higher magnification of the same lesion showing cellular atypia and mitotic figure. This degree of cellular atypia alone is not diagnostic of malignancy in the absence of local invasion or metastases. (H&E × 400, original)

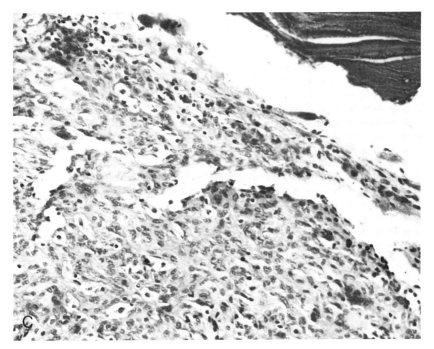

FIG. 6–41. *Continued.* **C:** Bone metastasis from the same patient shown in A and B. The metastatic lesion shows fewer lymphocytes than the primary tumor. (H&E × 100, original)

single patient with squamous cell carcinoma of the thymus and MG. Thomas and Manivel (292) reported a patient with a thymic carcinoma and aplastic anemia.

Squamous Cell Carcinoma of the Thymus

Squamous cell carcinomas are the most common variant of thymic carcinomas (18,294–296). They are most frequent in men in the sixth decade of life. There is no significant relationship to smoking. Patients present with weight loss, chest pain, cough, bloody sputum, and/or shoulder pain and have well-defined anterior mediastinal tumors on chest roentgenograms (18,294–296).

Squamous cell carcinomas of the thymus are partially encapsulated, firm, white–gray tumors with granular surfaces, small foci of necrosis and hemorrhage, and cystic spaces filled with brown fluid. They infiltrate adjacent soft tissues and mediastinal vascular structures, may extend into the pleura, lungs, and/or pericardium, and may metastasize to the anterior mediastinal lymph nodes. When the tumor extends into the pulmonary parenchyma, the lung appears to be pulled into the mediastinal mass. Bronchi are not involved by the neoplasm. These features allow the distinction of squamous cell carcinomas of the thymus from bronchogenic tumors.

Histologically these tumors have characteristic features of a squamous cell carcinoma with solid nests of polygonal cells with vesicular nuclei, distinct nucleoli, and eosinophilic cytoplasm separated by fibrous bands (Figs. 6-42 and 6-43). These cells

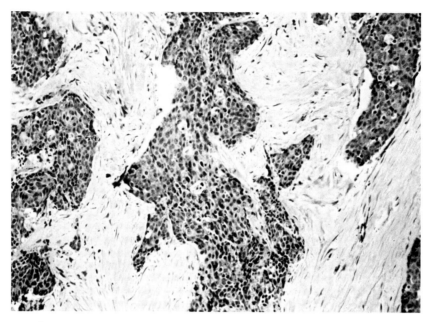

FIG. 6–42. Squamous cell carcinoma of the thymus showing solid nests of polygonal cells separated by fibrous bands. (H&E × 100, original)

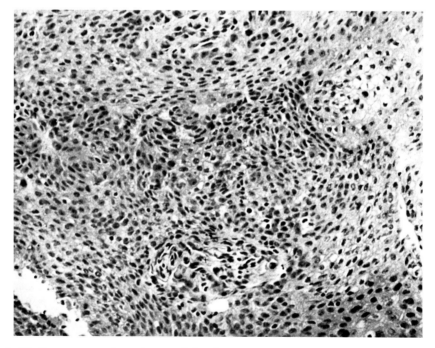

FIG. 6–43. Squamous cell carcinoma of the thymus showing solid sheets of polygonal cells with eosinophilic cytoplasm. (H&E × 100, original)

have intercellular bridges and may form keratotic pearls that may closely resemble Hassall's corpuscles.

Squamous cell carcinoma of the thymus may arise *de novo* or develop from a pre-existing thymoma. For example, a benign lymphoepithelial thymoma recurred 5 years after thymectomy in the form of a nonkeratinizing squamous cell carcinoma metastatic to a lymph node (297). Shimosato and associates (216) described a similar lymphoepithelial thymoma that had an area of squamous cell carcinoma at the periphery of the neoplasm. Morinaga and associates (288) reported an interesting patient with multiple nodules of a thymic neoplasm with mixed features of thymoma and squamous cell carcinoma.

Hassall's corpuscles may resemble squamous pearls in otherwise typical thymomas and should not be considered evidence of malignancy unless they are composed of cells with marked cytologic atypia and represent a significant proportion of the tumor. Shimosato and associates (216) have suggested that the presence of focal squamous cell differentiation in thymomas of epithelial type may indicate a more aggressive biologic potential of the lesion. This suggestion is based, however, on only two cases.

Squamous cell carcinomas of the thymus can have glandular areas (adenosquamous carcinoma) (298,299). The tumor cells usually exhibit immunoreactivity with antibodies to keratin (AE1/AE3) and epithelial membrane antigen (EMA) (283,284). They can also stain positively with antibodies to CEA and B72.3 antigen. Occasionally, S-100 reactive cells are also present, admixed with the tumor cells.

Squamous cell carcinomas of the thymus are biologically less aggressive neoplasms than similar tumors arising from the lung, larynx, or other primary sites. They are usually aggressive locally and in most patients do not metastasize widely. They are radiosensitive and can respond to chemotherapy with cyclophosphamide, doxorubicin, cisplatin, and prednisone (300).

Therapy, including surgery and radiotherapy, has relatively good results, particularly when the lesions are initially completely resectable. For example, of the eight patients of Shimosato and associates, two died with metastatic tumor 11 and 21 months after diagnosis, respectively, whereas the other six survived 1 to 12 years after surgery without evidence of disease (216).

In a recent review of the literature, DiMario and associates (283) reported a 22% recurrence rate at 5 years and less than 50% survival at 10 years for patients with squamous cell carcinoma of the thymus.

Lymphoepithelioma-like Carcinoma

Thymic neoplasms may be composed of solid sheets of large epithelial cells with open nuclei, small nucleoli, and indistinct cytoplasm admixed with prominent lymphoid infiltrates (Fig. 6-44) (4,280,293). These tumors have identical morphologic features to lymphoepitheliomas of the nasopharyngeal area (Schmincke's tumor) (301).

Patients with nasopharyngeal carcinomas frequently have elevated titers to Epstein–Barr virus (EB virus) (302). It has been suggested that the EB virus plays a role in the pathogenesis of lymphoepithelioma and other malignant tumors such as Burkitt's lymphoma. We studied a 19-year-old patient with a lymphoepithelioma-like

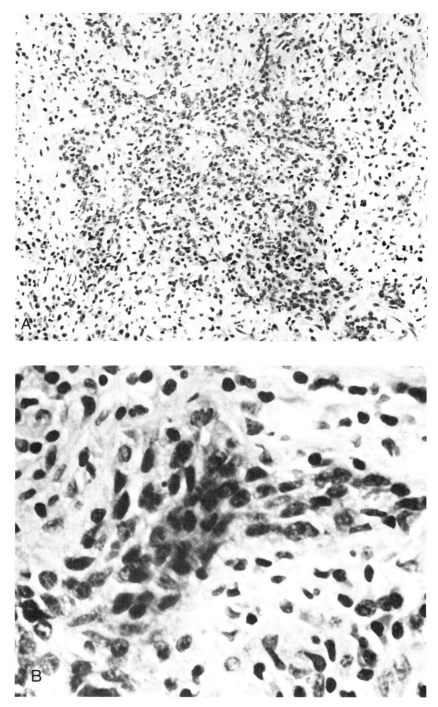

FIG. 6–44. A: Lymphoepithelioma-like carcinoma of the thymus. Note the presence of clusters of large, undifferentiated epithelial cells. (H&E × 100, original) **B:** Higher magnification showing a cluster of hyperchromatic epithelial cells. (H&E × 400, original)

carcinoma of the anterior mediastinum who had elevated serum levels of antibodies to EB virus (Fig. 6-44). He did not have a nasopharyngeal lesion; this was documented by careful clinical and radiologic examination and multiple blind biopsies of the area.

The viral genome can also be detected in the tumor specimen utilizing Southern blot analysis (211).

Lymphoepitheliomas of the thymus are difficult to distinguish from squamous cell carcinomas and are considered by some authors to be variants of the latter tumor (299).

Basaloid Carcinomas

Basaloid primary thymic carcinomas present as well-circumscribed masses in the anterior mediastinum measuring up to 8 cm in greatest diameter (299). One of the two tumors reported by Snover and associates (18) was partly solid and partly cystic. The other was predominantly cystic and multiloculated. The solid areas of both tumors consisted of solid nests and trabeculae of small, uniform polygonal cells exhibiting prominent palisading near the basement membrane in a pattern similar to that seen in basal cell carcinomas of the skin. The lesions had abundant mitotic figures, focal areas of squamous differentiation, and numerous gland-like spaces containing mucicarmine and alcian blue–periodic acid-Schiff (PAS)-positive material. Larger cystic spaces were also lined by tumor cells. The tumor cells of basaloid carcinomas were similar to those of oat-cell carcinomas of the thymus and had round to oval nuclei with finely stippled chromatin and inconspicuous nucleoli. Ultrastructural studies, however, have failed to demonstrate neurosecretory dense-core granules in the cytoplasm of basaloid carcinoma cells.

In both lesions the authors demonstrated benign cysts lined by squamous epithelium adjacent to the tumors. This finding suggests an origin from pre-existing benign thymic cysts.

The biologic behavior of these lesions is unknown. One of the two cases was followed for 1 year without evidence of residual disease after surgery. The other patient was lost to follow-up.

Mucoepidermoid Carcinoma

Tanaka and associates (276) and Snover and associates (18) reported rare instances of mucoepidermoid carcinomas of the thymus. These tumors are similar in cell morphology to their salivary gland counterparts and have squamous, mucinous, and intermediate cells.

The presence of mucinous differentiation in thymic neoplasms is not surprising. Indeed, mucinous epithelium can be found occasionally in the normal human thymus and in human thymomas (215). It is more frequently seen in the thymus of dogs and other animals and reflects the potential of the thymic epithelium to differentiate along multiple cell lines (276).

Mucoepidermoid carcinomas of the thymus can be aggressive neoplasms. One patient, for example, died of cardiac tamponade caused by tumor invasion 5 years after partial resection, postoperative radiotherapy, and chemotherapy with mitomycin (276). At autopsy the tumor was in the thymic areas, sternum, regional lymph nodes, pleura, and pericardium. Another patient, however, had no evidence of disease 2 years after surgery (18).

Oat-Cell Carcinoma

Oat-cell carcinoma of the thymus is an unusual but well-recognized variant of thymic malignant tumors (277–279).

This tumor may be identical to small-cell carcinomas of the lung and other organs. Indeed, confirmation as a primary malignancy of the thymus can be made only by the exclusion of other primary lesions either during life or at autopsy.

The tumors are large, well-circumscribed anterior mediastinal masses composed of soft gray tissue with areas of hemorrhage and necrosis (277). Histologically they have nests and trabeculae of small anaplastic cells in an organoid pattern with nests of cells separated by connective tissue septa (Fig. 6-45). The tumor cells have scanty cytoplasm with indistinct cell borders and round, oval, or spindle nuclei with a stippled chromatin pattern and inconspicuous nucleoli. The tumor cells can exhibit chromogranin immunoreactivity (299). Ultrastructurally these cells have prominent dense-core neurosecretory granules, abundant aggregates of cytoplasmic fibrils, and numerous desmosomes. Not infrequently, differentiated areas of carcinoid tumor can be found in the mediastinal mass (279).

Oat-cell carcinomas of the thymus are aggressive and can metastasize widely in a manner similar to their pulmonary counterparts. However, they respond to chemotherapy with single agents. There are at least two documented cases of oat-cell carcinoma of the thymus in prolonged remission after chemotherapy (277–279).

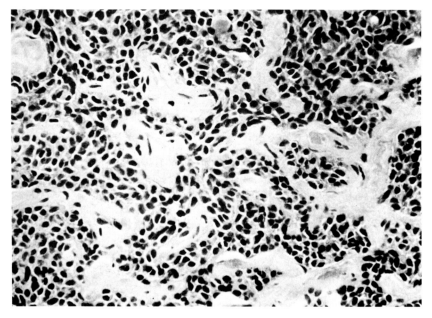

FIG. 6–45. Oat-cell carcinoma of the thymus with nests and anastomosing trabeculae of small cells with scanty cytoplasm. (H&E × 400, original)

The embryogenesis of these tumors has been the subject of controversy (303,304). Oat-cell carcinomas of the thymus are often associated with endocrine neoplasms of various organs (Multiple Endocrine Neoplasm type I syndrome), and they are themselves considered to be neuroendocrine neoplasms (279). Indeed, the tumor cells have histochemical and ultrastructural characteristics of amine precursor uptake and decarboxylation (APUD) cells including intracytoplasmic amines (serotonin) and neurosecretory dense-core granules (304). Such APUD cells have been thought to be of neural crest (ectoderm) origin.

This theory of an exclusive ectodermal origin of neuroendocrine cells has been disputed after careful embryologic and pathologic studies established that other neoplasms composed of cells with characteristics of APUD cells in the lung and intestine were most likely of endodermal origin (303).

It has been suggested that neuroendocrine tumors that exhibit prominent desmosomes and numerous aggregates of intracytoplasmic fibrils are probably of endodermal origin (305). These features are present in oat-cell carcinomas of the thymus (298).

Mixed Small-Cell (Oat-Cell)–Squamous Cell Carcinoma

Snover and associates (18) reported three instances of large mediastinal tumors exhibiting histologically combined features of oat-cell and squamous cell carcinoma. Although argyrophil stains were negative in these cases, ultrastructural studies demonstrated numerous cytoplasmic dense-core granules in the small-cell component of the tumors. The three patients died with metastatic tumor 9 months to 5 years after initial diagnoses in spite of surgical resection of their primary lesions and chemotherapy.

Other Forms of Thymic Carcinoma

Isolated cases of clear-cell carcinomas of the thymus and sarcomatoid carcinoma of the thymus have been described (18).

The patient with clear-cell carcinoma of the thymus presented with a firm, gray tumor composed of sheets of uniform polygonal cells with clear cytoplasm. The cells were separated by occasional fibrovascular septa. The morphology of the tumor was similar to that of a renal cell carcinoma. The patient was well for 9 years after surgical excision of the lesion but died 13 years after initial diagnosis with multiple metastases.

Moriyama and associates (289) reported a patient with a multicystic thymic tumor with areas of papillotubular adenocarcinoma arising from a cystic space.

The patient with sarcomatoid carcinoma of the thymus had a large, well-circumscribed, solid gray anterior mediastinal mass composed of large spindle cells arranged in fascicles or in a storiform pattern. Immunohistochemical studies showed the presence of myoglobin and keratin in their cytoplasm. Ultrastructural studies demonstrated myoid differentiation at all stages of development, ranging from isolated myofilaments to well-formed sarcomeres. The patient died with extensive tumor metastasis 13 months after initial diagnosis in spite of early resection and multiple-agent chemotherapy.

Undifferentiated Carcinomas

Occasionally, thymic carcinomas are composed of solid sheets of large, bizarre cells with marked pleomorphism (Fig. 6-46).

Differential Diagnosis Between Thymoma and Thymic Carcinoma

The distinction between thymomas and thymic carcinoma can be difficult to establish, particularly in small biopsy materials or in tumors that exhibit mixed histopathological features. The diagnosis of carcinoma rests on the presence of morphologic features of marked cytologic atypia, including large cell size, large nucleoli, high nuclear/cytoplasmic ratio, frequent mitotic figures, and foci of necrosis (299). Immunocytochemical studies and electron microscopy are of limited value for the differential diagnosis as thymomas and thymic carcinomas share similar immunohistochemical and ultrastructural features (Table 5). However, immunocytochemical methods can be helpful by detecting CEA in squamous or clear-cell carcinomas of the thymus or chromogranin in small-cell carcinomas, for example (299). Neuroendocrine granules are also present in small-cell carcinomas of the thymus.

Familial Thymic Tumors

It is not unusual for neuroendocrine thymic tumors (thymic carcinoid, oat-cell carcinoma) to have a high incidence in certain families (279). These patients frequently have other nonthymic endocrine neoplasms (MEN type I syndrome).

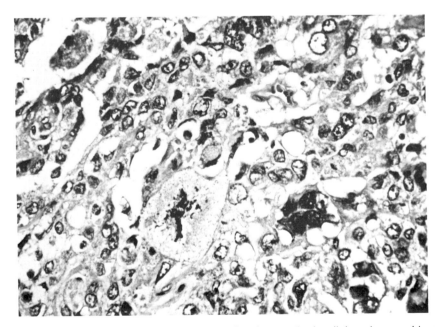

FIG. 6–46. Undifferentiated thymic carcinoma showing marked cellular pleomorphism with atypical mitosis. (H&E × 400, original)

TABLE 5. *Immunohistochemical features of thymic carcinoma: comparison with thymoma and the normal thymus*

	Keratin	EMA	CEA	B72.3	Leu-7	Chromogranin
Normal thymus*	+	+	+	+	+/−	−
Thymoma	+	+	−	−	+/−	−
Squamous cell carcinoma	+	+	+/−	+/−	−	−
Small-cell carcinoma	+	+	−	+/−	+/−	+/−
Clear-cell carcinoma	+	+	+	−	−	−
Adenosquamous carcinoma	+	+	−	+	+	−

Modified from Truong et al (299).
*Hassall's corpuscles

It is unusual, however, to find multiple thymic neoplasms in a family. Indeed, there are to our knowledge, only two reports of thymic neoplasia in siblings (305,306). In one instance, for example, a 56-year-old man had a thymic, poorly differentiated squamous cell carcinoma, and his younger brother had a spindle cell invasive thymoma with associated hypogammaglobulinemia (305). An explanation for the occurrence of the neoplasms in the two brothers could not be offered, but both tumors are so infrequent in the general population that the association may not be by chance.

Thymomas in Children

Thymomas have been reported in children as young as 8 months of age and present several distinct clinical features in patients younger than 15 years of age (307–316).

Thymomas are infrequent in children. They account for 12% to 20% of all mediastinal tumors in adults but only 5% of mediastinal neoplasms in children (311,317,318). Most mediastinal tumors in patients younger than 15 years of age are teratomas or lymphoid tumors (317).

The clinical presentation of the thymic neoplasm may also be different in young patients. Thymomas are frequently symptomatic, and patients present with signs and symptoms of respiratory and/or vascular compression including cough, dyspnea, cyanosis, wheezing, and superior vena cava syndrome (313,319). Except for a few isolated reports of MG, aplastic anemia, or leukemia, most children with the tumor have had no associated systemic disease (309,310,320).

The pathologic features of childhood thymomas are somewhat different from those of adults (Fig. 6-47). Dehner and associates (311) suggest that these tumors in young patients lack the typical features of thymomas in adults, such as the distinct lobulation, and that they are usually composed of proliferating bands of epithelium containing numerous Hassall's corpuscles, lymphocytes, and connective tissue septa. These differences probably fall, however, within the wide spectrum of morphologic features that can be found in thymomas.

Thymomas in children have a higher incidence of invasiveness than their counterparts in adult patients. For example, of 12 patients with thymoma reviewed at Children's Hospital Medical Center in Boston, 43% had malignant variants (313). This incidence of invasiveness is higher than the 7% to 33% encountered in adults (1).

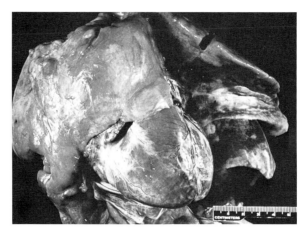

FIG. 6–47. Invasive thymoma infiltrating the lung parenchyma in a child.

Indeed, childhood thymomas may be more aggressive than their adult counterparts. Most lesions reported have followed a rapid clinical course with progression to death within 6 months of onset of symptoms (311). Bowie and associates (319), for example, in a review of 20 patients from the literature and their own experience, reported a 78% mortality in children with thymoma. This survival rate compares with an overall 65% 5-year survival rate of adult patients with thymoma (1).

Other authors have had much better therapeutic results and have indicated that the prognosis of thymomas in children is not necessarily dismal if patients are treated with aggressive surgical excision and adjuvant radiotherapy and chemotherapy (313). The Boston Children's Hospital patients were staged clinically according to the scheme of Bergh and associates (253). All patients underwent excision of their primary lesions and satellite nodules. Patients at stages II and III received adjuvant radiotherapy and/or chemotherapy. Four of these patients with more advanced disease survived 15 months to 9 years following onset of symptoms. The approximate long-term survival in this series is 60%, similar to that reported in adults with thymomas.

SPECIAL STUDIES ON THYMOMAS

Ultrastructural Studies

The ultrastructural characteristics of thymomas have been well defined in several studies (1,179,181–188,321). These studies have characterized the nature of the tumor cells and described diagnostic criteria for the distinction of thymomas from other lesions such as thymic carcinoids, lymphomas, and germ cell tumors.

In daily practice, ultrastructural studies are particularly useful when dealing with small samples of tissue obtained by needle biopsy. In these small specimens, the distinction of a thymoma from a well-differentiated lymphocytic lymphoma or a spindle cell tumor may be all but impossible without the aid of the electron microscope.

Thymomas mimic, at the ultrastructural level, the structure of the normal thymus gland (1). Although various histologic variants and different growth patterns are seen at the light microscopic level, the tumors are all composed of irregular sheets of epithelial–reticular cells of different sizes and shapes and lymphocytes when examined ultrastructurally (Figs. 6-48 and 6-49). Epithelial–reticular cells have characteristic long cytoplasmic processes connected by desmosomal attachments and form irregular sheets with multiple spaces in which lymphocytes lay (Fig. 6-50).

The epithelial cells of thymomas are oval, polyhedral, spindle, or irregular in shape and have multiple elongated cell processes measuring up to 20 μm in length (Figs. 6-51 and 6-52). These cord-like processes can be best seen with scanning electron microscopy and give the epithelial cells a markedly irregular cell contour (179). The elongated cell processes of epithelial cells are in close contact with basement membrane material and become attached to adjacent epithelial cells by well-formed macula–adherens-type junctions (desmosomes) (Fig. 6-53). In this way, the tumor cells become interlocked in a complex pattern of cell-to-cell relationships.

The cytoplasm of epithelial cells of thymomas has characteristic prominent tonofilaments, which form branching and interconnecting bundles measuring about 70 nm in thickness and up to 2 μm in length (179) (Fig. 6-54). These tonofilaments frequently extend into the cellular membrane and establish contact with desmosomes through thickenings of the subplasmalemmal regions. They become particularly prominent in epithelial cells exhibiting keratinization.

In addition, epithelial cells of thymomas have other cytoplasmic organelles, including large numbers of mitochondria, moderately well-developed Golgi apparatus,

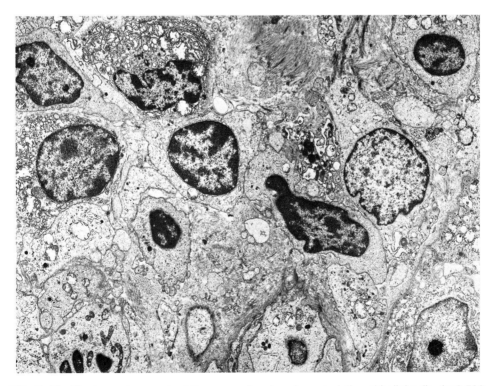

FIG. 6–48. Electron micrograph of thymoma showing characteristic epithelial cells. (×2,500, original)

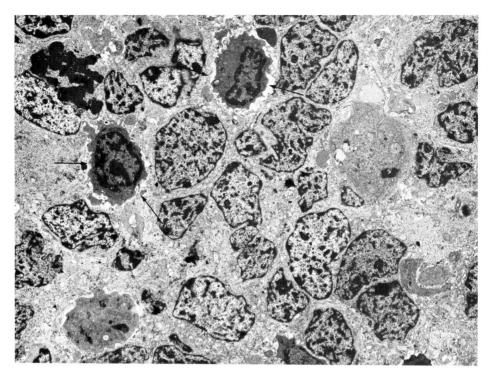

FIG. 6–49. Electron micrograph of thymoma showing clusters of epithelial cells with irregular nuclei. Note presence of lymphocytes (*arrows*) in tissue spaces. (×1,300, original)

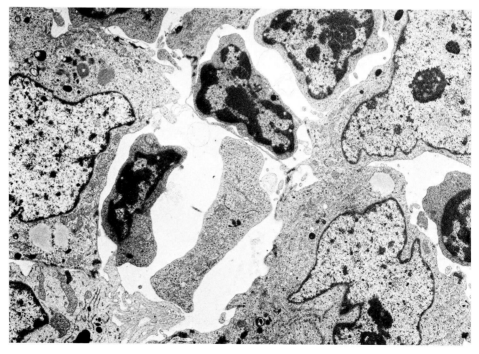

FIG. 6–50. Electron micrograph of lymphoepithelial thymoma showing lymphocytes in spaces lined by epithelial cells. (×2,600, original)

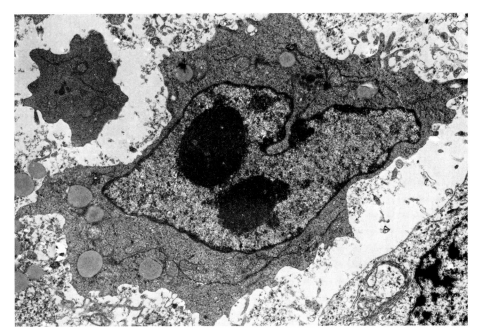

FIG. 6–51. Electron micrograph of epithelial cell of lymphoepithelial thymoma. The cell has an irregular nucleus with prominent nucleoli and long cytoplasmic processes. The cytoplasm contains lipid inclusions. (×5,000, original)

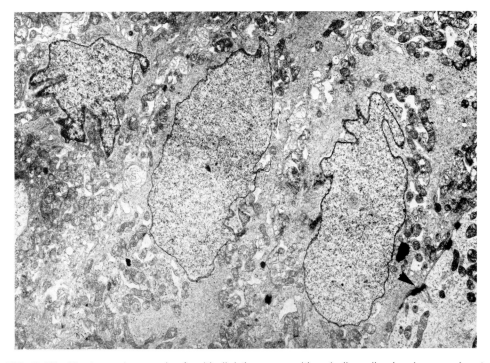

FIG. 6–52. Electron micrograph of epithelial thymoma with spindle cells showing prominent cytoplasmic processes and focal desmosomes (*arrowhead*). (×3,300, original)

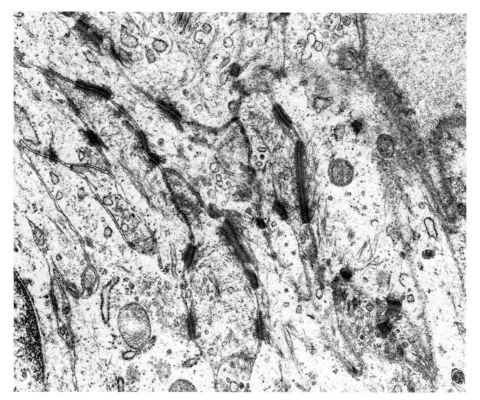

FIG. 6–53. Electron micrograph of thymoma showing epithelial cells with prominent desmosomes, tonofilaments, complex interlocking cellular processes, and focal basal lamina. (Courtesy of Dr. H. Sobel, New Jersey.)

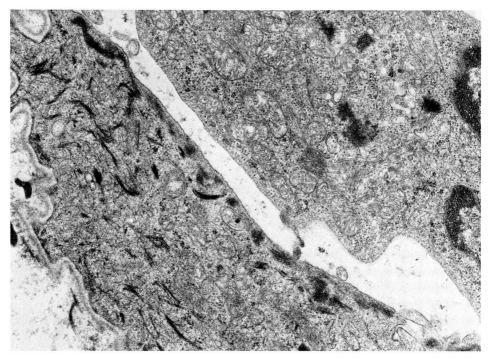

FIG. 6–54. Electron micrograph of epithelial cell of thymoma showing prominent intracytoplasmic tonofilaments. ($\times 8,300$, original)

centriole, pino/cytotic vesicles, scanty rough endoplasmic reticulum, lysosomes, occasional lipid droplets, and rare cilia (Figs. 6-55, 6-56, and 6-57). In some instances, they also have prominent cytoplasmic vacuoles lined by a smooth membrane. These probably represent a degenerative phenomenon and are present in thymomas that exhibit clear cells with light microscopy.

The nucleus of the epithelial cells of thymomas is round or oval and has a smooth or indented contour (Fig. 6-58). Heterochromatin is condensed beneath the nuclear membrane, and there are well-formed nucleoli with moderately developed nucleololemmas.

The epithelial cells of thymomas may become organized in structures already described at the light microscopic level. They can form gland-like spaces lined by cuboidal or flattened cells connected by desmosomes and arranged around a space filled with electron-dense amorphous material. These epithelial cells have prominent microvilli, which project into the lumen (179).

Occasionally, epithelial cells become concentrically arranged around a central area composed of degenerating and necrotic cells (Hassall's corpuscles). The epithelial cells of thymomas can also grow around vascular structures and establish a close relationship with capillaries, forming perivascular spaces characteristic of thymomas (Fig. 6-59) (179). These dilated spaces are present between the basal lamina of endothelial cells of capillaries and those of epithelial cells growing around the vessel. The central vessel is composed of endothelial cells with abundant cytoplasm. The epithelial cells are flattened or columnar and have basal nuclei and desmosomal attachments. The perivascular spaces contain fibrous long-spacing collagen, plasma,

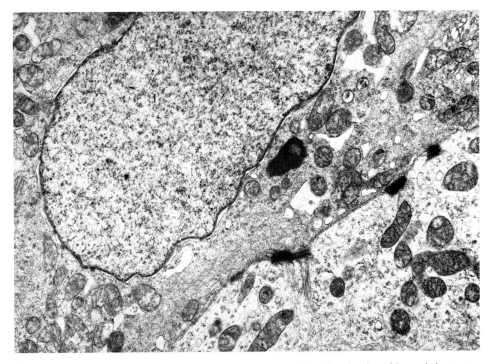

FIG. 6–55. Electron micrograph of epithelial thymoma cells with mitochondria and desmosomal attachment. ($\times$ 8,300, original)

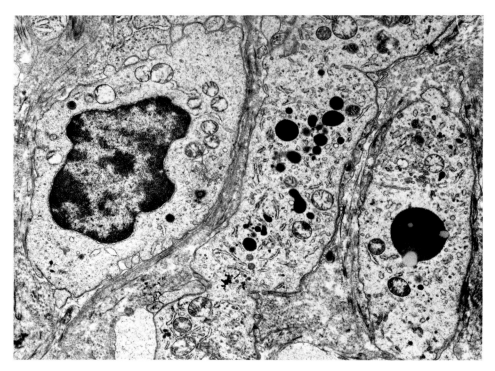

FIG. 6–56. Electron micrograph of epithelial thymoma cells with prominent lysosomal granules. (×5,000, original)

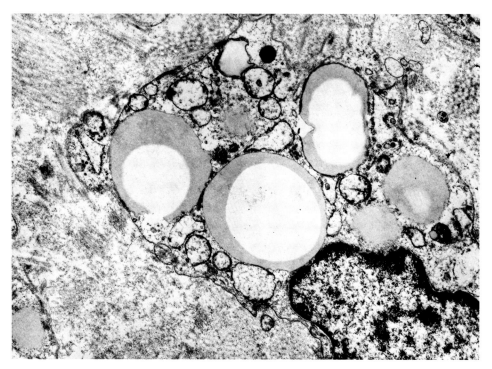

FIG. 6–57. Electron micrograph showing epithelial cell of thymoma with intracytoplasmic lipid vacuoles. (×5,000, original)

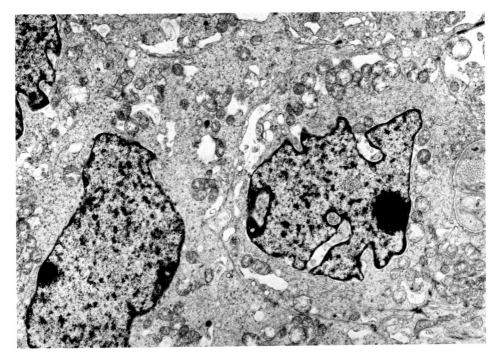

FIG. 6–58. Electron micrograph of thymoma showing epithelial cell with smooth oval nucleus adjacent to another tumor cell with convoluted nuclear morphology. Heterochromatin is condensed beneath the nuclear membrane. Nucleoli are present. (×5,000, original)

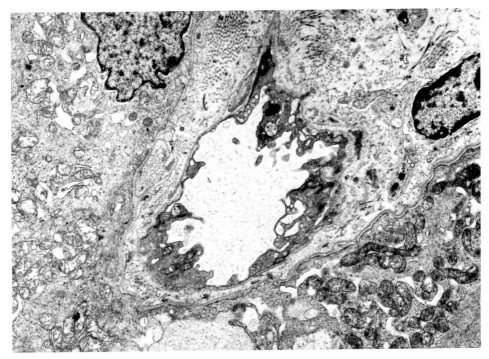

FIG. 6–59. Electron micrograph of perivascular space in a thymoma showing epithelial cells with well-formed basal lamina arranged around a capillary. (×4,000, original)

a variable number of lymphocytes, occasional red blood cells, macrophages, and/or mesenchymal cells. Lymphocytes can occasionally be seen migrating across the epithelial basal lamina into the epithelial site and can probably cross the endothelial basement membrane, as demonstrated in the animal thymus.

The lymphocytes of thymomas have been the subject of numerous studies (322–325). Indeed, it has been controversial whether they are a neoplastic or reactive component of the tumors. The lymphocytes of thymomas exhibit at the ultrastructural level variable morphologic features ranging from those of small resting cells to those of large transformed lymphocytes (186). In general, they have a smooth surface with few microvilli, as seen in T lymphocytes. These features are in contrast with the ruffled plasma membrane and abundant microvilli usually seen in transformed B lymphocytes.

The nucleus of the thymoma lymphocytes is usually round or slightly indented with abundant heterochromatin and a small nucleolus. The cytoplasm is scanty, with few mitochondria and moderate numbers of ribosomes. Larger lymphocytes have increased euchromatin, electron lucency of mitochondria, an increased number of polyribosomes and rare nuclear blebs. These features are characteristic of transformed lymphocytes. In comparison, malignant lymphomas of the thymus have lymphoid cells with a markedly irregular nuclear membrane and numerous nuclear blebs, a sign of aneuploidy.

The finding of lymphocytes at different stages of transformation in thymomas has led to the hypothesis that these cells represent a reactive or hyperplastic component of the tumor and may even be the result of a cell-mediated immune response to the neoplastic thymic epithelial cells (188).

Histochemical Studies

Special histochemical staining techniques are of little practical value for the diagnosis of thymomas. They only accentuate features that can be seen by careful examination of histologic sections stained with hematoxylin and eosin (H&E). For example, reticulin stains are useful to bring about perivascular spaces, and trichrome stains demonstrate clearly the typical lobulation of thymomas. Periodic acid–Schiff stains are negative in thymomas. Except for rare instances with mucinous cells, only occasional thymic epithelial cells exhibit intracytoplasmic PAS and diastase-resistant PAS granules (1). The gland-like spaces encountered in some thymomas also have bright PAS-positive material in their lumen.

Immunofluorescence and/or peroxidase–antiperoxidase (PAP) techniques for the detection of keratin utilizing antikeratin antibodies can be of great value for the diagnosis of thymomas (Fig. 6-60), especially when dealing with small samples of tissue in which the typical growth pattern of the tumor cannot be assessed (Color fig. 7) (188).

Phenotypic Features of the Various Cells of Thymomas

Several studies of thymomas with monoclonal antibodies have revealed that the majority of the lymphoid cells have phenotypic features of T cells (326). Cortical lymphocytes exhibit immunoreactivity with antibodies to TdT, Leu-6, Leu-5, Leu-4, Leu-3a, Leu-1, Leu-9, Leu-2a, Leu-M3, OKT-10, and T200 (327–332). Medullary

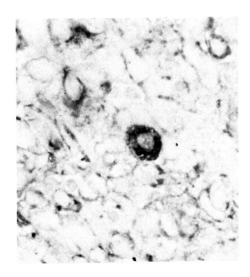

FIG. 6–60. Thymoma. Epithelial cell exhibits intracytoplasmic keratin immunoreactivity. (PAP method, ×400, original)

thymocytes are TdT−, Leu-6−, Leu-4+, Leu-3a−, Leu-1+, Leu-9+, Leu-2a−, Leu-M3−, OKT-10−, and T200+.

Recent studies of the lymphoid component of thymomas with molecular biology techniques have also shown that these cells exhibit polyclonal rearrangement of the T-cell receptor (TCR), providing genotypic evidence that supports the concept that they are nonneoplastic (332–334).

Kornstein and Kay (335) have recently described six thymomas with germinal centers interspersed throughout the tumors. The presence of B cells in these tumors was confirmed with immunoperoxidase studies utilizing LN1, LN2, and L26 antibodies. Only three of these patients had associated MG.

Epithelial Cells

The epithelial component of thymomas has been studied with various antibodies (336). The tumor cells can exhibit immunoreactivity with antibodies to keratin (CAM 5.2 and AE1/3), epithelial membrane antigen, A2B5, TE-4, anti-p19, PE-35, HLA class 1 and 2, Te-3, UH-1, and Leu-7, according to the proportion of cortical and medullary cells in the lesion. Thymomas with predominant medullary differentiation and squamous cell carcinomas of the thymus stain negatively with antibodies to Leu-7 (337). Takahashi and associates (338) reported the use of a PE-35 mouse monoclonal antibody that reacted with medullary thymomas. In their study with a panel of monoclonal antibodies, the tumor cells exhibited various phenotypes, suggesting the presence of different subsets of thymic epithelial cells within the neoplasm or tumor cells at different stages of differentiation. Hirokawa and associates (339) reported the presence of a monoclonal (UH-1) antibody in cortical thymomas.

Acetylcholine receptor (AChR) epitopes have also been detected immunocytochemically in the epithelial cells of thymomas, utilizing monoclonal antibodies to the cytoplasmic site of the alpha-chain of the receptor (338,340). However, there is no evidence, to our knowledge, of AChR activity in thymomas, and studies by Geuder and associates (341) reported that thymomas had no detectable messenger RNA coding for the AChR. In a recent study, Marx and associates (342) described a protein (p153) in human thymomas that shares antigenic determinants with the nicotinic AChR of muscle cells.

Most of these antibodies can be utilized only with frozen tissue and are of limited value in daily surgical pathology (343–348). Stains for the presence of keratin immunoreactivity, however, can be very helpful for the diagnosis of thymoma in biopsy materials. The presence of intracytoplasmic immunoreactivity in the tumor cells must be interpreted with caution, as the positive cells may represent epithelial cells of nonneoplastic thymic tissue "trapped" by a neoplasm other than a thymoma.

Other Cells

In addition to lymphocytes and epithelial cells, thymomas can have scattered macrophages that exhibit the PAM-1+/MAC+, HLA-DR− phenotype, interdigitating reticulum cells with the CD4+, CD45+, HLA-DR+, S-100 protein+ phenotype, and Langerhans cells with the OKT6+, S-100+ phenotype (349–351). As thymomas with medullary differentiation can have scattered interdigitating cells, immunostains with antibodies to S-100 protein can be helpful to detect them (347). Rare myoid cells that can be detected with light and electron microscopy and with antibodies to myoglobin, CPK-mm, and beta-enolase also have been described in thymomas with medullary differentiation (352). The presence of immunoreactivity with antibodies to muscle antigens must be interpreted with caution as they have been described in thymic epithelial cells (352).

The Extracellular Matrix

Mizuno and associates (353) have recently studied the distribution of fibronectin and laminin in human thymomas. In their experience, spindle cell thymomas exhibit a diffuse or partially intricate network of extracellular fibers with immunoreactivity to fibronectin and laminin. Thymomas with other cellular types exhibited a different pattern of staining with fibers surrounding blood vessels and are present in the fibrous septa and in perivascular spaces.

The detection of intracytoplasmic keratin in the epithelial cells of thymomas allows the pathologist to differentiate these cells from histocytes and spindle mesenchymal cells (354).

More recent studies by Palestro and associates (331) have demonstrated that cortical thymomas lack α-naphthylacetate esterase (ANAE) activity, whereas medullary thymomas exhibit strong enzymatic activity.

Pathogenesis of Myasthenia Gravis in Patients with Thymoma

Myasthenia gravis is an autoimmune disease characterized by the presence of circulating anti-AChR in over 90% of patients (355,356). The receptor has four subunits (alpha, beta, gamma, and delta), and its tridimensional structure is known (344). The antibodies to AChR are thought to play a role in the pathogenesis of the disease by various mechanisms, including activation of complement with destruction of the postsynaptic muscle membrane, antigenic modulation resulting in increased degradation of the receptor, and pharmacologic block of the receptor (356). As the thymus has rare myoid cells, it has been postulated that autoantibodies develop in response to the intrathymic release of AChR antigens by degenerating myoid cells (see Chapter 5).

Indeed, the number of myoid cells is smaller in the thymus of patients with MG (352).

However, recent studies by Marx and associates (344) have described that thymomas exhibit a protein (p153) that shares antigenic epitopes with the α-subunit of the AChR. These authors postulated that MG in these patients results from the activation of autoantibodies to the p153 protein, which cross-react with the AChR of skeletal muscle cells.

The pathogenesis of MG may be heterogeneous, and patients with thymoma may develop the disease as a result of different mechanisms than those activated in individuals with thymic hyperplasia. Experiments with monoclonal antibodies have indicated that the spectrum of anti-AChR antibodies is different in both patient populations (356). There is no presupposition regarding gender or human leukocyte antigen (HLA) for patients with MG associated with thymoma. However, female patients with the HLA-B8/DR3 haplotype are more likely to develop thymic hyperplasia associated with MG (357). Furthermore, thymoma patients with MG very frequently have antistriated muscle autoantibodies that are only seldom seen in patients with thymic hyperplasia (356). These antibodies are thought to develop as the result of autosensitization to cytoskeletal contractile proteins such as myosin, alpha actinin, or actin (243,356). These epitopes have been detected on epithelial cells from thymomas (358,359) that share a common epitope, defined by monoclonal antibodies, with skeletal muscle. These antibodies do not cross-react with the normal thymus, except for rare Hassall's corpuscles, label a large number of cells in thymomas, and recognize cross-striations from skeletal muscle cells (358).

Immunohistochemical techniques have also been utilized by several authors for the detection of thymic hormones such as thymosin and serum thymic factor (FTS) in the cytoplasm of thymic epithelial cells (360,361). The antisera to these hormones are not widely available, however, for routine use in the pathology laboratory.

Immunologic and Enzymatic Studies

As discussed in Chapter 4, the thymus gland is a central organ of the immune system and plays a very important role in the development and maturation of immune competent cells. Precursor bone marrow cells circulate through the thymic cortex and medulla during fetal life in a complex process in which they mature to become circulating T cells by acquiring or losing antigenic cell surface markers, enzymatic characteristics, and functional properties (360).

Several authors have studied with immunologic and enzymatic techniques the characteristics of the lymphocytic component of thymomas in efforts to determine the origin, functional properties, role, and nature of these cells (188,322–324).

These studies have determined that the lymphocytes of thymomas exhibit functional and antigenic characteristics of T cells such as the capacity to form rosettes with sheep erythrocytes (E rosettes).

Both the normal thymus gland and thymomas have lymphocytic subpopulations that differ from peripheral T cells in certain antigenic characteristics (324). For example, thymocytes have human T-lymphocyte differentiation (HTL) antigens that are absent on peripheral T lymphocytes. Moreover, cell suspensions of normal thymus and of thymomas have two distinct subpopulations of thymocytes: (a) a major population of mainly cortical lymphocytes able to form stable E rosettes that become agglutinated in contact with peanut agglutinin (PNA positive) and exhibit poor proliferative responses to phytohemagglutinin (PHA negative) and to allogeneic (foreign) cells in mixed lymphocyte cultures (MLC) and (b) a smaller population of mainly medullary thymocytes that are unable to form stable E rosettes and are PHA positive and PNA negative. The latter cells are thought to be a more advanced stage of maturation as discussed in Chapter 4.

Thymomas with a predominance of cortical epithelial cells have an admixture of cortical thymocytes with small- to medium-sized nuclei and large round or convoluted nuclei with open chromatin, small nucleoli, and scanty basophilic cytoplasm (lymphoblasts) (198). Medullary thymomas have a predominance of small pleomorphic thymocytes.

Thymomas with a high lymphocyte/epithelial (L/E) ratio have a high percentage of E-rosette-positive, PNA-positive, PHA-negative cells (323). Thymomas with low L/E ratios exhibited only small numbers of PNA-positive, PHA-negative cells and have instead a higher proportion of lymphoid cells with increased expression of surface receptors for the Fc portion of IgM. These lymphocytes are more mature and differentiated, suggesting that thymomas with low L/E ratios have a more mature population of thymocytes than their counterparts with high L/E ratios. It may be that tumors with higher densities of epithelial cells have a higher probability of intimate contact between these cells and lymphocytes, resulting in the maturation of thymocytes (323).

The distribution of ANAE activity has been studied by Palestro and associates (362) in the normal thymus, in the thymus of patients with MG, and in thymomas with quantitative histochemical and cytochemical techniques (324); ANAE is a known T-cell marker that is present preferentially in peripheral T lymphocytes (363). It is considered as a marker of matured T cells. Esterase-positive thymocytes are found in the thymic medulla and corticomedullary junction of thymus glands (362). However, only a relatively small proportion of thymocytes from normal thymuses exhibited positive enzyme activity. The thymuses of patients with MG and the thymomas exhibited increased proportions of ANAE-positive cells, suggesting that in these conditions lymphocytes are at a more advanced stage of maturation than those in the normal thymic cortex. Whether the thymocytes in thymomas or in MG have matured in response to intrathymic autoantigens or in response to hormonal secretion by thymic epithelial cells is not known.

Secretory Activities of Thymomas

The thymus gland epithelium secretes various hormones that modulate the development and maturation of immune competent cells. They include thymosin, prothymosin alpha, thymosin beta-4, FTS, thymopoietin, and others (360,361,364,365). Thymosin alpha-1, thymosin beta-3, and other markers have been localized to epithelial cells in immunocytochemical studies (339). They have been discussed in Chapter 4.

There are only a few patients with thymomas in whom serum levels of some of these thymic hormones have been studied (366,367).

Kirkpatrick and associates (367) described four patients with thymomas and chronic mucocutaneous candidiasis in whom plasma levels of thymopoietin-like activity were determined on several occasions. One patient with a malignant epithelial thymoma had elevated plasma levels of the hormone. The other three patients had normal plasma levels of the hormone. The authors suggested that the syndromes of immune deficiency and chronic mucocutaneous candidiasis that can be encountered in patients with thymomas are probably not related to a deficiency of thymopoietin.

The patient of Chollet and associates (366) with malignant epithelial thymoma had elevated plasma levels of FTS, a hormone that is not detectable in the serum of normal individuals. The elevated levels of FTS decreased markedly after treatment of the tumor with radiotherapy and combined chemotherapy. The patient also had hypergammaglobulinemia with a monoclonal IgG protein in serum and increased numbers of circulating T cells prior to therapy. The authors suggested that the inappropriate hypersecretion of FTS by the tumor contributed to these immunologic abnormalities. Lymphokines such as interleukin 1 (IL 1), and IL 2 and IL 1–induced IL 2–receptor have also been described in thymoma cell lines (365). These lymphokines are active in immune modulation and T-cell differentiation.

Hormone Receptors in Thymomas

Glucocorticoid Receptors

Several investigators have demonstrated the presence of a specific receptor system for glucocorticoids in the mammalian and human thymus (368). Glucocorticoid receptors have also been described in human thymic hyperplasia (369).

Ranelletti and associates (368) studied cell-free preparations from four lympho-epithelial and one epithelial thymoma utilizing a dextran-coated charcoal assay for the presence of receptor macromolecules capable of binding triamcinolone acetonide with high affinity and specificity. They were able to demonstrate receptors for this corticosteroid in all tumors studied, including the purely epithelial lesion. Moreover, the concentration of specific binding sites was greater in the tumors than in thymic hyperplasia.

These studies suggest that corticosteroids may have a role in the treatment of thymomas.

Estrogen Receptors

Hammar (370) and others (371,372) have discovered the antagonistic hormonal relationships between the thymus gland and the gonads. For example, gonadectomy is followed by thymic hyperplasia in animals, whereas treatment with testosterone and/or estrogen results in marked thymic atrophy in ovariectomized rats (371).

More recent studies by Ranelletti and associates (372) have demonstrated the presence of a receptor macromolecule for 17β-estradiol in human thymomas. This receptor is distinct from the receptor macromolecule capable of binding triamcinolone acetonide with high affinity and specificity.

Analysis of Nuclear DNA in Thymomas

The nuclear DNA content of thymomas has been studied by static microphotometry and by flow cytometry (290,373–375). The results with flow cytometry are controversial. Sauter and associates (290) reported no significant differences in patients with benign and malignant thymomas in whom DNA indices and S-phase fraction were measured by flow cytometry. Davies and associates (375), in a similar study, reported that DNA aneuploidy was predictive of tumor recurrence and was a prognostic variable independent of stage and cell type. Studies with cytofluorometry and morphometry by Asamura and associates (374) and Okada and associates (373) report an increase in the number of tumor cells with increased DNA content in invasive thymomas and thymic carcinoma. However, these studies demonstrate that benign thymomas can exhibit abnormal DNA histograms and that the methods cannot be used with certainty for diagnosis of prognosis of an individual patient.

Cytogenetic Studies in Thymomas

Kristoffersson and associates (376) recently reported two thymomas that have been studied with banding techniques and demonstrated in both lesions abnormal karyotypes.

Molecular Biology Studies in Thymomas

Mukai and associates (377) recently studied 21 thymomas with immunohistochemistry and immunoblot for the presence of ras oncogene p21 and reported an increased concentration of the product in the neoplastic cells. An increased amount of a p21 molecule with abnormal electrophoretic mobility was detected in metastatic thymomas.

Morphometric Analysis of Thymomas

Nomori and associates (378) have evaluated the epithelial cells of thymomas with morphometric techniques and demonstrated that the nuclear areas of the epithelial cells of invasive thymoma were larger than those of noninvasive tumors. The neoplastic cells of noninvasive thymomas were larger than those seen in thymic hyperplasias and normal thymuses. Noninvasive thymomas from patients with MG had larger cells than similar lesions from patients that had no associated neuromuscular disease. In a more recent study, Nomori and associates (379) demonstrated that cortical thymomas, which are more frequently invasive and associated with MG than medullary thymomas, had larger cells than medullary lesions.

SPONTANEOUS THYMOMAS IN ANIMALS: EXPERIMENTAL MODELS OF THYMOMA

A detailed description of the extensive experimental work performed in the field of thymic pathology is beyond the scope of this volume. Thus, we provide only a brief description of some important developments in the experimental pathology of thymomas.

Spontaneously occurring and experimentally induced tumors of the thymus have been described in sheep, cattle, goats, dogs, buffalo rats, transgenic mice, and other animals (380–405). It is not always clear whether these animal tumors were indeed thymomas or malignant lymphomas of the thymus gland (1). However, there are several documented instances of spontaneous thymomas in animals (385–391).

For example, Matsuyama and associates (392,393) have studied a very interesting model of spontaneous thymomas in BUF/Mna rats using histological, ultrastructural, biochemical, tissue culture, and physiologic methods. Nearly 100% of the animals developed spontaneous thymomas, and some animals developed atrophy of leg muscles and nephrotic syndrome. In a recent study, Matsuyama and associates (398) demonstrated that the development of tumors may be related to the rat nude gene (rnu), as the animals with $+/+$ genotype developed the tumors in 94% of instances.

Thymomas can also be induced experimentally by exposing mice to whole-body X-irradiation (392). The animals developed thymomas and radiation-induced leukemia several months after exposure. Mice can also develop thymomas after exposure to single sublethal doses of alkylating agents such as N-ethyl-N-nitrourea or infection with polyoma virus (388,400). Rats can develop thymomas after infection with the Moloney murine leukemia virus (401,402). Squamous cell carcinomas of the thymus have been induced in mice utilizing alkylating carcinogens (405).

The availability of these experimental models has enabled investigators to study possible etiologic agents involved in the development of thymomas, the biologic activities of the tumors, and has led to several studies in which specific thymoma cell lines have been kept in tissue culture and studied with biochemical, immunologic, and molecular biology techniques (397–405).

For example, mouse EL-4 thymoma cells have been grown in tissue culture and have been demonstrated to secrete T-cell growth factor (interleukin 2) (389). Interleukin 2 is a 30,000-dalton protein capable of enhancing several immune functions of mouse lymphocytes *in vitro*. In another experiment, two murine thymoma cell lines were cultured, and a new variant of murine thymoma that is supersensitive to dexamethasone was characterized (390).

The studies may eventually elucidate some of the fundamental questions regarding the origin, development, biologic aspects, and treatment of thymomas.

REFERENCES

1. Rosai J, Levine GD: Tumors of the thymus. *Atlas of Tumor Pathology,* Fasc 13, ser 2. Washington, Armed Forces Institute of Pathology, 1976.
2. Gray GF, Gutowski WT: Thymoma. A clinicopathologic study of 54 cases. *Am J Surg Pathol* 1979;3:235–249.
3. Wilkins EW Jr, Castleman B: Thymoma: A continuing survey at the Massachusetts General Hospital. *Ann Thorac Surg* 1979;28:252–256.
4. Levine GD, Rosai J: Thymic hyperplasia and neoplasia: a review of current concepts. *Hum Pathol* 1978;9:495–515.
5. Seybold WD, McDonald JR, Clagett OT, et al: Tumors of the thymus. *J Thorac Cardiovasc Surg* 1950;20:195–214.
6. Bernatz PE, Harrison EG, Clagett OT: Thymoma: a clinicopathologic study. *J Thorac Cardiovasc Surg* 1961;42:424–444.
7. Hasner E, Westengard E: Thymomas. *Acta Chir Scand* 1963;126:58–65.

8. Oldham HN Jr, Sabiston DC Jr: Primary tumors and cysts of the mediastinum. *Monogr Surg Sci* 1967;4:243–279.
9. Murray M: Discussion of Lattes R, Jonas S: pathological and clinical features in 80 cases of thymoma. *Bull NY Acad Med* 1957;33:145–147.
10. Videbaek A, Thomsen G: Tumours of the thymic region. Follow-up on 36 operated cases. *Acta Radiol (Stockh) [Suppl.]* 1959;188:261–275.
11. Dyer NH: Cystic thymomas and thymic cysts. A review. *Thorax* 1967;22:408–421.
12. Friedman NB: Tumors of the thymus. *J Thorac Cardiovasc Surg* 1967;53:163–182.
13. Smith WF, DeWall RA, Krumholz RA: Giant thymoma. *Chest* 1970;58:383–385.
14. Lattes R: Thymoma and other tumors of the thymus. An analysis of 107 cases. *Cancer* 1962;15:1224–1260.
15. Effler DB, McCormack LJ: Thymic neoplasms. *J Thorac Cardiovasc Surg* 1956;31:60–82.
16. Sellors TH, Thackray AC, Thomson AD: Tumours of the thymus. A review of 88 operation cases. *Thorax* 1967;22:193–220.
17. Batata MA, Martini N, Huvos AG, et al: Thymomas: clinicopathologic features, therapy, and prognosis. *Cancer* 1974;34:389–396.
18. Snover DC, Levine GD, Rosai J: Thymic carcinoma. Five distinct histological variants. *Am J Surg Pathol* 1982;6:451–470.
19. Benjamin SP, McCormack LJ, Effler DB, et al: Primary tumors of the mediastinum. *Chest* 1972;62:297–303.
20. Salyer WR, Eggleston JC: Thymoma: a clinical and pathological study of 65 cases. *Cancer* 1976;37:229–249.
21. Le Golvan DP, Abell MR: Thymomas. *Cancer* 1977;39:2142–2157.
22. Pascuzzi RM, Sermas A, Phillips LH, et al: Familial autoimmune myasthenia gravis and thymoma: occurrence in two brothers. *Neurology* 1986;36:423–437.
23. Jansen JD, Johnson FE: Fatal ectopic thymoma. *Ann Thorac Surg* 1990;50:469–470.
24. Fukuda T, Itami M, Sawa H, et al: A case of thymoma arising from undescended thymus. High uptake of thallium-201 chloride. *Eur J Nucl Med* 1980;5:465–468.
25. Ridenhour CE, Henzel JH, DeWeese MS, et al: Thymoma arising from undescended cervical thymus. *Surgery* 1970;67:614–619.
26. Cosío-Pascal M, González-Méndez A: Left hilar thymoma. Report of a case. *Dis Chest* 1967;51:647–649.
27. Perera HW, Wilson JR: Anterior inferior mediastinal thymoma—case report. *Br J Dis Chest* 1962;56:44–46.
28. Cooper GN Jr, Narodick BG: Posterior mediastinal thymoma. Case report. *J Thorac Cardiovasc Surg* 1972;63:561–563.
29. McBurney RP, Clagett OT, McDonald JR: Primary intrapulmonary neoplasm (thymoma?) associated with myasthenia gravis: report of a case. *Mayo Clinic Proc* 1951;26:345–353.
30. Yeoh CB, Ford JM, Lattes R, et al: Intrapulmonary thymoma. *J Thorac Cardiovasc Surg* 1966;51:131–136.
31. Green WR, Pressoir R, Gumbs RV, et al: Intrapulmonary thymoma. *Arch Pathol Lab Med* 1987;111:1074–1076.
32. Wadon von A: Thymoma intratracheale. *Zentralbl Allg Pathol* 1934;60:308–312.
33. Asamura H, Morinaga S, Shimosato Y, et al: Thymoma displaying endobronchial polypoid growth. *Chest* 1988;94:647–649.
34. Jain U, Frable WJ: Thymoma: analysis of benign and malignant criteria. *J Thorac Cardiovasc Surg* 1974;67:310–321.
35. Mottet NK: Malignant thymoma. *Am J Clin Pathol* 1964;41:61–71.
36. Yoshida A, Shigematsu T, Mori H, et al: Non-invasive thymoma with widespread blood borne metastatis. *Virchows Arch [Pathol Anat]* 1981;390:121–126.
37. Andritsakis GD, Sommers SC: Criteria of thymic cancer and clinical correlations of thymic tumors. *J Thorac Cardiovasc Surg* 1959;37:273–290.
38. Hellwig CA: Malignant thymoma. Clinical-pathological study of eight cases. *Surg Gynecol Obstet* 1941;73:851–863.
39. Bernatz PE, Khonsari S, Harrison EG Jr, et al: Thymoma: factors influencing prognosis. *Surg Clin North Am* 1973;53:885–892.
40. Honma K, Mishina M, Watanabe Y: Polypoid endobronchial extension from invasive thymoma. *Virchows Arch* 1988;413:469–474.
41. Atsmon A, Pinkhas J, Djaldetti M: Sudden death caused by pressure of thymoma on the right atrium. *Arch Intern Med* 1962;110:295–298.
42. Soorae AS, Stevenson HM: Cystic thymoma simulating pulmonary stenosis. *Br J Dis Chest* 1980;74:193–197.
43. Schloss M, Kronzon I, Gelber PM, et al: Cystic thymoma simulating constrictive pericarditis. The role of echocardiography in the differential diagnosis. *J Thorac Cardiovasc Surg* 1975;70:143–146.

44. Battaglia S, Barbolini G, Botticelli AR: Thymoma mimicking Hodgkin's disease of the thymus. *Pathol Res Pract* 1981;172:205–210.
45. Weigert C: Pathogisch-Anatomischer Beirtrag zur Erbschen Krankheit (myasthenia gravis). *Neurol Zentralbl* 1901;20:597.
46. Kimura J, van Allen MW: Postthymectomy myasthenia gravis. Report of a case of ocular myasthenia gravis after total removal of a thymoma and review of the literature. *Neurology (Minneap)* 1967;17:413–420.
47. Bell ET: Tumors of the thymus in myasthenia gravis. *J Nerv Ment Dis* 1917;45:130–143.
48. Guillan RA, Zelman S, Smalley RL, et al: Malignant thymoma associated with myasthenia gravis, and evidence of extra-thoracic metastases. An analysis of published cases and report of a case. *Cancer* 1971;27:823–830.
49. Goldman AJ, Herrmann C Jr, Keesey JC, et al: Myasthenia gravis and invasive thymoma. A 20 year experience. *Neurology (Minneap)* 1975;25:1021–1025.
50. Namba T, Brunner NG, Grob D: Myasthenia gravis in patients with thymoma, with particular reference to onset after thymectomy. *Medicine* 1978;57:411–433.
51. Osserman KE, Genkins G: Studies in myasthenia gravis. Review of a twenty-year experience in over 1200 patients. *Mt Sinai J Med* 1971;38:497–537.
52. Slater G, Papatestas AE, Genkins G, et al: Thymomas in patients with myasthenia gravis. *Ann Surg* 1978;188:171–174.
53. Goldstein G, Mackay IR: Thymic tumors and systemic diseases associated with thymoma, in: *The Human Thymus*. St. Louis, Warren H Green, 1969, pp 194–227.
54. Hannon GT, Bennington JL, Haber SL: Malignant thymoma with myasthenia and embolic metastasis. Report of a case. *Dis Chest* 1966;50:645–648.
55. Lauritzen M, Smith T, Fischer-Hansen B, et al: Eaton–Lambert syndrome and malignant thymoma. *Neurology (NY)* 1980;30:634–638.
56. Laforet EG, Norton CP, Sampson RJ: Disabling neuropathy associated with thymoma. Reversal by excision. *J Thorac Cardiovasc Surg* 1974;67:164–166.
57. Kuroiwa Y, Yamada A, Ikebe K, et al: Myotonic dystrophy and thymoma: a necropsy case report. *J Neurol Neurosurg Psychiatry* 1981;44:173–175.
58. Beard MEJ, Krantz SB, Johnson SAN, et al: Pure red cell aplasia. *Q J Med* 1978;187:339–348.
59. Korn D, Gelderman A, Cage G, et al: Immune deficiencies, aplastic anemia and abnormalities of lymphoid tissue in thymoma. *N Engl J Med* 1967;276:1333–1339.
60. Barnes RDS, O'Gorman P: Two cases of aplastic anaemia associated with tumors of the thymus. *J Clin Pathol* 1962;15:264–268.
61. Böttiger LE, Rausing A: Pure red cell anemia; immunosuppressive treatment. *Ann Intern Med* 1972;76:593–597.
62. Burrows S, Carroll R: Thymoma associated with pancytopenia. *Arch Pathol* 1971;92:465–468.
63. DiGiacomo J, Furst SW, Nixon DD: Primary acquired red cell aplasia in the adult. *J Mt Sinai Hosp* 1966;33:382–395.
64. Eisemann G, Dameshek W: Splenectomy for "pure red-cell" hypoplastic (aregenerative) anemia associated with autoimmune hemolytic disease. Report of a case. *N Engl J Med* 1954;251:1044–1048.
65. Hirst E, Robertson TI: The syndrome of thymoma and erythroblastopenic anemia. A review of 56 cases including 3 case reports. *Medicine* 1967;46:225–264.
66. Jepson JH, Vas M: Decreased *in vivo* and *in vitro* erythropoiesis induced by plasma of ten patients with thymoma, lymphosarcoma, or idiopathic erythroblastopenia. *Cancer Res* 1974;34:1325–1334.
67. Kuang DT, Cech RF, Peterson RE: Benign thymoma and erythroid hypoplasia: thirteen-year "cure" following thymectomy. *Cancer* 1968;22:445–450.
68. Tiber C, Casimir M, Nogeire C, et al: Thymoma with red cell aplasia and hemolytic anemia. *South Med J* 1981;74:1164–1165.
69. Krantz SB: Pure red-cell aplasia. *N Engl J Med* 1974;291:345–350.
70. Remigio PA: Granulomatous thymoma associated with erythroid hypoplasia. *Am J Clin Pathol* 1971;55:68–72.
71. Roland AS: The syndrome of benign thymoma and primary aregenerative anemia. An analysis of forty-three cases. *Am J Med Sci* 1964;247:719–731.
72. Zeok JV, Todd EP, Dillon M, et al: The role of thymectomy in red cell aplasia. *Ann Thorac Surg* 1979;28:257–260.
73. Degos L, Faille A, Housset M, et al: Syndrome of neutrophil agranulocytosis, hypogammaglobulinemia and thymoma. *Blood* 1982;60:968–972.
74. Dawson MA: Thymoma associated with pancytopenia and Hashimoto's thyroiditis. *Am J Med* 1972;52:406–410.
75. Sündstrom C: A case of thymoma in association with erythrocytosis. *Acta Pathol Microbiol Scand (A)* 1972;80:235–240.

76. Griffin JD, Aisenberg AC, Long JC: Lymphocytic thymoma associated with T cell lymphocytosis. *Am J Med* 1978;64:1075–1079.
77. Sündstrom C, Lundberg D, Werner I: A case of thymoma in association with megakaryocytopenia. *Acta Pathol Microbiol Scand (A)* 1972;80:487–490.
78. Lindstrom FD, Williams RC Jr, Brunning RD: Thymoma associated with multiple myeloma. *Arch Intern Med* 1968;122:526–531.
79. Adams JE: Leukemogenic thymoma. Report of a unique case. *Am J Clin Pathol* 1963;40:173–182.
80. Andersen V, Pedersen H: Thymoma and acute leukaemia. *Acta Med Scand* 1967;182:581–590.
81. Vilpo JA, Klemi P, Lassila O, et al: Malignant thymus tumour progressing into acute leukemia with non-specific esterase activity. *Acta Pathol Microbiol Scand (A)* 1981;89:223–226.
82. Waldmann TA, Broder S, Durm M, et al: Suppressor T cells in the pathogenesis of hypogammaglobulinemia associated with a thymoma. *Trans Assoc Am Physicians* 1975;88:120–134.
83. Montes LF, Ceballos R, Cooper MD, et al: Chronic mucocutaneous candidiasis, myositis, and thymoma. A new triad. *JAMA* 1972;222:1619–1623.
84. Kauffman CA, Linnemann CC Jr, Alvira MM: Cytomegalovirus encephalitis associated with thymoma and immunoglobulin deficiency. *Am J Med* 1979;67:724–728.
85. Beck S, Slater D, Harrington CI: Fatal chronic cutaneous herpes simplex associated with thymoma and hypogammaglobulinaemia. *Br J Dermatol* 1981;105:471–474.
86. Uhlin SR, Maiocco KJ, Bhatia SG: Pemphigus erythematosus and thymoma. *Cutis* 1980;25:177–180.
87. Cooper A, Wells JV: Pemphigus foliaceus, myasthenia gravis and thymoma in a patient with serological evidence of SLE. *Aust NZ J Med* 1981;11:277–280.
88. Kough RH, Barnes WT: Thymoma associated with erythroid aplasia, bullous skin eruption, and the lupus erythematosus cell phenomenon. Report of a case. *Ann Intern Med* 1964;61:308–315.
89. Alarcon-Segovia D, Galbraith RF, Maldonado JE, et al: Systemic lupus erythematosus following thymectomy for myasthenia gravis. Report of two cases. *Lancet* 1963;2:662–665.
90. Singh BN: Thymoma presenting with polyserositis and the lupus erythematosus syndrome. *Aust Ann Med* 1969;18:55–58.
91. Posner MR, Prout MN, Berk S: Thymoma and the nephrotic syndrome; a report of a case. *Cancer* 1980;45:387–391.
92. Varsano S, Bruderman I, Bernheim JL, et al: Minimal change nephropathy and malignant thymoma. *Chest* 1980;77:695–697.
93. Skinnider LF, Alexander S, Horsman D: Concurrent thymoma and lymphoma: A report of two cases. *Hum Pathol* 1982;13:163–166.
94. Gould TS, Tanguay PR, DeLellis RA: Thymoma and primary lymphoma of the small intestine. *Cancer* 1977;40:1755–1958.
95. Souadjian JV, Silverstein MN, Titus JL: Thymoma and cancer. *Cancer* 1968;22:1221–1225.
96. Vessey MP, Doll R: Thymectomy and cancer—a follow-up study. *Br J Cancer* 1972;26:53–58.
97. Maberry JD, Stone OJ: Kaposi's sarcoma with thymoma. *Arch Dermatol* 1967;95:210–213.
98. Ridell B, Larsson S: Coexistence of a thymoma and Hodgkin's disease of the thymus. A case report. *Acta Pathol Microbiol Scand (A)* 1980;88:1–4.
99. Lesser M, Mouli C, Jothikumar T: Hypertrophic osteoarthropathy associated with a malignant thymoma. *Mt Sinai J Med* 1980;47:24–30.
100. Palmer FJ, Sawyers TM: Hyperparathyroidism, chemodectoma, thymoma and myasthenia gravis. *Arch Intern Med* 1978;138:1402–1403.
101. Alpert LI, Papatestas A, Kark A, et al: A histologic reappraisal of the thymus in myasthenia gravis. A correlative study of thymic pathology and response to thymectomy. *Arch Pathol* 1971;91:55–61.
102. Levasseur P, Menestrier M, Gaud C, et al: Thymomas and associated diseases. Apropos of a series of 255 surgically treated thymomas. *Rev Mal Respir* 1988;5:173–178.
103. Monden Y, Uyama T, Taniki T, et al: The characteristics of thymoma with myasthenia gravis: a 28-year experience. *J Surg Oncol* 1988;38:151–154.
104. Piccolo G, Martino G, Moglia A, et al: Autoimmune myasthenia gravis with thymoma following the spontaneous remission of stiff-man syndrome. *Ital J Neurol Sci* 1990;11:177–180.
105. Oda K, Miyasaki K, Ohta M, et al: A case of myasthenia gravis associated with thymoma, multiple schwannomas and monoclonal IgA gammopathy. *Jpn J Med* 1987;26:223–225.
106. Bailey RO, Dunn HG, Rubin AM, et al: Myasthenia gravis with thymoma and pure red blood cell aplasia. *Am J Clin Pathol* 1988;89:6587–6593.
107. Conti JA, Colicchio AR, Howard LM: Thymoma, myasthenia gravis, and relapsing polychondritis. *Ann Intern Med* 1988;109:163–164.
108. Miller H, Shenstone BD, Joffe R, et al: A case of invasive thymoma associated with myasthenia gravis, myositis and demyelinating neuropathy. *Clin Exp Neurol* 1986;22:13–18.
109. Ohmi M, Ohuchi M: Recurrent thymoma in patients with myasthenia gravis. *Ann Thorac Surg* 1990;50:243–247.

110. Lewis JE, Wick MR, Scheithauer BW, et al: Thymoma. A clinicopathologic review. *Cancer* 1987;60:2727–2743.

111. Maggi G, Giaccone G, Donadio M, et al: Thymomas. A review of 169 cases, with particular reference to results of surgical treatment. *Cancer* 1986;58:765–776.

112. Stoll DB, Lublin F, Brodovsky H, et al: Association of subacute motor neuronopathy with thymoma. *Cancer* 1984;54:770–772.

113. Tabbaa MA, Leshner RT, Campbell WW: Malignant thymoma with dysautonomia and disordered neuromuscular transmission. *Arch Neurol* 1986;955–957.

114. Ben-Shahar M, Rosenblatt E, Green J, et al: Malignant thymoma associated with progressive systemic sclerosis. *Am J Med Sci* 1987;294:262–267.

115. McArdle JP, Millingen KS: Limbic encephalitis associated with malignant thymoma. *Pathology* 1988;20:292–295.

116. Witt NJ, Bolton CF: Neuromuscular disorders and thymoma. *Muscle Nerve* 1988;11:398–405.

117. Masaoka A, Hashimoto T, Shibata K, et al: Thymomas associated with pure red cell aplasia. Histologic and follow-up studies. *Cancer* 1989;64:1872–1878.

118. Insler MS, Shelin RG: Sjögren's syndrome and thymoma. *Am J Ophthalmol* 1987;104:90–91.

119. Voigt S: Polycytaemia vera associated with thymoma. Case report. *Acta Pathol Microbiol Immunol Scand (A)* 1986;94:351–352.

120. Weir AB, Dow LW: Response of agranulocytosis to thymectomy in a patient with thymoma and chronic lymphocytic leukemia. *Med Pediatr Oncol* 1989;17:58–61.

121. Davila DG, Ryan DH: Thymoma, hypogammaglobulinemia, and pernicious anemia. *South Med J* 1986;79:904–906.

122. Ackland SP, Bur ME, Adler SS, et al: White blood cell aplasia associated with thymoma. *Am J Clin Pathol* 89:260–263.

123. Lyonnais J: Thymoma and pancytopenia. *Am J Hematol* 1988;28:195–196.

124. Fitzmaurice RJ, Gardner D: Thymoma with bone marrow eosinophilia. *J R Soc Med* 1990;83:270–271.

125. Mathieson PW, O'Neill JH, Durrant ST, et al: Antibody-mediated pure neutrophil aplasia, recurrent myasthenia gravis and previous thymoma: case report and literature review. *Q J Med* 1990;74:57–61.

126. Marks P, Marks C: Thymoma and aregenerative anemia. *South Med J* 1988;81:1182–1184.

127. Watts RG, Kelly DR: Fatal varicella infection in a child associated with thymoma and immunodeficiency (Good's syndrome). *Med Pediatr Oncol* 1990;18:246–251.

128. Rothberg MS, Eisenbud L, Griboff S: Chronic mucocutaneous candidiasis-thymoma syndrome. A Case report. *Oral Surg* 1989;68:411–413.

129. McGuire LJ, Huang DP, Teoh R, et al: Epstein–Barr virus genome in thymoma and thymic lymphoid hyperplasia. *Am J Pathol* 1988;131:385–390.

130. Inghirami G, Chilosi M, Knowles DM: Western thymomas lack Epstein–Barr virus by Southern blotting analysis and by polymerase chain reaction. *Am J Pathol* 1990;136:1429–1436.

131. Teoh R, McGuire L, Wong K, et al: Increased incidence of thymoma in Chinese myasthenia gravis: possible relationship with Epstein–Barr virus. *Acta Neurol Scand* 1989;80:221–225.

132. Perronne C, Ooka T, Decaussin G, et al: Antibodies to Epstein–Barr virus in 50 patients with thymic tumor. *JAMA* 1990;264:570–571.

133. Gibson LE, Muller SA: Dermatologic disorders in patients with thymoma. *Acta Derm Venereol* 1987;67:351–356.

134. Thorlacius S, Aarli JA, Riise T, et al: Associated disorders in myasthenia gravis: autoimmune diseases and their relation to thymectomy. *Acta Neurol Scand* 1989;80:290–295.

135. Fournel P, Emonot A, Claudy AL, et al: Thymoma and lupus: apropos of a case with recurrences and histological dedifferentiation. *Rev Pneumol Clin* 1987;43:98–101.

136. Colburn KK, Cao JD: Thymoma associated with rheumatoid arthritis in a patient taking methotrexate. *J Rheumatol* 1986;13:437–439.

137. Sawai T, Tuchikawa K: Kaposi's sarcoma developed in a patient with a thymoma in the setting of excess numbers of CD8-positive cells in the peripheral blood. *Arch Pathol Lab Med* 1990;114:611–613.

138. Byrne DJ, Gunn A, Davidson DL, et al: Parathyroid hyperplasia associated with thymoma. *Postgrad Med J* 1989;65:310–311.

139. Brown LR, Muhm JR, Gray JE: Radiographic detection of thymoma. *Am J Roentgenol* 1980;134:1181–1188.

140. Lin SR, Freundlich IM: Malignant thymoma with radiographic evidence of distant intrathoracic implantation. Report of five cases. *Radiology* 1970;94:135–138.

141. Baron RL, Lee JKT, Sagel SS, et al: Computed tomography of the abnormal thymus. *Radiology* 1982;142:127–134.

142. Fon GT, Bein ME, Mancuso AA, et al: Computed tomography of the anterior mediastinum in myasthenia gravis. A radiologic-pathologic correlative study. *Radiology* 1982;142:135–141.

143. Zerhouni EA, Scott WW Jr, Baker RR, et al: Invasive thymomas: diagnosis and evaluation by computed tomography. *J Comput Assist Tomogr* 1982;6:92–100.
144. Chen JL, Weisbrod GL, Herman SJ: Computed tomography and pathologic correlation of thymic lesions. *J Thorac Imaging* 1988;3:61–65.
145. Davis RD Jr, Oldham HN Jr, Sabiston DC Jr: Primary cysts and neoplasms of the mediastinum: recent changes in clinical presentation, methods of diagnosis, management, and results. *Ann Thorac Surg* 1987;44:229–237.
146. Ferguson MK, Lee E, Skinner DB, et al: Selective operative approach for diagnosis and treatment of anterior mediastinal masses. *Ann Thorac Surg* 1987;44:583–586.
147. Frija J, Amadmsbaum C, Hacein-Bey L, et al: Efficacy of x-ray computed tomography in the diagnosis of tumors of the mediastinum. 103 cases. *J Radiol* 1988;69:473–483.
148. Rendina EA, Pescarmona EO, Venuta F, et al: Thymoma: a clinico-pathologic study based on newly developed morphologic criteria. *Tumori* 1988;74:79–84.
149. Juliani G: Radiological diagnosis of thymoma in myasthenia gravis (MG). Review of a series of 523 surgically controlled patients. *Clin Imaging* 1990;14:48–54.
150. Blegvad S, Lippert H, Simper LB, et al: Mediastinal tumours. A report of 129 cases. *Scand J Thorac Cardiovasc Surg* 1990;24:39–42.
151. Wilson RL, Cowan RJ: Tc-99m pertechnate uptake in a thymoma: case report. *Clin Nucl Med* 1982;7:149–150.
152. Swick HM, Preston DF, McQuillen MP: Gallium scans in myasthenia gravis. *Ann NY Acad Sci* 1976;274:536–554.
153. Lamke LO, Bergdahl L, Lamke B: Intrathoracic goitre: a review of 29 cases. *Acta Chir Scand* 1979;145:83–86.
154. van der Geld H, Feltkamp TEW, van Loghem JJ, et al: Multiple antibody production in myasthenia gravis. *Lancet* 1963;2:373–375.
155. Aarli JA, Tönder O: Antiglobulin consumption test with sera from patients with myasthenia gravis. *Clin Exp Immunol* 1970;7:11–21.
156. Aarli JA: Myasthenia gravis antibodies to an acid-soluble antigen in striated muscle. *Clin Exp Immunol* 1972;10:453–461.
157. Aarli JA: Localization and properties of an acid soluble muscle antigen reacting with antibodies in myasthenia gravis sera. *Acta Pathol Microbiol Scand (B)* 1972;80:453–459.
158. Aarli JA, Lefvert AK, Tönder O: Thymoma specific antibodies in sera from patients with myasthenia gravis demonstrated by indirect haemagglutination. *J Neuroimmunol* 1981;1:421–427.
159. Aarli JA, Thunold S: Serological detection of thymoma in myasthenia gravis. *Eur Neurol* 1981;20:380–387.
160. Oosterhuis HJGB, Bethlem J, Feltkamp TEW: Muscle pathology, thymoma and immunological abnormalities in patients with myasthenia gravis. *J Neurol Neurosurg Psychiatry* 1968;31:460–463.
161. Weiner LB, Osserman KE: Studies in myasthenia gravis: demonstration of presence of immunofluorescence in serum correlated with clinical findings. *Ann NY Acad Sci* 1966;135:644–655.
162. Keesey J, Bein M, Mink J, et al: Detection of thymoma in myasthenia gravis. *Neurology (NY)* 1980;30:233–239.
163. Shulman S, Lang R, Beutner E, et al: Precipitation of autoantibody in serum from patients with myasthenia gravis. *Immunology* 1966;10:289–303.
164. Cikes N, Momoi MY, Williams CL, et al: Striational autoantibodies: quantitative detection by enzyme immunoassay in myasthenia gravis, thymoma, and recipients of D-penicillamine or allogeneic bone marrow. *Mayo Clin Proc* 1988;63:474–481.
165. Aarli JA, Gilhus NE, Hofstad H: CA-antibody: an immunological marker of thymic neoplasia in myasthenia gravis. *Acta Neurol Scand* 1987;76:55–57.
166. Ohta M, Ohta K, Itoh N, et al: Anti-skeletal muscle antibodies in the sera from myasthenic patients with thymoma: identification of anti-myosin, actomyosin, actin and alpha-actinin antibodies by a solid phase radioimmunoassay and a Western blotting analysis. *Clin Chem Acta* 1990;187:255–264.
167. Gilhus NE, Pandey JP, Gaarder PI, et al: Immunoglobulin allotypes in myasthenia gravis patients with a thymoma. *J Autoimmun* 1990;3:299–305.
168. Rosenberger A, Adler O: Fine needle aspiration in the diagnosis of mediastinal lesions. *Am J Roentgenol* 1978;131:239–242.
169. Adler O, Rosenberger A: Invasive radiology in the diagnosis of mediastinal masses. *Radiologe* 1979;19:169–172.
170. Haaga JR: New techniques in CT-guided biopsies. *Am J Roentgenol* 1979;133:633–641.
171. Pak HY, Yokota SB, Friedberg HA: Thymoma diagnosed by transthoracic fine needle aspiration. *Acta Cytol* 1982;26:210–216.
172. Sajjad SM, Lukeman JM, Llamas L, et al: Needle biopsy diagnosis of thymoma. A case report. *Acta Cytol* 1982;26:503–506.

173. Sterrett G, Whitaker D, Shilkin KB, et al: The fine needle aspiration cytology of mediastinal lesions. *Cancer* 1983;51:127–135.
174. Spahr J, Frable WJ: Pulmonary cytopathology of an invasive thymoma. *Acta Cytol* 1981;25:163–166.
175. Martigne C, Velly JF, Clear P, et al: Value and current role of anterior mediastinotomy in the diagnosis of mediastinal diseases. Apropos of a series of 100 cases. *Ann Chir* 1989;43:171–173.
176. Saito T, Kobayashi H, Sugama Y, et al: Ultrasonically guided needle biopsy in the diagnosis of mediastinal masses. *Am Rev Respir Dis* 1988;138:679–684.
177. Battifora H, Sun TT, Bahu RM, et al: The use of antikeratin antiserum as a diagnostic tool: Thymoma versus lymphoma. *Hum Pathol* 1980;11:635–641.
178. Nabarra B, Manganella G, Savino W: Differential diagnosis between undifferentiated tumor and thymoma by electron microscopy and immunohistochemical labelling. *Pathol Res Pract* 1989;185:257–263.
179. Levine GD, Rosai J, Bearman RM, et al: The fine structure of thymoma, with emphasis on its differential diagnosis. A study of 10 cases. *Am J Pathol* 1975;81:49–86.
180. Rosai J: The value of electron microscopy in diagnostic pathology. Case 9. *Ultrastruct Pathol* 1980;1:121–126.
181. Pedraza MA: Thymoma immunological and ultrastructural characterization. *Cancer* 1977;39:1455–1461.
182. Cossman J, Deegan MJ, Schnitzer B: Thymoma, an immunologic and electron microscopy study. *Cancer* 1978;41:2183–2191.
183. Bloodworth JMB Jr, Hiratsuka H, Hickey RC, et al: Ultrastructure of the human thymus, thymic tumors and myasthenia gravis. *Pathol Annu* 1975;10:329–391.
184. Toker C: Thymoma: an ultrastructural study. *Cancer* 1968;21:1157–1163.
185. Kameya T, Watanabe Y: Electron microscopic observations on human thymus and thymoma. *Acta Pathol Jpn* 1965;15:223–246.
186. Kay S: Comparative ultrastructural studies on three thymic lesions. *Arch Pathol* 1970;90:416–422.
187. Levine GD, Bensch KG: Epithelial nature of spindle-cell thymoma. An ultrastructural study. *Cancer* 1972;30:500–511.
188. Levine GD, Polliack A: The T-cell nature of the lymphocytes in two human epithelial thymomas: a comparative immunologic, scanning and transmission electron microscopic study. *Clin Immunol Immunopathol* 1975;4:199–208.
189. Pinkus GS: Diagnostic immunocytochemistry of paraffin-embedded tissues. *Hum Pathol* 1982;13:411–415.
190. Isaacson P, Wright DH, Jones DB: Malignant lymphoma of true histiocytic (monocyte/macrophage) origin. *Cancer* 1983;51:80–91.
191. van Sonnenberg E, Casola G, Ho M, et al: Difficult thoracic lesions: CT guided biopsy experience in 150 cases. *Radiology* 1988;167:457–461.
192. Linder J, Olsen GA, Johnston WW: Fine needle aspiration biopsy of the mediastinum. *Am J Med* 1986;81:1005–1008.
193. Millar J, Allen R, Wakefield JS, et al: Diagnosis of thymoma by fine-needle aspiration cytology: light and electron microscopic study of a case. *Diagn Cytopathol* 1987;3:166–169.
194. Sherman ME, Black-Schaffer S: Diagnosis of thymoma by needle biopsy. *Acta Cytol (Baltimore)* 1990;341:63–68.
195. Taccagni G, Cantaboni A, Dell'Antonio G, et al: Electron microscopy of fine needle aspiration biopsies of mediastinal and paramediastinal lesions. *Acta Cytol* 1988;32:868–879.
196. Casamassima F, Di Lollo S, Arganini L, et al: CT-guided percutaneous fine-needle biopsy in the histological characterization of mediastinal-pulmonary lesions. *Radiol Med* 1988;76:438–442.
197. Finley JL, Silverman JF, Strausbauch PH, et al: Malignant thymic neoplasms: diagnosis by fine-needle aspiration biopsy with histologic, immunocytochemical, and ultrastructural confirmation. *Diagn Cytopathol* 1986;2:118–125.
198. Müller-Hermelink HK, Marino M, Palestro G: Pathology of thymic epithelial tumors. *Curr Top Pathol* 1986;207–268.
199. Verley JM, Silbert D, Hollmann KH, et al: Histopathology and prognosis of thymomas. Statistical analysis of 200 cases. *Rev Mal Respir* 1988;5:179–185.
200. Monden Y, Tanioka T, Maeda M, et al: Malignancy and differentiation of neoplastic epithelial cells of thymoma. *J Surg Oncol* 1986;31:130–138.
201. Marino M, Müller-Hermelink HK: Thymoma and thymic carcinoma. Relation of thymoma epithelial cells to the cortical and medullary differentiation of thymus. *Virchows Arch [Pathol Anat]* 1985;407:119–149.
202. Rendina EA, Venuta F, Ceroni L, et al: Computed tomographic staging of anterior mediastinal neoplasms. *Thorax* 1988;43:441–445.
203. Elert O, Buchwarld J, Wolf K: Epithelial thymus tumors—therapy and prognosis. *Thorac Cardiovasc Surg* 1988;36:109–113.

204. Ricci C, Rendina EA, Pescarmona EO, et al: Correlations between histological type, clinical behaviour, and prognosis in thymoma. *Thorax* 1989;44:455–460.
205. Takacs L, Savino W, Monostori E, et al: Cortical thymocyte differentiation in thymomas: an immunohistologic analysis of the pathologic microenvironment. *J Immunol* 1987;138:687–698.
206. Kirchner T, Schalke B, Marx A, et al: Evaluation of prognostic features in thymic epithelial tumors. *Thymus* 1989;14:195–203.
207. Pescarmona E, Rendina EA, Venuta F, et al: The prognostic implication of thymoma histologic subtyping. A study of 80 consecutive cases. *Am J Clin Pathol* 1990;93:190–195.
208. Kornstein MJ, Curran WJ Jr, Turrisi AT, et al: Cortical versus medullary thymomas: a useful morphologic distinction? *Hum Pathol* 1988;19:1335–1339.
209. Nomori H, Kobayashi K, Ishihara T, et al: A case of multiple thymoma; the possibility of intra-thymic metastasis. *Jpn J Clin Oncol* 1990;20:209–211.
210. Fisher ER: Thymus, in Bloodworth JMB Jr (ed): *Endocrine Pathology.* Baltimore, Williams & Wilkins, 1968, pp 206–207.
211. Dimery IW, Lee JS, Blick M, et al: Association of the Epstein–Barr virus with lymphoepithe-lioma of the thymus. *Cancer* 1988;61:2475–2480.
212. Ribet M, Voisin C, Gosselin B, et al: Lympho-epithelial thymoma. Anatomo-clinical and thera-peutic study of 113 cases. *Rev Mal Respir* 1988;5:53–60.
213. Masaoka A, Nagaoka Y, Maeda M, et al: Study on the ratio of lymphocytes to epithelial cells in thymoma. *Cancer* 1977;40:1222–1228.
214. Henry K: An unusual thymic tumour with a striated muscle (myoid) component (with a brief review of the literature on myoid cells). *Br J Dis Chest* 1972;66:291–299.
215. Henry K: Mucin secretion and striated muscle in the human thymus. *Lancet* 1966;1:183–185.
216. Shimosato Y, Kameya T, Nagai K, et al: Squamous cell carcinoma of the thymus: an analysis of eight cases. *Am J Surg Pathol* 1977;1:109–121.
217. Tedeschi LG, Sherman JD, Tedeschi CG: Sclerosiderotic granulomatosis in thymoma. *Arch Pa-thol* 1965;80:235–240.
218. Wilkerson JA, Fonkalsrud EW, Richards W. Granulomatous thymoma in childhood. *Dis Chest* 1968;54:156–159.
219. Rosai J, Limas C, Husband EM: Ectopic hamartomatous thymoma. A distinctive lesion of lower neck. *Am J Surg Pathol* 1984;8:501–513.
220. Fetsch JF, Weiss SW: Ectopic hamartomatous thymoma: clinicopathologic, immunohistochem-ical, and histogenetic considerations in four new cases. *Hum Pathol* 1990;21:662–668.
221. Jansen JD, Johnson FE: Fatal ectopic thymoma. *Ann Thorac Surg* 1990;50:469–470.
222. MacLean G, Guberman A, Giulivi A: Late pseudo-exacerbation of myasthenia gravis due to ectopic thymoma invading lower cranial nerves. *Can J Neurol Sci* 1990;17:46–48.
223. Cocconi G, Boni C, Cuomo A: Long-lasting response to *cis*-platinum in recurrent malignant thymoma: case report. *Cancer* 1982;49:1985–1987.
224. Slater G, Papatestas AE, Kornfeld P, et al: Transcervical thymectomy for thymoma in myas-thenia gravis. *Am J Surg* 1982;144:254–256.
225. Appelqvist P, Kostiainen S, Franssila K, et al: Treatment and prognosis of thymoma: a review of 25 cases. *J Surg Oncol* 1982;20:265–268.
226. Wick MR, Nichols WC, Ingle JN, et al: Malignant, predominantly lymphocytic thymoma with central and peripheral nervous system metastases. *Cancer* 1981;47:2036–2043.
227. Jose B, Yu AT, Morgan TF, et al: Malignant thymoma with extrathoracic metastasis: a case report and review of literature. *J Surg Oncol* 1980;15:259–263.
228. Chahinian AP, Bhardwaj S, Meyer RJ, et al: Treatment of invasive or metastatic thymoma: report of eleven cases. *Cancer* 1981;47:1752–1761.
229. Needles B, Kemeny N, Urmacher C: Malignant thymoma: renal metastases responding to *cis*-platinum. *Cancer* 1981;48:223–226.
230. Nordstrom DG, Tewfik HH, Latourette HB: Thymoma: therapy and prognosis as related to op-erative staging. *Int J Radiat Oncol Biol Phys* 1979;5:2059–2062.
231. Collins JD, Pagani JJ: Thymoma metastatic to bone. *J Natl Med Assoc* 1979;71:773–774.
232. Evans WK, Thomson DM, Simpson WJ, et al: Combination chemotherapy in invasive thymoma, role of COPP. *Cancer* 1980;46:1523–1527.
233. Nickels J, Franssila K: Thymoma metastasizing to extrathoracic sites. A case report. *Acta Pa-thol Microbiol Scand (A)* 1976;84:331–334.
234. Wychulis AR, Payne WS, Clagett OT, et al: Surgical treatment of mediastinal tumors. A 40 year experience. *J Thorac Cardiovasc Surg* 1971;62:379–392.
235. Rosen VJ, Christiansen TW, Hughes RK. Metastatic thymoma presenting as a solitary pulmo-nary nodule. *Cancer* 1966;19:527–532.
236. Ericsson J, Hook O: Malignant thymoma with metastases. A report of three cases, two with myasthenia gravis. *J Neuropathol Exp Neurol* 1960;19:538–553.
237. Papatestas AE, Alpert LI, Osserman KE, et al: Studies in myasthenia gravis: effects of thymec-

tomy. Results on 185 patients with nonthymomatous and thymomatous myasthenia gravis, 1941–1969. *Am J Med* 1971;50:465–474.

238. Bergh NP, Rosengren B, Seeman T: Treatment of tumours of the thymus. *Scand J Thorac Cardiovasc Surg* 1968;2:65–69.
239. Fechner RE: Recurrence of noninvasive thymomas. Report of four cases and review of literature. *Cancer* 1969;23:1423–1427.
240. Gravanis MB: Metastasizing thymoma. Report of a case and review of the literature. *Am J Clin Pathol* 1968;49:690–696.
241. Rachmaninoff N, Fentress V: Thymoma with metastasis to the brain. *Am J Clin Pathol* 1964;41:618–625.
242. Green JD, Forman WH: Response of thymoma to steroids. *Chest* 1974;65:114–116.
243. Williams CL, Lennon VA: Thymic B lymphocyte clones from patients with myasthenia gravis secrete monoclonal striational autoantibodies reacting with myosins, alpha actinin or actin. *J Exp Med* 164;1043:1986.
244. Korobkin M, Gasano VA: Intracaval and intracardiac extension of malignant thymoma: CT diagnosis. *J Comput Assist Tomogr* 1989;13:348–350.
245. Penn CRH, Hope-Stone HF: The role of radiotherapy in the management of malignant thymoma. *Br J Surg* 1972;59:533–539.
246. Marks RD Jr, Wallace KM, Pettit HS: Radiation therapy control of nine patients with malignant thymoma. *Cancer* 1978;41:117–119.
247. Boston B: Chemotherapy of invasive thymoma. *Cancer* 1976;38:49–52.
248. Almog C, Pik A, Weisberg D, et al: Regression of malignant thymoma with metastases after treatment with adrenocortical steroids. *Isr J Med Sci* 1978;14:476–480.
249. Ariaratnam LS, Kalnicki S, Mincer F, et al: The management of malignant thymoma with radiation therapy. *Int J Radiat Oncol Biol Phys* 1979;5:77–80.
250. Kornfeld P, Genkins G, Papatestas AE, et al: Steroid therapy in myasthenia gravis associated with thymoma. *Mt Sinai J Med* 1978;45:106–115.
251. Shellito J, Khandekar JD, McKeever WP, et al: Invasive thymoma responsive to oral corticosteroids. *Cancer Treat Rep* 1978;62:1397–1400.
252. Arriagada R, Gerard-Marchant R, Tubiana M, et al: Radiation therapy in the management of malignant thymic tumors. *Acta Radiol (Oncol)* 1981;20:167–172.
253. Bergh NP, Gatzinsky P, Larsson S, et al: Tumors of the thymus and thymic region: I. Clinicopathological studies on thymomas. *Ann Thorac Surg* 1978;25:91–98.
254. Masaoka A, Monden Y, Nakahara K, et al: Follow-up study of thymomas with special reference to their clinical stages. *Cancer* 1981;48:2485–2492.
255. Denayer MA, Rao KR, Wirz D, et al: Hepatic metastatic thymoma and myasthenia gravis twenty-two years after the apparent cure of an invasive thymoma. A case report and review of the literature. *J Neurol Sci* 1986;76:23–30.
256. Curran WJ Jr, Kornstein MJ, Brooks JJ, et al: Invasive thymoma: the role of mediastinal irradiation following complete or incomplete surgical resection. *J Clin Oncol* 1988;6:1722–1727.
257. Dahan M, Gaillard J, Mary H, Renella-Coll J, Berjaud J: Long-term survival of surgically treated lympho-epithelial thymomas. *Rev Mal Respir* 1988;5:159–165.
258. Donovan PJ, Foley JF: Chemotherapy in invasive thymomas: five case reports. *J Surg Oncol* 1986;33:14–17.
259. Dy C, Calvo FA, Mindan JP, Aparicio LA, Algarra SM, Gil A, Gonzalez F, Harguindey S: Undifferentiated epithelial-rich invasive malignant thymoma: complete response to cisplatin, vinblastine, and bleomycin therapy. *J Clin Oncol* 1988;6:536–542.
260. Fornasiero A, Daniele O, Ghiotto C, Sartori F, et al: Chemotherapy of invasive thymoma. *J Clin Oncol* 1990;8:1419–1423.
261. Goldel N, Boning L, Fredrik A, Holzel D, Hartenstein R, Wilmanns W: Chemotherapy of invasive thymoma. A retrospective study of 22 cases. *Cancer* 1989;15:1493–1500.
262. Guerin RA: Radiotherapy of thymomas. *Rev Mal Respir* 1988;5:167–171.
263. Jaretzki A, Penn AS, Younger DS, Wolff M, Olarte MR, Lovelace RE, Rowland LP: "Maximal" thymectomy for myasthenia gravis results. *J Thorac Cardiovasc Surg* 1988;95:747–757.
264. Kosmidis PA, Iliopoulos E, Pentea S: Combination chemotherapy with cyclophosphamide, adriamycin, and viscristine in malignant thymoma and myasthenia gravis. *Cancer* 1988;61:1736–1740.
265. Krueger JB, Sagerman RH, King GA: Stage III thymoma: results of postoperative radiation therapy. *Radiology* 1988;168:855–858.
266. Loehrer PJ Sr, Perez CA, Roth LM, Greco A, et al: Chemotherapy for advanced thymoma. Preliminary results of an intergroup study. *Ann Intern Med* 1990;113:520–524.
267. Nakagawa K, Sakaki S, Oka Y, Matsuoka K: Malignant thymoma with intracranial metastases. *No Shinkei Geka* 1988;16:589–595.
268. Nakahara K, Ohno K, Hashimoto J, Maeda H, Miyoshi S, Sakurai M, Monden Y, Kawashima

Y: Thymoma: results with complete resection and adjuvant postoperative irradiation in 141 consecutive patients. *J Thorac Cardiovasc Surg* 1988;95:1041–1047.

269. Ohara K, Okumura T, Sugahara S, Akisada M, et al: The role of preoperative radiotherapy for invasive thymoma. *Acta Oncol* 1990;29:425–429.

270. Papatestas AE, Pozner J, Genkins G, Kornfeld P, Matta RJ: Prognosis in occult thymomas in myasthenia gravis following transcervical thymectomy. *Arch Surg* 1987;122:1352–1356.

271. Ring NP, Addis BJ: Thymoma: an integrated clinicopathological and immunohistochemical study. *J Pathol* 1986;149:327–337.

272. Yamashita C, Nakamura K, Okada M, Ishii N, Oota T, Oobo H, Okada A, Tsubota N: Surgical treatment of stage III and IV thymoma. *Nippon Kyoby Geka Gakkai Zasshi* 1989;37:391–395.

273. Kirschner PA: Reoperation for thymoma: report of 23 cases. *Ann Thorac Surg* 1990;49:550–554.

274. Arakawa A, Yasunaga T, Saitoh Y, Uozumi H, Takada C, Baba Y, Yoshizumi K, Takahashi M: Radiation therapy of invasive thymoma. *Int J Radiat Oncol Biol Phys* 1990;18:529–534.

275. Couture MM, Mountain CF: Thymoma. *Semin Surg Oncol* 1990;6:110–114.

276. Tanaka M, Shimokawa R, Matsubara O, et al: Mucoepidermoid carcinoma of the thymic region. *Acta Pathol Jpn* 1982;32:703–712.

277. Wick MR, Scheithauer BW: Oat-cell carcinoma of the thymus. *Cancer* 1982;49:1652–1657.

278. Duguid JB, Kennedy AM: Oat-cell tumours of mediastinal glands. *J Pathol Bacteriol* 1930;33:93–99.

279. Rosai J, Levine G, Weber WR, et al: Carcinoid tumours and oat cell carcinomas of the thymus. *Pathol Annu* 1976;11:201–226.

280. Thompson AD, Thackray AC: The histology of tumours of the thymus. *Br J Cancer* 1957;11:348–357.

281. Conkle DM, Adkins RB Jr: Primary malignant tumors of the mediastinum. *Ann Thorac Surg* 1972;14:553–567.

282. Alguacil-Garcia A, Halliday WC: Thymic carcinoma with focal neuroblastoma differentiation. *Am J Surg Pathol* 1987;11:474–479.

283. DiMario FJ Jr, Lisak RP, Kornstein MJ, Brooks JJ: Myasthenia gravis and primary squamous cell carcinoma of the thymus: a case report. *Neurology* 1988;38:580–582.

284. Herczeg E, Kahn LB: Primary thymic carcinoma. An unusual case originating in a lymphocytic rich thymoma. *Virchows Arch A* 1986;409:163–169.

285. Ishimaru H, Shibata Y, Ohkawara S, Ohshima H, Kihara S: Lymphoepithelial cystic lesion related to adenocarcinoma in the mediastinum. *Am J Clin Pathol* 1989;92:808–813.

286. Lagrange W, Dahm HH, Karstens J, Feichtinger J, Mittermayer C: Melanocytic neuroendocrine carcinoma of the thymus. *Cancer* 1987;59:484–488.

287. Matsuno Y, Mukai K, Noguchi M, Sato Y, Shimasato Y: Histochemical and immunohistochemical evidence of glandular differentiation in thymic carcinoma. *Acta Pathol Jpn* 1989;39:433–438.

288. Morinaga S, Sato Y, Shimosato Y, Sinkai T, Tsuchiya R: Multiple thymic squamous cell carcinomas associated with mixed type thymoma. *Am J Surg Pathol* 1987;11:982–988.

289. Moriyama S, Shimizy N, Kurita A, Teramoto S, Taguchi K: A case of adenocarcinoma of the thymus. *Nippon Kyobu Geka Gakkai Zasshi* 1989;37:717–722.

290. Sauter ER, Sardi A, Hollier LH, Cooper ES, Bolton JS: Prognostic value of DNA flow cytometry in thymomas and thymic carcinomas. *South Med J* 1990;83:656–659.

291. Taylor HG, Butler WM, Karcher DS, Zaloznik AJ: Thymic carcinoma: clinical findings in two patients with extrathoracic metastases. *South Med J* 1988;81:664–666.

292. Thomas CV, Manivel JC: Thymic carcinoma and aplastic anemia: report of a previously undocumented association. *Am J Hematol* 1987;25:333–335.

293. Hartmann CA, Roth C, Minck C, et al: Thymic carcinoma. Report of five cases and review of the literature. *J Cancer Res Clin Oncol* 1990;16:69–82.

294. Frank HA, Reiner L, Fleischner FG: Co-occurrence of large leiomyoma of the esophagus and squamous-cell carcinoma of the thymus. Report of a case with roentgenologic, pathological and clinical discussion. *N Engl J Med* 1956;255:159–164.

295. Maezawa M, Mikami J, Ooami H: An autopsy case of squamous cell carcinoma of possible thymic origin. *Lung Cancer* 1974;14:91–97.

296. Watson RR, Weisel W, O'Connor TM: Thymic neoplasm. A surgical enigma. *Arch Surg* 1968;97:230–238.

297. Nagaoka Y: Histological and clinical study on thymoma. *Nihon Kyobu Geka Gakkai Zasshi* 1973;21:768–793.

298. Kuo T, Chang J-P, Lin F-J, et al: Thymic carcinomas: histopathological varieties and immunohistochemical study. *Am J Surg Pathol* 1990;14:24–34.

299. Truong LD, Mody DR, Cagle PT, et al: Thymic carcinoma. A clinicopathologic study of 13 cases. *Am J Surg Pathol* 1990;14:151–166.

300. Umsawadi T, Chong C, Weedn VW, et al: Squamous cell carcinoma of the thymus: a case report of rapid response to cyclophosphamide, doxorubicin, cisplatin, and prednisone. *Med Pediatr Oncol* 1986;14:338–341.

301. Carbone A, Micheau C. Pitfalls in microscopic diagnosis of undifferentiated carcinoma of naso-pharyngeal type (lymphoepithelioma). *Cancer* 1982;50:1344–1351.
302. Henle G, Henle W: Epstein–Barr virus-specific IgA serum antibodies as an outstanding feature of nasopharyngeal carcinoma. *Int J Cancer* 1976;17:1–7.
303. Sidhu GS: The endodermal origin of digestive and respiratory tract APUD cells. Histopathologic evidence and a review of the literature. *Am J Pathol* 1979;96:5–20.
304. Pearse AGE, Takor T: Embryology of the diffuse neuroendocrine system and its relationship to the common peptides. *Fed Proc* 1979;38:2288–2294.
305. Wick MR, Scheithauer BW, Dines DE: Thymic neoplasia in two male siblings. *Mayo Clin Proc* 1982;57:653–656.
306. Matani A, Dritsas C: Familial occurrence of thymoma. *Arch Pathol* 1973;95:90–91.
307. Deshpande GN, Fisher JE, Jewett TC Jr, et al: Malignant thymoma in an eight-month-old boy. *J Surg Oncol* 1981;18:61–66.
308. Halpern SR, Schoelzel E, Johnson RB: Thymoma in a young child producing symptoms of asthma. *Am J Dis Child* 1966;111:99–104.
309. Talerman A, Amigo A: Thymoma associated with aregenerative and aplastic anemia in a five-year-old child. *Cancer* 1968;21:1212–1218.
310. Wasserman P, Epstein JW: Congenital carcinoma of the thymus with extensive generalized me-tastases. *J Pediatr* 1939;14:798–804.
311. Dehner LP, Martin SA, Sumner HW: Thymus related tumors and tumor-like lesions in childhood with rapid clinical progression and death. *Hum Pathol* 1977;8:53–66.
312. Chatten J, Katz SM: Thymoma in a 12-year-old boy. *Cancer* 1976;37:953–957.
313. Welch KJ, Tapper D, Vawter GP: Surgical treatment of thymic cysts and neoplasms in children. *J Pediatr Surg* 1979;14:691–698.
314. Shibata K, Koga Y, Onitsuka T, et al: Primary malignant thymoma in a 6-year-old boy. *Jpn J Surg* 1986;439–442.
315. Mineo TC, Francioni F, Cristino B, et al: Cysts and primary tumors of the mediastinum in child-hood. *Minerva Chir* 1988;54:1161–1167.
316. Mullen B, Richardson JD: Primary anterior mediastinal tumors in children and adults. *Ann Thorac Surg* 1986;42:338–345.
317. Pokorny WJ, Sherman JO: Mediastinal masses in infants and children. *J Thorac Cardiovasc Surg* 1974;68:869–875.
318. Wychulis AR, Payne WS, Clagett OT, et al: Surgical treatment of mediastinal tumors. A 40 year experience. *J Thorac Cardiovasc Surg* 1971;62:379–391.
319. Bowie PR, Teixeira OHP, Carpenter B: Malignant thymoma in a nine-year-old boy presenting with pleuro pericardial effusion. *J Thorac Cardiovasc Surg* 1979;77:777–781.
320. Furman WL, Buckley PJ, Green AA, et al: Thymoma and myasthenia gravis in a 4-year-old child. Case report and review of the literature. *Cancer* 1985;56:2703–2706.
321. Galil-Ogly GA, Ingberman IaKH, Berschchanskaia AM: Comparative ultrastructural character-istics of epithelial cells of the parenchyma of the thymus gland and thymoma. *Arkh Patol* 1988;50:51–60.
322. Shirai T, Miyata M, Nakase A, et al: Lymphocyte subpopulation in neoplastic and non-neoplastic thymus and in blood of patients with myasthenia gravis. *Clin Exp Immunol* 1976;26:118–123.
323. Lauriola L, Maggiano N, Marino M, et al: Human thymoma: immunologic characteristics of the lymphocytic component. *Cancer* 1981;48:1992–1995.
324. Lauriola L, Piantelli M, Carbone A, et al: Subpopulations of lymphocytes in human thymomas. *Clin Exp Immunol* 1979;37:502–506.
325. Musiani P, Lauriola L, Maggiano N, et al: Functional properties of human thymoma lympho-cytes: role of subcellular factors in blastic activation. *J Natl Cancer Inst* 1982;69:827–831.
326. Sato Y, Watanabe S, Mukai K, et al: An immunohistochemical study of thymic epithelial tumors. II. Lymphoid component. *Am J Surg Pathol* 1986;10:862–870.
327. Suster S, Rosai J: Histology of the normal thymus. *Am J Surg Pathol* 1990;14:284–303.
328. Chilosi M, Iannucci A, Menestrina F, et al: Immunohistochemical evidence of active thymocyte proliferation in thymoma. Its possible role in the pathogenesis of autoimmune diseases. *Am J Pathol* 1987;128:464–470.
329. Hofmann WJ, Palesen G, Moller P, et al: Expression of cortical and medullary thymic epithelial antigens in thymomas. An immunohistological study of 14 cases including a characterization of the lymphocytic compartment. *Histopathology* 1989;14:447–463.
330. Musiani P, Maggiano N, Aiello FB, et al: Phenotypical characteristics and proliferative capabil-ities of thymocyte subsets in human thymoma. *Clin Immunol Immunopathol* 1986;40:385–392.
331. Palestro G, Valente G, Novero D, et al: Relationship between structure and T-lymphocyte mat-uration in human thymomas. Enzyme histochemical and immunohistological studies. *Virchows Arch [Cell Pathology]* 1987;52:389–402.
332. Katzin WE, Fishleder AJ, Linden MD, et al: Immunoglobulin and T-cell receptor genes in thy-

momas: genotypic evidence supporting the nonneoplastic nature of the lymphocytic component. *Hum Pathol* 1988;19:323–328.

333. Scarpa A, Chilosi M, Capelli P, et al: Expression and gene rearrangement of the T-cell receptor in human thymomas. *Virchows Arch [Cell Pathology]* 1990;58:235–239.

334. Ito M, Taki T, Miyake M, et al: Lymphocyte subsets in human thymoma studied with monoclonal antibodies. *Cancer* 1988;61:284–287.

335. Kornstein MJ, Kay S: B cells in thymomas. *Mod Pathol* 1990;3:61–63.

336. Le PT, Tuck DT, Dinarello CA, et al: Human thymic epithelial cells produce interleukin 1. *J Immunol* 1987;138:2520–2526.

337. Kodama T, Watanabe S, Sato Y, et al: An immunohistochemical study of thymic epithelial tumors. I. Epithelial component. *Am J Surg Pathol* 1986;10:26–33.

338. Takahashi T, Ueda R, Nishida K, et al: Immunohistological analysis of thymic tumors with PE-35 monoclonal antibody reactive with medullary thymic epithelium. *Cancer Res* 1988;48:1896–1903.

339. Hirokawa K, Utsuyama M, Moriizumi E, et al: Immunohistochemical studies in human thymomas. Localization of thymosin and various cell markers. *Virchows Arch [Cell Pathology]* 1988;55:371–380.

340. Papadopoulos T, Kirchner T, Marx A, et al: Primary cultures of human thymic epithelial tumors. Morphological and immunocytochemical characterization. *Virchows Arch [Cell Pathology]* 1989;56:363–370.

341. Geuder KI, Schoepfer R, Kirchner T, et al: The gene of the alpha-subunit of the acetylcholine receptor: molecular organization and transcription in myasthenia-associated thymomas. *Thymus* 1989;14:179–186.

342. Marx A, O'Connor R, Tzartos S, et al: Acetylcholine receptor epitope in proteins of myasthenia gravis-associated thymomas and non-thymic tissues. *Thymus* 1989;14:171–178.

343. Dardenne M, Savino W, Bach JF: Thymomatous epithelial cells and skeletal muscle share a common epitope defined by a monoclonal antibody. *Am J Pathol* 1987;126:194–198.

344. Marx A, O'Connor R, Geuder KI, et al: Characterization of a protein with an acetylcholine receptor epitope from myasthenia gravis-associated thymomas. *Lab Invest* 1990;62:279–286.

345. Caillaud JM, Carlu C, Bretel JJ, et al: Immunohistochemical study of 11 epithelial tumors of the thymus or thymomas with anti-keratin antibodies: KL-1. *Rev Mal Respir* 1988;5:153–157.

346. Eimoto T, Teshima K, Shirakusa T, et al: Heterogeneity of epithelial cells and reactive components in thymomas: an ultrastructural and immunohistochemical study. *Ultrastruct Pathol* 1986;10:157–173.

347. Lee D, Wright DH: Immunohistochemical study of 22 cases of thymoma. *J Clin Pathol* 1988;41:1297–1304.

348. Willcox N, Schluep M, Ritter MA, et al: Myasthenic and nonmyasthenic thymoma. An expansion of a minor cortical epithelial cell subset? *Am J Pathol* 1987;127:447–460.

349. Ruco LP, Rosali S, Monardo F, et al: Macrophages and interdigitating reticulum cells in normal thymus and in thymoma: an immunohistochemical study. *Histopathology* 1989;14:37–45.

350. Suster S, Rosai J: Histology of the normal thymus. *Am J Surg Pathol* 1990;14:284–303.

351. Kraus VB, Harden EA, Wittels B, et al: Demonstration of phenotypic abnormalities of thymic epithelium in thymoma including two cases with abundant Langerhans cells. *Am J Pathol* 1988;132:552–562.

352. Sato T, Tamaoki N: Myoid cells in the human thymus and thymoma revealed by three different immunohistochemical markers for striated muscle. *Acta Pathol Jpn* 1989;39:509–519.

353. Mizuno T, Hashimoto T, Masaoka A: Distribution of fibronectin and laminin in human thymoma. *Cancer* 1990;65:1367–1374.

354. Nagle RB, McDaniel KM, Clark VA, et al: The use of antikeratin antibodies in the diagnosis of human neoplasms. *Am J Clin Pathol* 1983;79:458–466.

355. Rouse RV, Weiss LM: Human thymomas: evidence of immunohistologically defined normal and abnormal microenvironmental differentiation. *Cell Immunol* 1988;111:94–106.

356. Hohlfeld R: Myasthenia gravis and thymoma: paraneoplastic failure of neuromuscular transmission. *Lab Invest* 1990;62:241–242.

357. Compston DAS, Vincent A, Newsom-Davis J, et al: Clinical, pathological, HLA antigen and immunological evidence for disease heterogeneity in myasthenia gravis. *Brain* 1980;103:579.

358. Gilhus NE, Aarli JA, Christensson B, et al: Rabbit antiserum to citric acid extract of human skeletal muscle staining thymomas from myasthenia gravis patients. *J Neuroimmunol* 1984;7:55–64.

359. Kirchner T, Hoppe F, Muller-Hermelink HK, et al: Acetylcholine receptor epitopes on epithelial cells of thymoma in myasthenia gravis. *Lancet* 1987;1:218.

360. Wara DW: Thymic hormones and the immune system. *Adv Pediatr* 1981;28:229–270.

361. Bach J-F: Thymic hormones. *J Immunopharmacol* 1979;1:277–310.

362. Palestro G, Valente G, Micca FB, et al: Detection and distribution of alpha-naphthyl acetate

esterase activity in thymocytes of normal, myasthenic thymus and thymoma. Histochemical and cytochemical study in relation to E-rosetting. *Virchows Arch [Cell Pathol]* 1980;35:33–43.

363. Knowles DM II, Hoffman T, Ferrarini M, et al: The demonstration of acid alpha naphthyl acetate esterase activity in human lymphocytes: usefulness as a T-cell marker. *Cell Immunol* 1978;35:112–123.

364. Low T: Biochemical characterization of thymic hormones in thymoma tissues. *Thymus* 1990;15:93–105.

365. von Hoegen I, Falk W, Kojouharoff G, et al: Internalization of interleukin 1 (IL 1) correlates with IL 1-induced IL 2 receptor expression and IL 2 secretion of EL4 thymoma cells. *Eur J Immunol* 1989;19:329–334.

366. Chollet P, Plagne R, Fonck Y, et al: Thymoma with hypersecretion of thymic hormone. *Thymus* 1981;3:321–334.

367. Kirkpatrick CH, Greenberg LE, Chapman SW, et al: Plasma thymic hormone activity in patients with chronic mucocutaneous candidiasis. *Clin Exp Immunol* 1978;34:311–317.

368. Ranelletti FO, Iacobelli S, Carmignani M, et al: Glucocorticoid receptors and *in vitro* cortico-sensitivity in human thymoma. *Cancer Res* 1980;40:2020–2025.

369. Ranelletti FO, Carmignani M, Iacobelli S, et al: Glucocorticoid binding components in human thymus hyperplasia. *Cancer Res* 1978;38:516–520.

370. Hammar JA: *Die Normal-Morphologische Thymusforschung*, Barth, Leipzig 1936.

371. Sobhon P, Jirasattham C: Effect of sex hormones on the thymus and lymphoid tissue of ovariec-tomized rats. *Acta Anat* 1974;89:211–225.

372. Ranelletti FO, Carmignani M, Marchetti P, et al: Estrogen binding by neoplastic human thymus cytosol. *Eur J Cancer* 1980;16:951–955.

373. Okada K, Hoshino K, Hitomi S: Analysis of nuclear DNA histograms in thymomas. *Nippon Ganka Gakkai Zasshi* 1988;89:416–422.

374. Asamura H, Nakajima T, Mukai K, et al: Degree of malignancy of thymic epithelial tumors in terms of nuclear DNA content and nuclear area. An analysis of 39 cases. *Am J Pathol* 1988;133:615–622.

375. Davies SE, Macartney JC, Camplejohn RS, et al: DNA flow cytometry of thymomas. *Histopathology* 1989;15:77–83.

376. Kristoffersson U, Heim S, Mandahl N, et al: Multiple clonal chromosome aberrations in two thymomas. *Cancer Genet Cytogenet* 1989;41:93–98.

377. Mukai K, Sato Y, Hirohashi S, et al: Expression of ras p21 protein by thymoma. *Virchows Arch [Cell Pathol]* 1990;59:11–16.

378. Nomori H, Horinouchi H, Kaseda S, et al: Evaluation of the malignant grade of thymoma by morphometric analysis. *Cancer* 1988;61:982–988.

379. Nomori H, Ishihara T, Torikata C: Malignant grading of cortical and medullary differentiated thymoma by morphometric analysis. *Cancer* 1989;64:1694–1699.

380. Ghadially FN, Illman O: Naturally occurring thymomas in the European hamster. *J Pathol* 1965;90:465–469.

381. Hall GA, Howell J McC, Lewis DG: Thymoma with myasthenia gravis in a dog. *J Pathol* 1972;108:177–180.

382. Kurokawa Y, Fujii K, Suzuki M, et al: Spontaneous tumors of the thymus in mastomys *(Rattus natalensis). Gann* 1968;59:145–150.

383. Langerlöff B: The ultrastructure of virus- and radiation-induced thymomas of C57B1 mice. *Acta Pathol Microbiol Scand (A)* 1968;74:495–513.

384. Rappaport H, Baroni C: A study of the pathogenesis of malignant lymphoma induced in the Swiss mouse by 7,12-dimethylbenz(*a*)anthracene injected at birth. *Cancer Res* 1962;22:1067–1074.

385. Sandison AT, Anderson LJ: Tumors of the thymus in cattle, sheep, and pigs. *Cancer Res* 1969;29:1146–1150.

386. Boniver J: Pathogenesis of thymic lymphomas in C57BL mice. *Pathol Res Pract* 1981;171:268–278.

387. Maisin JR, Leonard A, Mattelin G: Preleukemic cells and radiation-induced thymoma. *Biomedicine* 1980;33:47–49.

388. Frei JV, Lawley PD: Thymomas induced by simple alkylating agents in C57BL/Cbi mice: kinetics of the dose response. *J Natl Cancer Inst* 1980;64:845–852.

389. Farrar JJ, Fuller-Farrar J, Simon PL, et al: Thymoma production of T-cell growth factor (interleukin 2). *J Immunol* 1980;125:2555–2558.

390. Mermod J-J, Intrière L, MacLeod CL, et al: Characterization of a new type of thymoma variants supersensitive to dexamethasone. *J Steroid Biochem* 1981;15:25–34.

391. Spanopoulou E, Early A, Elliott J, et al: Complex lymphoid and epithelial thymic tumours in Thy1-myc transgenic mice. *Nature* 1989;342:185–189.

392. Matsuyama M, Suzuki H, Yamada S, et al: Ultrastructure of spontaneous and urethan-induced thymomas in buffalo rats. *Cancer Res* 1975;35:2771–2779.

393. Matsuyama M, Amo H: Host origin of lymphoid cells in thymomas developed from subcutaneous thymus grafts in buffalo rats. *Gann* 1977;68:293–300.

394. Kato F, Watanabe M: Motor dysfunction in thymoma rats: comparison between fast and slow muscles. *J Pharm Dyn* 1982;5:1005–1011.

395. Kato F, Watanabe M, Matsuyama M: Nephrotic syndrome in spontaneous thymoma rats, Buffalo/Mna. *Biom Res* 1983;4:105–110.

396. Kato F, Watanabe M: Biochemical study on spontaneous thymoma rats with motor dysfunction. *J Pharm Dyn* 1983;6:275–279.

397. Masuda A, Amo H, Matsuyama M: Cytological characteristics of cultured epithelial cells from thymomas in BUF/Mna rats. *Virchows Arch [Cell Pathol]* 1984;46:283–296.

398. Matsuyama M, Yamada C, Kojima A: Possible single dosage effects of the nude gene: suppression of spontaneous development of thymoma and nephropathy in BUF/Mna-rnu/+ rats. *Jpn J Cancer Res* 1987;78:40–44.

399. Bandyopadhyay SK, D'Andrea E, Fleissner E: Expression of oncogenes: unrearranged c-myc gene but altered promoter usage in radiation-induced thymoma. *Oncogene Res* 1989;4:311–318.

400. Hoot GP, Kettman JR: Primary polyoma virus-induced murine thymic epithelial tumors. A tumor model of thymus physiology. *Am J Pathol* 1989;135:679–695.

401. Vijaya S, Steffen DL, Kozak C, et al: Dsi-1, a region with frequent proviral insertions in Moloney murine leukemia virus-induced rat thymomas. *J Virol* 1987;61:1164–1170.

402. Lazo PA, Tsichlis PN: Recombination between two integrated proviruses, one of which was inserted near c-myc in a retrovirus-induced rat thymoma: implications for tumor progression. *J Virol* 1988;62:788–794.

403. von Hoegen I, Falk W, Kojouharoff G, et al: Internalization of interleukin 1 (IL 1) correlates with IL 1-induced IL 2 receptor expression and IL 2 secretion of EL4 thymoma cells. *Eur J Immunol* 1989;19:329–334.

404. Nairn RS, McIntyre BW, Richie ER, et al: Characterization of env gene recombination in x-ray-induced thymomas of C57BL/6 mice. *Mol Carcinog* 1989;2:126–130.

405. Segal A, Seidman I, Melchionne S: Induction of thymic lymphomas and squamous cell carcinomas following topic application of isopropyl methanesulfonate to female Hsd:(IC)BR mice. *Cancer Res* 1987;47:3402–4505.

7

Other Tumors of the Thymus

The thymus gland can be the organ of origin of carcinoids, thymolipomas, germ cell tumors, malignant lymphomas, histiocytosis, and lymphangiomas (1). In the past, these neoplasms were included under the generic name of thymoma, but they are now recognized as distinct and separate entities from the thymic epithelium tumors.

THYMIC CARCINOID TUMORS

In 1972, Rosai and associates (2) reported 11 patients with carcinoid tumors of the thymus and proposed diagnostic criteria for their distinction from thymomas.

Thymic carcinoid tumors presumably have a different embryologic origin from thymomas (3–11). Thymomas are derived from endodermal thymic epithelial cells, whereas carcinoid tumors are of neural crest origin. This view is supported by morphologic and ultrastructural similarities between carcinoid tumors and neuroendocrine cells with biochemical characteristics of amine precursor uptake and decarboxylation (APUD) cells and by the presence of multiple endocrine neoplasms (MEN) in patients with these neoplasms (1,5,11). However, APUD cells have not been described in the normal human thymus, although ultrastructural studies have identified them in other mammals (1).

Clinical Features

Thymic carcinoids are unusual neoplasms that have distinct clinical, pathologic, and biologic characteristics (12–22).

Thymic carcinoids are more frequent in male patients (3:1) in their fifth decade of life (median age of diagnosis, 43 years; age range: 9 to 87 years old); either they are discovered on routine chest roentgenograms or patients present with nonspecific systemic, local, and/or endocrine symptoms (12,21). Nonspecific systemic symptoms are of little help for the diagnosis of thymic carcinoids and include fatigue, malaise, fever, and, rarely, polyarthropathy, digital clubbing, proximal myopathy, and peripheral myopathy (4). No association with myasthenia gravis, aplastic anemia, hypogammaglobulinemia, or other systemic syndromes encountered in patients with thymomas has been described (12).

Local thoracic symptoms are caused by displacement of mediastinal structures by the neoplasm and include chest or interscapular back pain, dyspnea, cough, and/or manifestations of the superior vena cava syndrome (1,12). Rarely, mediastinal carcinoids rupture with hemorrhage resulting in hemothorax and mediastinal enlargement (13).

Endocrine abnormalities are frequent in patients with thymic carcinoids. About 50% of patients present with endocrine disturbances including Cushing's syndrome, inappropriate ADH secretion, hyperparathyroidism, or MEA syndrome (1,22–28).

Cushing's syndrome, caused by hypersecretion of ACTH by the neoplasm, is the most frequent abnormality, and several studies have confirmed the presence of the hormone in tumor extracts and in tumor cells (24–27). Occasionally, tumor extracts of patients with thymic carcinoids and Cushing's syndrome exhibit the presence of several other polypeptide hormones including α-MSH, β-endorphin, Met-enkephalin, and somatostatin when studied with radioimmunoassay (14,15,23,24).

About 19% of patients with thymic carcinoids present with manifestations of MEA type I (Wermer's syndrome) (12). This condition is inherited as an autosomal dominant trait with variable penetrance and is characterized by the presence of hyperparathyroidism resulting from parathyroid adenomas (multiple or single) or hyperplasia, islet cell tumors of the pancreas, pituitary adenoma, and, less frequently, carcinoid tumors of the lung, intestine, and/or thymus (1). These patients can also have adrenal neoplasms (adenomas or carcinomas), thyroid adenomas, and multiple lipomata.

Rarely, patients with thymic carcinoids have medullary carcinoma of the thyroid and other neoplasms encountered in MEA type II (Sipple's syndrome) (28) (Figs. 7-1, 7-2, and 7-3).

Our patient with thymic carcinoid and incomplete Sipple's syndrome had medullary carcinoma of the thyroid, parathyroid hyperplasia, carcinoid tumors in multiple organs (including the intestine, stomach, and gallbladder), and an adrenal neuroma.

Anterior mediastinal aggressive carcinoid tumors can arise after initially successful treatment of a germ cell tumor (18).

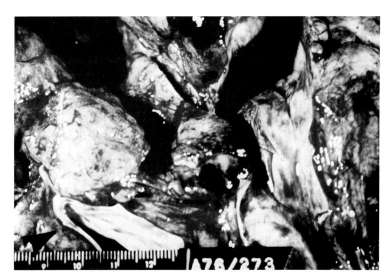

FIG. 7–1. Thymic carcinoid compressing the superior vena cava. Patient also had other manifestations of the MEA type II syndrome.

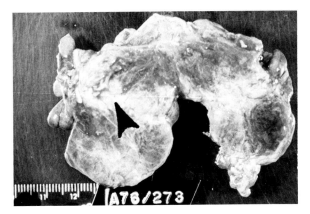

FIG. 7–2. Medullary carcinoma of the thyroid (*arrowhead*) associated with thymic carcinoid.

Roentgenologic Features

Thymic carcinoids are usually large, solid, lobulated anterior mediastinal masses that occasionally exhibit focal stippled calcification (12). Computed tomographic scans may show the infiltrative character of the lesion. Bone scans and roentgenograms are useful in detecting metastases, which are usually multifocal and osteoblastic (12).

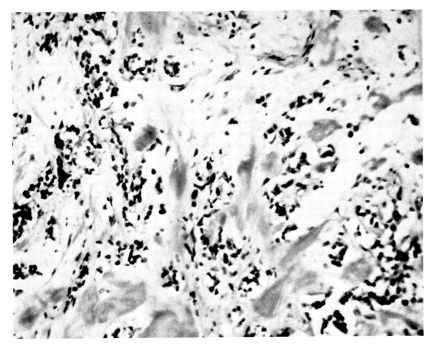

FIG. 7–3. Medullary carcinoma of the thyroid with amyloid stroma in a patient with incomplete MEA II syndrome. (H&E × 100, original)

Pathologic Features

Thymic carcinoids are solid, usually large, lobulated tan–gray neoplasms with focal areas of calcification that give the surface a "sandy," gritty appearance. They are frequently invasive locally and do not have the typical encapsulation and compartmentalization characteristic of thymomas. Thymic carcinoids can have areas of hemorrhage and yellow foci of necrosis. They usually do not undergo cystic degeneration, a frequent finding in thymomas (1).

Histologically, thymic carcinoids are composed of cords, anastomosing ribbons and festoons, islands ("balls"), and/or rosette-like formations composed of oval to round cells with amphophilic or eosinophilic cytoplasm and uniform nuclei, inconspicuous nucleolus, and stippled chromatin pattern (Figs. 7-4, 7-5, and 7-6). The tumor cells have argyrophilic intracytoplasmic granules that can be detected in preparations stained with the Grimelius double-impregnation silver technique or the Sevier–Munger stain. However, argentaffin stains are negative. Formalin-induced fluorescence and α-glycerophosphate dehydrogenase can also be demonstrated in thymic carcinoids (5).

Levine and Rosai (29) reported instances of thymic carcinoids composed predominantly of spindle cells. The neuroendocrine nature of these tumors was suspected on the basis of the distinctive "serpiginous or organoid" arrangement of neoplastic cells, but the diagnosis was established only with the aid of electron microscopy. The diagnosis of spindle cell thymic carcinoid should be suspected in thymic neo-

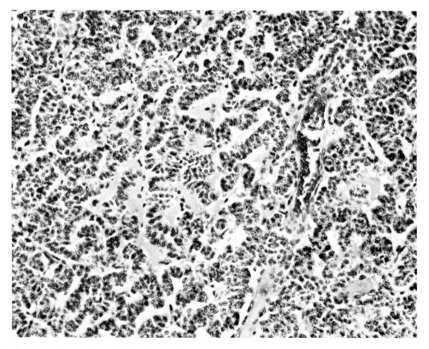

FIG. 7–4. Thymic carcinoid. The tumor is composed of anastomosing cords of small uniform round cells. (H&E × 100, original)

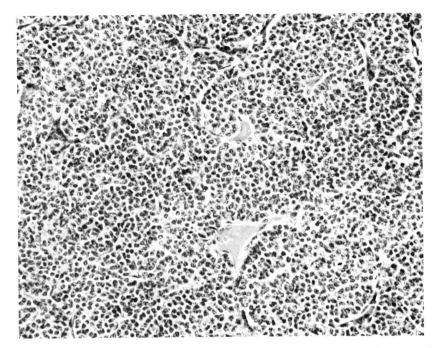

FIG. 7–5. Thymic carcinoid. The tumor is composed of solid nests of small uniform round cells. (H&E × 100, original)

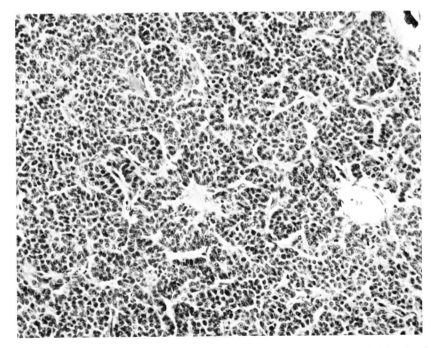

FIG. 7–6. Thymic carcinoid. The tumor has a typical "endocrine" pattern with islands of small uniform round cells surrounded by a fine fibrovascular stroma. (H&E × 100, original)

plasms that lack a significant lymphocytic component, perivascular spaces, compartmentalization, rosettes, and other features encountered in thymomas.

Several studies reported another unusual feature in thymic carcinoids: the presence of prominent pigmentation in the lesions. Ho and Ho (30) reported a pigmented carcinoid in which melanin was demonstrated histochemically and ultrastructurally in the cytoplasm of nonneoplastic cells that probably represented hyperplastic thymic melanoblasts stimulated by the neoplasm. Wick and associates (31) reported thymic carcinoids with other unusual morphologic features including a prominent cribriform pattern, sclerotic stroma, and tumor cells growing in an Indian file arrangement or in solid sheets. One of the tumors in their study was brown–gray and was composed of pigmented cells containing intracytoplasmic lipofuscin. However, no melanin was found.

Immunocytochemical Features

Immunocytochemical stains for the detection of peptide immunoreactivity in the cytoplasm of tumor cells can be useful to confirm the endocrine nature of a thymic tumor and to correlate the pathologic with the clinical findings.

Wick and associates (31) recently reported 13 thymic carcinoids stained with antisera to serotonin, gastrin, ACTH, and calcitonin utilizing a PAP technique. Four tumors in their study exhibited ACTH-like immunoreactivity, and three of these patients had Cushing's syndrome (31). Two tumors exhibited focal serotonin-like immunoreactivity; no gastrin or calcitonin was found in any of the thymic carcinoids.

In a more recent study, Herbst and associates (19) reported cholecystokinin, neurotensin, ACTH, calcitonin, chromogranin A, and neuron-specific enolase immunoreactivity in carcinoid tumors of the thymus. The study also demonstrated that each tumor reacted slightly differently with the various markers, emphasizing the need for the use of a panel of reagents for diagnostic purposes. In addition, the presence of peptide immunoreactivity in the tumor cells did not correlate well with endocrine symptoms in several patients.

Ultrastructural Features

Ultrastructural studies are very helpful to establish the diagnosis of thymic carcinoid. Indeed, in a study at the Mayo Clinic, 4 of 11 tumors that were initially classified as thymic carcinoids on the basis of light microscopic features had to be reclassified as thymomas after ultrastructural studies demonstrated the lack of neurosecretory granules in the cytoplasm of the tumor cells, which exhibited, instead, numerous desmosomes, tonofilaments, and cytoplasmic processes (12). Thymic carcinoids have ultrastructurally a population of polyhedral and/or spindle cells with clear cytoplasm admixed with smaller electron-dense ("dark") cells (1). The latter are probably undergoing degeneration. The tumor cells have a round to oval nucleus with a central small nucleolus and fine chromatin pattern. The cytoplasm has a well-developed Golgi apparatus, granular endoplasmic reticulum, polyribosomes, microtubules, characteristic membrane-bound dense-core neurosecretory granules ranging in size from 100 to 300 nm, easily discernible smooth endoplasmic reticulum, rare exocytoses of neurosecretory granules, and rare rudimentary cilia (15).

Larger pleomorphic granules measuring up to 450 nm in diameter can also be seen (Fig. 7-7). The cytoplasm can also have intracellular type I and II microfilaments measuring 5 to 7 nm that are arranged in whorls and are usually closely associated with dense-core granules. In unusual instances, they can become so prominent in thymic carcinoids as to be visible by light microscopy as 1- to 4-μm eosinophilic argyrophilic intracytoplasmic inclusions (32).

Fetissof and associates (32) classified a lesion with those features as microfilamentous carcinoid of the thymus. This tumor had numerous intermediate-type 10-nm filaments arranged in whorls and bundles associated with neurosecretory granules.

Similar filaments have been designated as type II microfilaments and have been described in normal endocrine cells of the gastroenteropancreatic system (D cells secreting somatostatin) and in carcinoid tumors of the lung, stomach, rectum, and duodenum that are now believed to have an endodermal origin (15,33–35).

The presence of intracytoplasmic whorls of microfilaments in thymic carcinoids has been suggested to be evidence that these tumors may also have an endodermal origin (32).

Differential Diagnosis Between Thymic Carcinoid Tumor, Thymoma, and Other Neoplasms

Thymic carcinoid tumors should be distinguished from thymomas, thymic carcinomas, germ cell tumors, and malignant lymphomas. The neuroendocrine lesions are usually not encapsulated as thymomas and lack their lobular configuration. Histologically, they exhibit the organoid features described previously and lack the presence of a prominent lymphoid component. The cells of carcinoid tumors are smaller and less pleomorphic than those of germ cell tumors and thymic carcinomas. Immunocytochemical studies with a battery of markers, particularly chromogranin, neuron-specific enolase, and neuropeptides can be very helpful to confirm the epithelial and neuroendocrine nature of thymic carcinoids. Ultrastructurally, thymic carcinoids exhibit prominent dense-core granules, smooth endoplasmic reticulum, and type I and II microfilaments (15). Although it is rare, thymic carcinomas can have ultrastructural features similar to those to carcinoid tumors (15); however, these tumors are more pleomorphic under light microscopy and probably represent more primitive carcinomas with neuroendocrine differentiation.

Treatment and Prognosis

Thymic carcinoids are malignant tumors that invade contiguous mediastinal structures in 50% of patients and metastasize in 30% to 40% of instances (15,19).

They are treated primarily by wide local excision. Postoperative radiotherapy can be of value in instances of persistent or recurrent disease, but adjuvant chemotherapy has shown little value in controlling metastatic disease (31).

In a study of 15 patients with thymic carcinoids followed at the Mayo Clinic for up to 25 years, Wick and associates (31) reported metastasis in 73% of patients. Metastatic sites included mediastinal and cervical lymph nodes, liver, bone, skin, and lungs. Bone metastases were usually osteoblastic. The overall cure rate in patients followed for at least 5 years was 13%. The mean survival rate of patients with

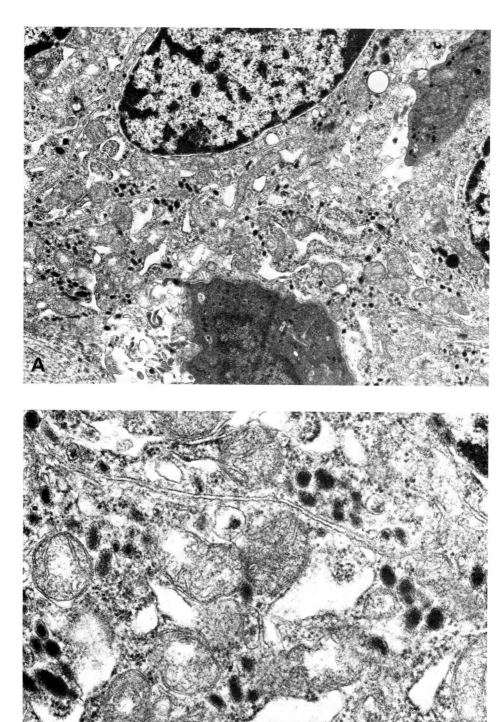

FIG. 7–7. A: Electron micrograph of thymic carcinoid showing numerous intracytoplasmic neurosecretory granules. (×8,300, original) **B:** Higher magnification of dense-core neurosecretory granules with halo and single membrane. (×26,000, original)

metastasis was 3 years after the diagnosis of extrathymic disease. Adjuvant chemotherapy did not influence the prognosis.

Patients with thymic carcinoids have a very prolonged clinical course and need to
be followed for many years before they are considered cured. For example, the patient shown in Fig. 7-1 developed metastatic and invasive disease that resulted in her
death 10 years after the initial diagnosis.

Patients with thymic carcinoids and associated endocrine syndromes such as
Cushing's or MEA type I have a worse prognosis (1). Most individuals reported in
the literature with these associations died with tumor and/or metabolic abnormalities
secondary to the secretory activities of the endocrine neoplasms (31).

THYMOLIPOMA

In 1916, Lange (36) reported a patient with an unusual large mediastinal tumor
composed of lobules of fat and thymic tissue and classified the lesion as a lipoma of
the thymus. In 1948, Hall (37) proposed the term "thymolipoma" for the diagnosis
of these unusual tumors. Thymolipomas comprise 2% to 9% of all thymic neoplasms
(38–60).

Clinical Features

Thymolipomas exhibit no sex predilection and occur in patients whose ages range
from 3 to 60 years (44). They are more frequent, however, in adolescents and young
adults (mean age of occurrence, 22 years old) (45).

Patients are asymptomatic in 50% of instances and are found to have large anterior
mediastinal masses on chest roentgenograms or present with symptoms related to
compression of mediastinal structures by the tumor mass, including cough, dyspnea,
hemoptysis, and/or paroxysmal atrial tachycardia. However, thymolipomas can
grow to a large size and compress mediastinal structures without causing clinical
symptoms (38–60).

Rarely, patients with thymolipoma have associated systemic diseases including
Grave's disease, aplastic anemia, and myasthenia gravis (44,47,59,60). The association of the mediastinal tumor with the latter condition is of particular interest and
has been well documented in seven instances, but it is not clear whether the thymolipomas played a role in the pathogenesis of myasthenia gravis (57,59,60). The
patient of Reintgen and associates (54), for instance, experienced marked improvement in the symptoms of myasthenia gravis following removal of his mediastinal
tumor, whereas the patient of Otto and associates (44) had only a transient remission
in his neuromuscular symptoms followed by aggravation of his condition 3 weeks
after thoracotomy.

Roentgenologic Features

The radiologic features of thymolipomas are variable (40). They present as areas
of mediastinal widening or as slowly enlarging anterior mediastinal masses that can
reach a very large size (Fig. 7-8). They are difficult to distinguish on plain chest
roentgenograms from other mediastinal tumors and from pleural tumors, basal atel-
ectasis, and pericardial tumors or cysts. In addition, 40% of thymolipomas mimic

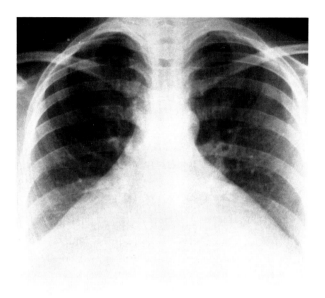

FIG. 7–8. Thymolipoma simulating cardiomegaly.

cardiomegaly on chest roentgenograms (45,55). Indeed, in only 5 of 20 instances of mediastinal thymolipomas studied with conventional chest roentgenograms and reviewed by Benton and Gerard (46) was the correct diagnosis suggested pre-operatively.

Barium esophagograms, diagnostic pneumomediastinum, tomograms, and particularly CT scans are useful for the differential diagnosis of thymolipoma. Indeed, most lesions can now be diagnosed accurately preoperatively with the latter technique (Fig. 7-9). Adipose tissue has a characteristic coefficient of X-ray attenuation

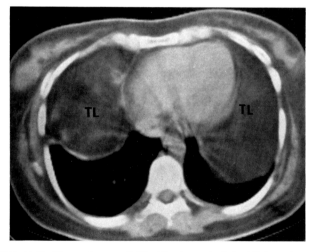

FIG. 7–9. Thymolipoma (*TL*) with characteristic bilobar shape.

that can be identified and quantitated by CT scan (52). Thymolipomas can also be distinguished from mediastinal lipomas located outside the thymus (mediastinal lipomatosis) on the basis of their characteristic bilobate shape, which is usually absent in extrathymic lesions (52).

Pathologic Features

Thymolipomas are well encapsulated and resemble an enlarged thymus with two lobes and an isthmus (Fig. 7-10). They can vary in size from 90 to 3,000 g but are usually quite large (44).

Moigneteau and associates (56) have described the largest thymolipoma on record weighing 12 kg. On section, thymolipomas are soft, tan–yellow, and lobulated. Histologically, they are composed of large lobules of mature adipose tissue with interspersed islands of thymic tissue (Fig. 7-11). The latter usually comprise less than 10% of the tumor mass and consist of epithelial cells, lymphocytes, and Hassall's

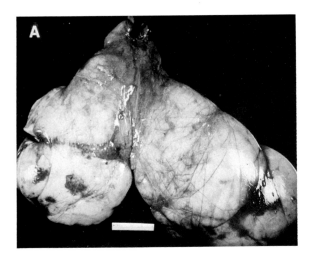

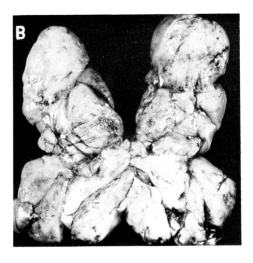

FIG. 7–10. A: Large thymolipoma with well-formed capsule and soft yellow uniform surface. **B:** Cut surface of thymolipoma showing a lobulated appearance.

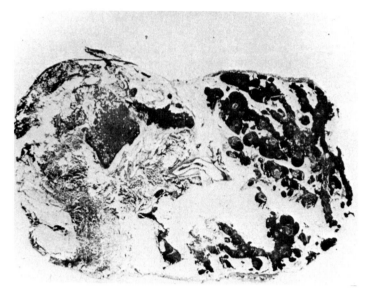

FIG. 7–11. Thymolipoma composed of adipose tissue and islands of thymic tissue. (H&E, whole mount)

corpuscles as seen in the normal thymus. Indeed, some thymolipomas contain distinct areas of thymic cortex and medulla.

Iseki and associates (58) reported the presence of clusters of striated myoid cells in a thymolipoma. These cells exhibited myoglobin, desmin, and vimentin immunoreactivity and Z band structures observed by electron microscopy.

Otto and associates (44) described IgG-positive plasma cells in the thymolipoma of a myasthenia gravis patient. Whether this histologic finding has prognostic value is not known.

Thymolipomas exhibit no features of malignancy. They can adhere, however, to the pleura and/or pericardium and compress mediastinal structures, but they never invade adjacent organs.

Patients are cured by excision of their lesions. To our knowledge, no instances of malignant transformation of a thymolipoma have been reported.

Pathogenesis

The nature of thymolipomas is unknown and has been the subject of controversy (44,45). Thymolipomas may represent lipomas of the thymus, neoplasms of adipose and thymic tissue, or instances of massive thymic hyperplasia with subsequent involution of thymic tissue.

Several authors favor the concept that thymolipomas are lipomas of the thymus gland that develop as a result of a multifocal proliferation of benign perivascular adipose tissue that pull small particles of thymic tissue and incorporate them into the neoplasm during a slow process of tumor growth (44,45,50).

GERM CELL TUMORS

Germ cell tumors are a group of neoplasms that characteristically arise from the testes and ovaries. They are thought to arise from primitive cells that differentiate into embryonic and extraembryonic structures, resulting in a spectrum of benign and malignant neoplasms that are listed in Table 1 (61–75).

Germ cell tumors occasionally develop in extragonadal sites, usually located along the body midline and including the mediastinum, retroperitoneum, sacrococcygeal area, pineal body, stomach, liver, and other sites (76–87).

The mediastinum is the most frequent site of origin of extragonadal germ cell tumors. Indeed, these neoplasms account for approximately 20% of all anterior and superior mediastinal tumors and cysts and approximately 10% of primary mediastinal tumors (76–85). All pathologic variants of germ cell tumors have been encountered in the mediastinum; teratomas are the most frequent histologic type.

Pathogenesis of Mediastinal Germ Cell Tumors

Different hypotheses have been offered to explain the pathogenesis of extragonadal germ cell tumors. Friedman (63) proposed an origin from potentially biphasic germ cells left in the thymus during embryogenesis. Lattes (87) and Schlumberger (88) suggested an origin during embryogenesis from somatic cells in a maldeveloped thymic gland. These hypothesis are partially based on the fact that most mediastinal germ cell tumors are near the thymus or within its parenchyma. However, they do not explain the occurrence of germ cell tumors at extragonadal sites other than the mediastinum. An alternative hypothesis has suggested that mediastinal germ cell tumors arise from aberrant totipotential germ cells that migrate from the urogenital ridge into the mediastinum during embryogenesis (64). This theory is based on the fact that most extragonadal germ cell tumors arise from sites located near the body midline, where the aberrant germ cells are most likely to migrate during embryogenesis.

To our knowledge, there have been no descriptions of nonneoplastic germ cells in the normal thymus.

TABLE 1. *Histopathologic variants of germ cell tumors*

Teratoma
Mature, solid
Cystic (dermoid cyst)
Immature
Malignant (teratocarcinoma)
Mixed
Seminoma (germinoma)
Embryonal carcinoma
Endodermal sinus tumor (yolk-sac tumor)
Choriocarcinoma
Mixed germ cell tumor

Diagnosis of Mediastinal Germ Cell Tumors

Mediastinal germ cell tumors have identical pathologic features to their gonadal counterparts. Indeed, the presence of a primary mediastinal tumor can be established only after careful clinical examination of the ovaries or testes to rule out the presence of a small occult neoplasm. This task can be difficult in instances of small, yet highly malignant, germ cell tumors of the testes or ovaries, as these neoplasms metastasize widely from an occult primary site (68). Serial determinations of serum levels of tumor markers such as human chorionic gonadotropin (hCG), α-fetoprotein (AFP), and carcinoembryonic antigen (CEA) can be useful for the diagnosis and follow-up of these occult neoplasms (68,86,89).

Recently, Oosterhuis and associates (90) demonstrated differences in ploidy between mediastinal and gonadal malignant germ cell tumors in adult patients and suggested that this method may help to differentiate primary lesions in the mediastinum from metastasis to the area. In their experience, 6 of 19 primary mediastinal malignant germ cell tumors studies were near diploid. The remaining tumors had a median DNA index of 1.91 (near tetraploid). There were no significant differences between seminomas and nonseminomatous tumors. Testicular seminomas in adult patients are seldom diploid and are usually hypertriploid. Nonseminomatous germ cell tumors in adult patients are usually hypotriploid (90). Germ cell tumors in children have been reported to have ploidy patterns that are similar to those of mediastinal lesions (90).

Mediastinal Germ Cell Tumors and Congenital Syndromes

Patients with Klinefelter's syndrome, a congenital syndrome characterized by testicular atrophy, elevated gonadotropin levels, and at least one extra X chromosome (47,XXY) have a markedly increased incidence (7.7%) of teratomas and other non-seminomatous mediastinal germ cell tumors (91–93). Indeed, Lachman and associates (91) have calculated that the incidence rate of Klinefelter's syndrome among patients with mediastinal germ cell tumors is 30 to 40 times the incidence of the syndrome in the general population.

Mediastinal germ cell tumors have also been reported in patients with trisomy 8, isochromosome of chromosome 12, and other chromosomal abnormalities (94–96). Testicular seminomas also have been described in patients with Marfan's and Down's syndromes (80).

TERATOMAS

Teratomas are neoplasms composed of several tissue components that recapitulate abnormally the development of two or three of the embryonic layers (ectoderm, endoderm, and mesoderm). They account for most instances of mediastinal germ cell tumors (91,97–117).

The tissue components of teratomas can be histologically mature, immature, and/or malignant (Table 1).

Clinical Features

Mature teratomas represent up to 75% of all mediastinal germ cell tumors. They can occur in patients of all ages but are more frequent in young adults (104).

Mediastinal teratomas have been described as congenital intrauterine tumors resulting in nonimmune hydrops fetalis in newborns (93–95).

Mature teratomas exhibit no sex predilection and are frequently detected on routine chest roentgenograms or present with symptoms related to compression of mediastinal structures by a large tumor mass, such as cough, dyspnea, or chest pain (97,98). On rare occasions patients present with cough and sputum containing hair and oily material because of erosion of the trachea or a bronchus by the neoplasm and evacuation of the cyst contents through the respiratory tree. Life-threatening hemoptysis or recurrent pericarditis have also been described (106,107).

Immature teratomas account for fewer than 1% of mediastinal teratomas and are more frequent in children and adolescents (118). They have seldom been encountered in adult patients, in whom they have a more aggressive biologic behavior.

Patients are usually symptomatic at diagnosis and present with weight loss, fatigue, cough, dyspnea, and chest pain (100,118).

Malignant teratomas (teratocarcinomas) occur almost exclusively in male patients (76,77,104). They are usually symptomatic at the time of diagnosis as a result of compression of mediastinal structures by the aggressive and rapidly growing tumors.

Roentgenologic Features

Teratomas appear on chest roentgenograms as large, round, lobulated anterior mediastinal masses that displace adjacent structures such as the trachea, carina, great vessels, lungs, and others (64,65). They are often cystic and exhibit areas of calcification of their cyst walls. Occasionally, teratomas are found within the pericardial cavity and the posterior mediastinum (108,113).

Immature and malignant teratomas are also large and frequently involve adjacent mediastinal structures. Patients present with pleural or pericardial effusions and/or exhibit evidence of venous and/or arterial compression (118,119).

Pathologic Features

Mature teratomas are cystic in most instances (dermoid cysts of the mediastinum) but can be predominantly solid (Fig. 7-12). They are ovoid or globular, well encapsulated, with a gray, smooth surface. The capsule is frequently partially calcified. On section, mature teratomas have a unilocular or multilocular cavity filled with hair and white, yellow, or brown oily, sebaceous, or gelatinous material. Focal solid areas may be present in the cyst wall. Mature teratomas do not invade adjacent mediastinal structures but can be adherent to the pleura, pericardium, or phrenic nerves.

Histologically, mature teratomas exhibit a cyst lined by mature stratified squamous epithelium and containing various other tissues in its wall such as intestinal or bronchial epithelia, bone, cartilage, pancreatic islets, nervous tissue, apocrine glands, thyroid, and other components derived from two or three embryonal germinal layers (Figs. 7-13 to 7-15).

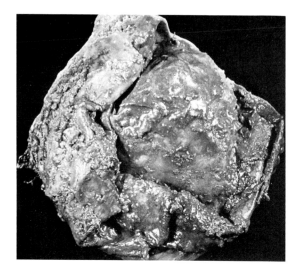

FIG. 7–12. Cystic teratoma (dermoid cyst of the mediastinum).

In addition, mediastinal teratomas frequently have well-differentiated pancreatic tissue with islets of Langerhans and exocrine elements (115). These tissues are functional, and patients with mature teratomas with pancreatic tissue elements can present with mild hypoglycemia and elevated serum amylase levels (115,116).

Occasionally, thymic tissue is found within the dermoid cyst wall. The cyst wall

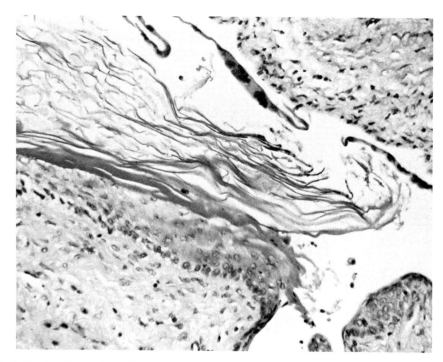

FIG. 7–13. Cystic teratoma lined by keratinizing mature squamous epithelium. (H&E × 100, original)

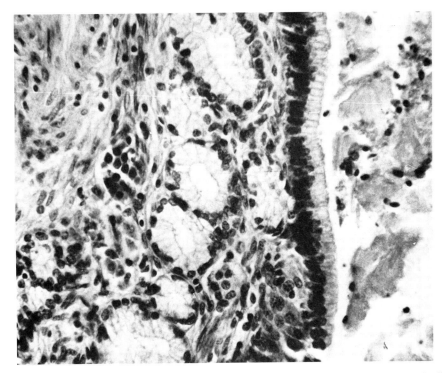

FIG. 7–14. Cystic teratoma containing mature mucinous glands. (H&E × 100, original)

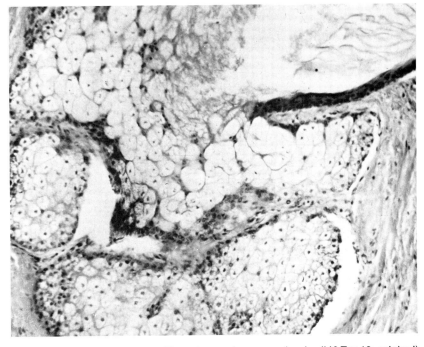

FIG. 7–15. Cystic teratoma with mature sebaceous glands. (H&E × 40, original)

of mature teratomas can also have areas of rupture. They appear histologically as areas of foreign body reaction to hair and lipid material and are usually accompanied by substantial fibrosis.

Immature teratomas are malignant neoplasms characterized by the presence of various tissues that resemble histologically several embryonal structures. They are large, predominantly solid, lobulated anterior mediastinal neoplasms that frequently invade or become adherent to adjacent structures (Fig. 7-16). They can weigh over 1,400 g and measure over 12 cm in diameter.

On section, immature teratomas have a variegated appearance with numerous small cysts interspersed with solid areas composed of bone, cartilage, soft yellow adipose tissue, and/or gray neural tissue. Areas of hemorrhage and necrosis are frequent. Histologically, they exhibit a wide variety of mature and immature tissues derived from all three germinal layers. Mature tissues include stratified squamous epithelium, apocrine glands, bone, cartilage, and others. Immature tissues include various types of embryonal epithelium of ectodermal or endodermal origin, immature cartilage, bone, skeletal muscle, and others (Figs. 7-17 to 7-22). The predominant component of immature teratomas is usually neural tissue, including glial elements as well as neuroepithelium forming tubules and rosettes (Figs. 7-23 to 7-25).

Thurlbeck and Scully (120) have proposed a classification of immature teratomas of the ovary into grades I to III according to the quantities of immature tissues, particularly of immature neuroepithelium, and to the degree of differentiation. This classification has prognostic value. Grade III tumors, for example, are almost invariably aggressive biologically and are associated with a poor prognosis (120,121).

Gonzalez-Crussi and associates (122) have utilized a similar prognostic system for the study of sacrococcygeal immature teratomas with a good correlation between histologic features and prognosis.

However, such a system has not been developed for the study of mediastinal immature teratomas. Indeed, in these tumors there is no clear correlation between histology and biologic behavior (118). Carter and associates (96), in a review of the literature and report of two patients with immature teratomas of the mediastinum, indicate that the best prognostic indicator of these lesions is the age of the patients. Well-encapsulated immature teratomas in children behave as biologically benign le-

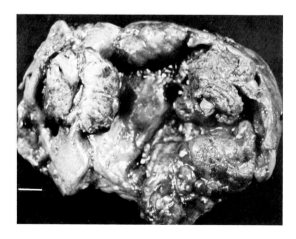

FIG. 7–16. Immature teratoma with solid and cystic areas exhibiting hemorrhage and necrosis. (Bar = 1 cm).

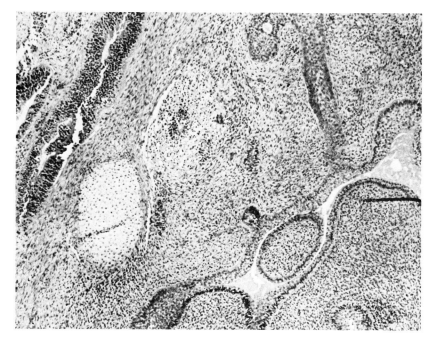

FIG. 7–17. Immature teratoma with epithelial-lined spaces, cartilage, mesenchyme, and neuroepithelium. Tissues resemble embryonal structures. (H&E × 40, original)

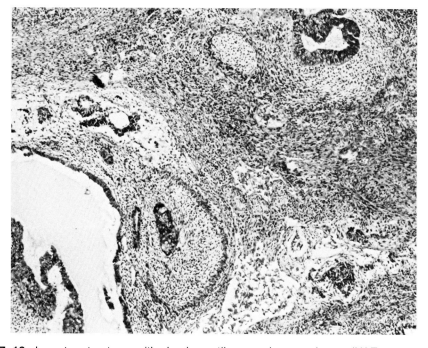

FIG. 7–18. Immature teratoma with glands, cartilage, and mesenchyme. (H&E × 40, original)

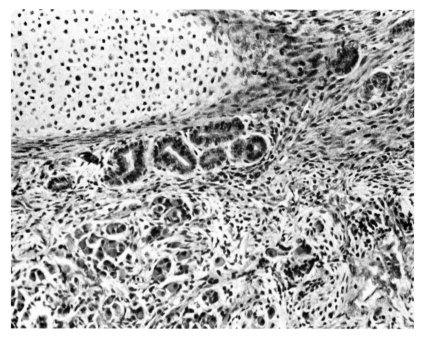

FIG. 7–19. Immature teratoma with mature cartilage and glands admixed with embryonal skeletal muscle. (H&E × 100, original)

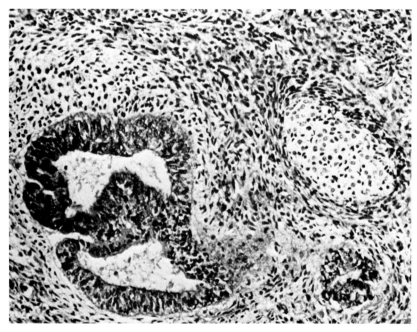

FIG. 7–20. Immature teratoma with embryonal glands, cartilage, and mesenchyme. (H&E × 100, original)

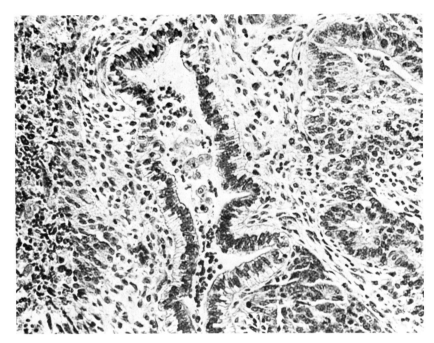

FIG. 7–21. Immature teratoma with glands and embryonal mesenchyme. (H&E × 100, original)

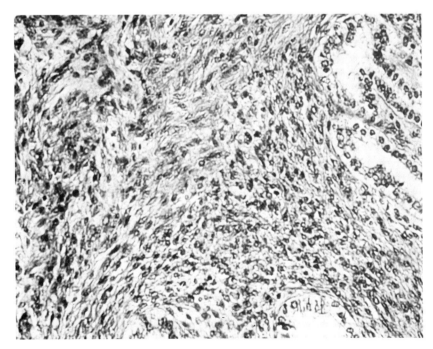

FIG. 7–22. Immature teratoma with cellular mesenchyme. (H&E × 100, original)

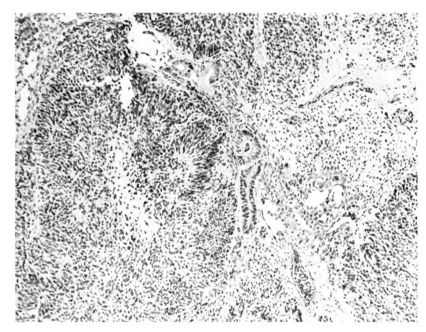

FIG. 7–23. Immature teratoma with abundant neuroectodermal tissue. (H&E × 40, original)

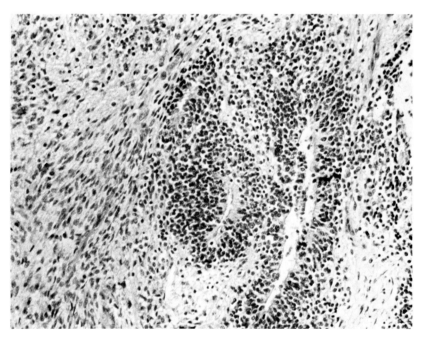

FIG. 7–24. Immature teratoma with neuroectodermal tissue forming tubules. (H&E × 100, original)

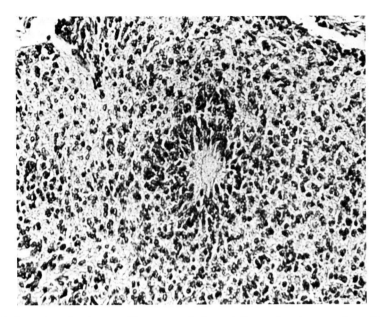

FIG. 7–25. Immature teratoma with neuroectodermal tissue forming rosettes. (H&E × 100, original)

sions, whereas lesions with similar morphology in adolescents or adults are highly malignant.

Irie and associates (86) detected with immunocytochemical methods and radioimmunoassay the presence of AFP, CEA, and hCG in an immature teratoma of the mediastinum. These markers were present in the immature glandular tissues of the teratoma and in the patient's serum. The elevated serum levels of AFP and hCG in this patient declined after treatment of the lesion with chemotherapy.

Further hormonal studies of immature teratomas of the mediastinum are needed to determine the prognostic value of these markers for the diagnosis and follow-up of these lesions.

Teratocarcinomas are malignant germ cell tumors in which a seminoma, embryonal carcinoma, choriocarcinoma, or endodermal sinus tumor develops from a mature or immature teratoma (76). The pathologic features of these neoplasms vary according to the malignant tumor component present in each instance.

Malignant transformation of mature cystic teratomas with development of squamous cell carcinoma or undifferentiated carcinoma has also been described in the mediastinum (1).

Treatment and Prognosis

Mature teratomas are benign tumors that do not infiltrate adjacent organs or metastasize. They may, however, result in life-threatening complications by virtue of reaching a large size and compressing vital mediastinal structures. They are treated surgically with good results, and there are only a few reports of patients dying of postoperative complications (76). The completely excised lesions do not recur.

Immature teratomas are malignant neoplasms with the capacity to infiltrate local structures and metastasize widely in adult patients (118). However, these tumors behave in a manner similar to mature teratomas when they occur in infants and children younger than 15 years old (118). All immature teratomas of the mediastinum in these young patients that are well encapsulated, noninfiltrative tumors at the time of initial diagnosis can be cured by complete surgical excision (111).

Immature teratomas behave as highly malignant neoplasms in patients 15 years of age or older because they are detected at a late stage of their disease or are more aggressive biologically in these individuals (75).

Teratocarcinomas of the mediastinum are also highly malignant neoplasms (76). They are usually large and infiltrative and/or metastatic at the time of initial diagnosis and not infrequently can only be biopsied initially or treated with limited surgical excision for reduction of the tumor mass. Patients usually receive postoperative radiotherapy and chemotherapy with poor results. For example, three of four patients with malignant teratomas reported by Bergh and associates (76) died with tumor 9 months after the initial diagnosis in spite of extensive surgery and radiotherapy. A patient with teratocarcinoma reported by Irie and associates (86) died within 3 months of hospitalization in spite of surgery, radiotherapy, and adjuvant chemotherapy with VAC (vincristine, actinomycin, and cyclophosphamide).

Wirtanen and associates (110) recently reported a patient who survived a malignant teratoma of the anterior mediastinum for 23 years after surgical resection and adjuvant therapy with intraarterial iododeoxyuridine and radiotherapy.

SEMINOMA

Mediastinal seminomas (germinomas) are germ cell tumors composed of large uniform cells that resemble germinal cells (123). They represent 25% to 30% of all malignant mediastinal germ cell tumors (124–133). Mediastinal seminomas are unusual neoplasms (134–139).

Clinical Features

Mediastinal seminomas occur most frequently in male patients in their third and fourth decades of life. Only a few have been described in women (124,129).

Patients are asymptomatic at the time of initial diagnosis and are found to have large mediastinal masses on routine chest roentgenograms or present with various symptoms including chest or shoulder pain, weight loss, fatigue, fever, dyspnea, cervical or supraclavicular lymphadenopathy, dysphagia, or manifestations of superior vena cava obstruction. The latter is the presenting feature in approximately 10% of patients with mediastinal seminoma (129).

Takahashi and associates (139) reported a patient with primary mediastinal seminoma with high serum levels of alkaline phosphatase (ALP) and angiotensin converting enzyme (ACE). These serum markers returned to normal values after therapy.

The tumors are considered primary mediastinal neoplasms in patients with no palpable testicular abnormalities and no roentgenologic evidence of a retroperitoneal neoplasm. Most authors agree with the concept that orchiectomy or testicular biopsy is not necessary in patients with mediastinal seminoma and no palpable testicular abnormality (124,131).

Radiologic Features

Mediastinal seminomas appear on chest roentgenograms as large, globular, non-calcified anterior mediastinal tumors (Fig. 7-26). A few instances have been reported in the posterior mediastinum (128).

Patients also have, in many instances, evidence of hilar lymphadenopathy or pleural, diaphragmatic, or pulmonary involvement. Venograms can demonstrate superior vena cava compression or invasion by the tumor. Lymphangiograms, CT scans, MRI, and sonograms of the abdomen demonstrate the presence or absence of tumor in the retroperitoneum.

Pathologic Features

Mediastinal seminomas are well circumscribed, soft, gray–white, and large, and they usually infiltrate into adjacent structures (Fig. 7-27). Their cut surface is usually homogeneous, glistening, and lobulated. Areas of hemorrhage and necrosis are not prominent except in very large lesions.

Histologically, they are composed of large polyhedral or round tumor cells with distinct cell borders and clear or granular cytoplasm that contains variable amounts of glycogen. The nucleus of these tumor cells is centrally located, round, and hyperchromatic with one or two prominent nucleoli. Mitotic figures are infrequent. The tumor cells exhibit minimal pleomorphism and are arranged in sheets or lobules supported by a delicate connective tissue stroma that usually contains a significant number of lymphocytes (Fig. 7-28). The tumor cells exhibit immunoreactivity with antibodies to ALP and are negative with AFP. Bailey and associates (135) reported the use of an antiseminoma monoclonal antibody to confirm the diagnosis of a mediastinal seminoma in an FNA specimen. The lymphoid infiltrates are thought to repre-

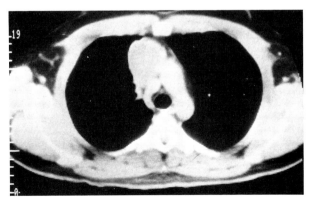

FIG. 7–26. Seminoma of the anterior mediastinum presenting as a large, round, well-circumscribed mass.

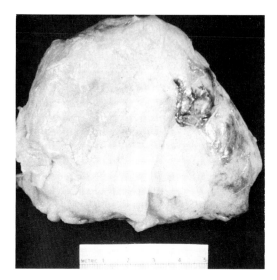

FIG. 7–27. Thymic seminoma.

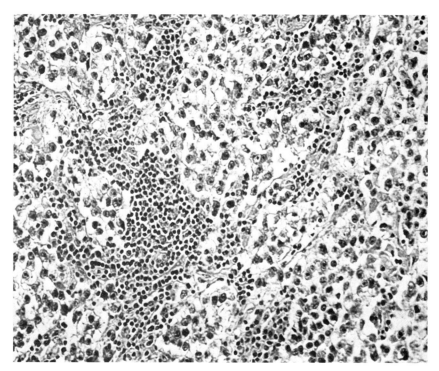

FIG. 7–28. Thymic seminoma with nests of uniform, large cells with open nuclei, prominent nucleoli, and clear cytoplasm. Stroma has abundant lymphoid infiltrates. (H&E × 100, original)

sent an immunologic reaction to the tumor cells and may become so prominent as to obscure the neoplastic cells. Occasionally, the stroma also exhibits a prominent granulomatous reaction.

Seminomas can also contain isolated, large, multinucleated tumor cells that closely resemble syncytiotrophoblasts (Fig. 7-29). These cells have an eosinophilic cytoplasm containing hCG that can be demonstrated in tissue sections utilizing immunocytochemical techniques. Large tumors also have focal or large areas of coagulative-type necrosis.

Special types of seminomas described in the testis, such as the spermatocytic or anaplastic variants, have not been described, to our knowledge, in the mediastinum (140).

Treatment and Prognosis

Mediastinal seminomas are malignant tumors that frequently metastasize within the thorax to the lungs and regional lymph nodes (124,129). They can also metastasize to the skeletal system, liver, spleen, adrenal system, central nervous system, and other sites.

Patients are treated with total surgical excision followed by radiation therapy to the mediastinum, supraclavicular, infraclavicular, and low cervical lymph nodes utilizing 3,000 to 5,000 rads (124). However, not infrequently, the mediastinal tumor is very large and difficult to resect, and radiotherapy becomes the primary therapeutic modality. Fortunately, seminomas are very radiosensitive (125).

Patients with metastatic disease are treated with radiotherapy and adjuvant che-

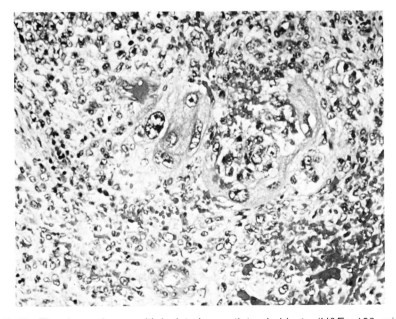

FIG. 7–29. Thymic seminoma with isolated syncytiotrophoblasts. (H&E × 100, original)

motherapy (128). Overall 5-year survival rates for patients with mediastinal semi-nomas are approximately 75% but vary from 40% to 100% (64,67,69,70). Mediastinal seminomas can recur as late as 19 years following initially successful therapy (137).

Hurt and associates (128), in a review of their experience at the Mayo Clinic with mediastinal seminomas, suggest that the following factors appear to be associated with a less favorable prognosis: age of the patient (older than 35 years old), lymph-adenopathy (hilar enlargement on chest roentgenograms, supraclavicular or cervical adenopathy), fever, and superior vena cava syndrome at the time of initial diagnosis (128).

In a recent study from a multiinstitutional study group, Kersch and associates (73) reported 100% actuarial 5-year survival in patients with mediastinal seminoma.

EMBRYONAL CARCINOMA

Embryonal carcinomas are highly malignant neoplasms (140). They are unusual in the mediastinum, where they can occur as pure embryonal carcinoma or in associ-ation with teratomas or other germ cell neoplasms (131,141–143).

The clinical features of embryonal carcinomas are similar to those described in patients with mediastinal seminomas (Fig. 7-30). Patients have, in addition, elevated serum levels of AFP and may have the clinical and chromosomal abnormalities of Klinefelter's syndrome (144,145).

Pathologic Features

Embryonal carcinomas are large, nonencapsulated neoplasms that frequently in-filtrate adjacent mediastinal structures (Fig. 7-31). Their cut surfaces have a varie-gated appearance with extensive areas of hemorrhage and necrosis (Fig. 7-32). His-tologically, they are composed of solid sheets, acini, anastomosing ducts and glands, tubules, or papillary structures composed of very large tumor cells with indistinct cell borders, amphophilic or vacuolated cytoplasm, and irregular round or oval nu-clei with prominent nucleoli (Figs. 7-33 and 7-34). The tumor cells exhibit marked

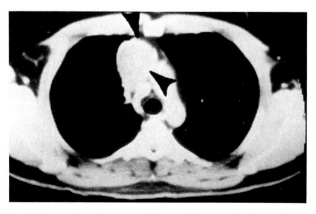

FIG. 7–30. Embryonal carcinoma of the anterior mediastinum (*arrowheads*).

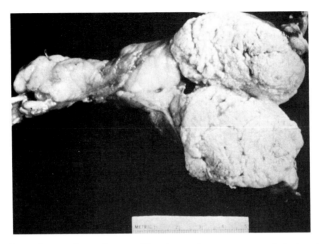

FIG. 7–31. Thymic embryonal carcinoma. The tumor is nonencapsulated, soft, gray–tan with areas of necrosis. Note presence of normal thymus.

pleomorphism and contain intracytoplasmic AFP that can be demonstrated in tissue sections with immunocytochemical techniques (Figs. 7-35 and 7-36).

In addition, embryonal carcinomas frequently have scattered multinucleated syncytiotrophoblastic tumor cells that contain intracytoplasmic hCG (Fig. 7-37).

The demonstration of AFP and hCG in histologic sections of embryonal cell car-

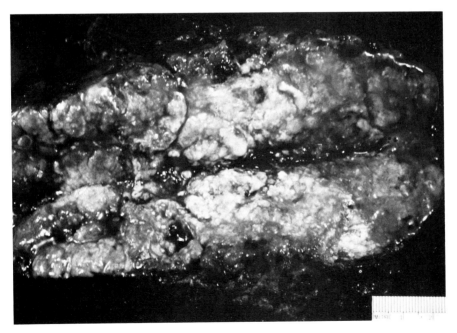

FIG. 7–32. Large embryonal carcinoma of the thymus with a variegated surface exhibiting extensive necrosis and hemorrhage.

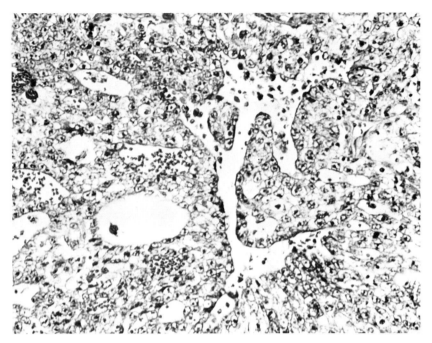

FIG. 7–33. Embryonal carcinoma of the thymus composed of broad sheets, papilla, and rudimentary glands formed by large cells with clear cytoplasm. (H&E × 100, original)

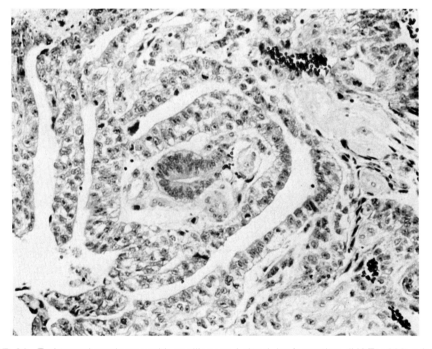

FIG. 7–34. Embryonal carcinoma with papillary and glandular formation. (H&E × 200, original)

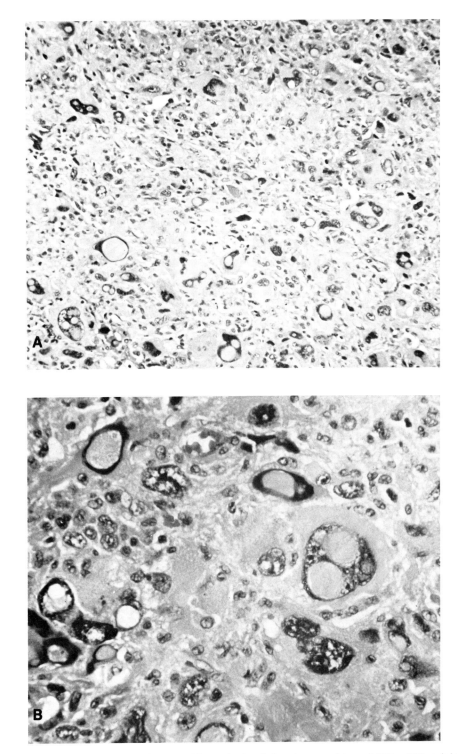

FIG. 7–35. A: Embryonal carcinoma with marked cellular pleomorphism. (H&E × 100, original)
B: Higher magnification of anaplastic cells. (× 400, original)

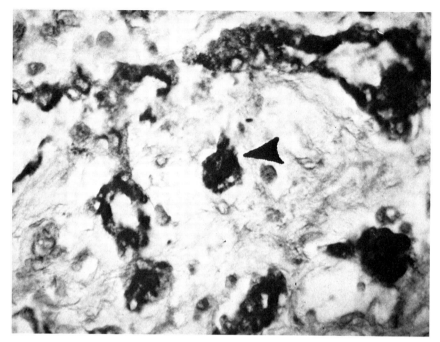

FIG. 7–36. Tumor cell of embryonal carcinoma with intracytoplasmic AFP immunoreactivity (*arrowhead*). (PAP method ×400, original)

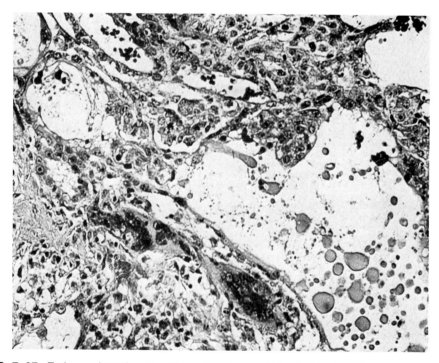

FIG. 7–37. Embryonal carcinoma with scattered syncytiotrophoblasts. (H&E × 100, original)

cinomas is useful for their diagnosis, as these markers are absent in other carcinomas that can be confused histologically with these tumors.

Embryonal carcinomas exhibit abundant mitotic figures and extensive areas of necrosis. The latter have to be sampled for histologic study to rule out the presence of an associated choriocarcinoma.

Treatment and Prognosis

Embryonal carcinomas of the mediastinum frequently infiltrate mediastinal structures and metastasize to the lungs, skeletal system, and other organs (144,145). Patients undergo resection of their lesions, but not infrequently the tumors cannot be resected completely and are treated with adjuvant chemotherapy. They are also radioresistant.

In a study by Burt and Javadpour (131) at the National Cancer Institute, the complete response rate of patients with nonseminomatous germ cell tumors in extragonadal locations was 36.4% compared to 55% for patients with testicular nonseminomatous germ cell tumors metastatic to the lung; the median survival of the patients with extragonadal neoplasms was only 10.5 months.

More recent studies of primary mediastinal nonseminomatous germ cell tumors utilizing intense cisplatin-based chemotherapy with adjunctive surgical debulking, when needed, report improved results, with a median survival of 64 months and a 50% to 57% 5-year survival rate (72,74).

Serial studies of serum levels of AFP and hCG are useful to monitor the response to therapy of patients with mediastinal embryonal carcinoma. These markers remain elevated in patients who have undergone incomplete response of their primary tumors and become elevated after recurrence of the neoplasms.

ENDODERMAL SINUS TUMOR

Endodermal sinus tumor (yolk-sac tumor) is a highly malignant germ cell neoplasm described in the gonads and extragonadal locations (146–156). It was first recognized as a distinct entity by Teilum (61) in 1959, who suggested that the tumor had morphologic features that reproduced the extraembryonic structures of the embryo such as the yolk-sac endoderm and the extraembryonic mesoblast.

Clinical Features

Approximately 76 patients with endodermal sinus tumors in the mediastinum have been reported (146–156). The tumor occurs mostly in male patients; only recently it has been described in a female (156). Most patients are in their third and fourth decades of life (mean age 27.4 years) (146–156).

Patients are usually symptomatic at initial diagnosis and present with dyspnea, cough, chest pain, pleural effusions, and a large mediastinal mass. Serum levels of AFP are markedly elevated, a useful finding to confirm the diagnosis of germ cell tumor and to support the hypothesis of yolk-sac differentiation.

Pathologic Features

Endodermal sinus tumors are unencapsulated, large, solid, soft, gray–yellow, and have prominent areas of cystic degeneration, hemorrhage, and/or necrosis.

Histologically, they exhibit a very characteristic reticular pattern with multiple communicating spaces lined by flattened tumor cells in papillary, tubular, and solid growth patterns (Fig. 7-38). Simple papillary structures containing a single central blood vessel and lined by columnar cells (Schiller–Duval bodies) project into the lumina and these spaces (Fig. 7-39). The tumors also have characteristic multiple intracellular and extracellular eosinophilic PAS-positive hyaline globules containing α_1-antitrypsin and AFP. Both tumor markers can be demonstrated in tissue sections by immunocytochemical techniques.

The tumors can also exhibit keratin and CEA immunoreactivity (154). Ultrastructurally, endodermal sinus tumors exhibit intracellular and extracellular basement membrane-like material, large multivesicular bodies, desmosomes, and microvilli (154).

Treatment and Prognosis

Endodermal sinus tumors of the mediastinum are highly malignant neoplasms that are usually unresectable at initial diagnosis and frequently metastasize to the lungs, brain, liver, and bones (150–156).

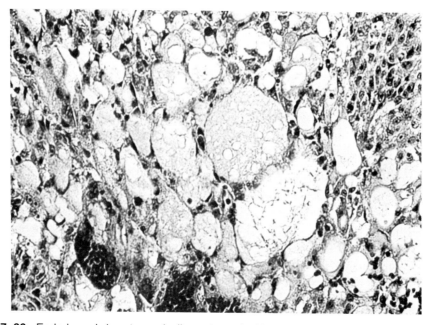

FIG. 7–38. Endodermal sinus tumor (yolk-sac tumor) with multiple intercommunicating spaces in a reticular pattern. (H&E × 100, original)

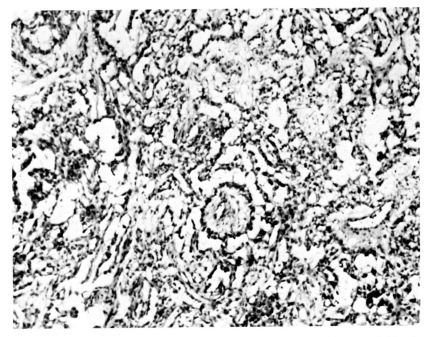

FIG. 7–39. Endodermal sinus tumor with Schiller–Duval body with central blood vessel. (H&E × 40, original)

Most patients reported have died with metastatic tumor within months of the initial diagnosis. However, recent studies have reported improved results in patients receiving cisplatin-based intensive chemotherapy with or without surgery and radiotherapy (72,74). In a recent report by Sham and associates (153) three patients survived between 17 and 40 months following diagnosis. According to Truong and associates (154), the most important prognostic indicator in patients with mediastinal endodermal sinus tumors is whether the neoplasm can be completely excised before or after chemotherapy.

CHORIOCARCINOMA

Rare instances of primary choriocarcinoma of the mediastinum have been reported in male and female patients in their third decade of life (157–162). Male patients frequently have gynecomastia and elevated hCG serum levels that result in positive pregnancy tests (158).

Choriocarcinoma is one of the germ cell tumors in which an extragonadal origin is most difficult to prove because it is well known that they can metastasize widely from small occult testicular or ovarian primaries, which measure only a few millimeters in size. However, the distinction between a choriocarcinoma primary in the gonads or in the mediastinum has little clinical value, as in both instances the neoplasms are treated with similar therapeutic protocols with identical prognosis.

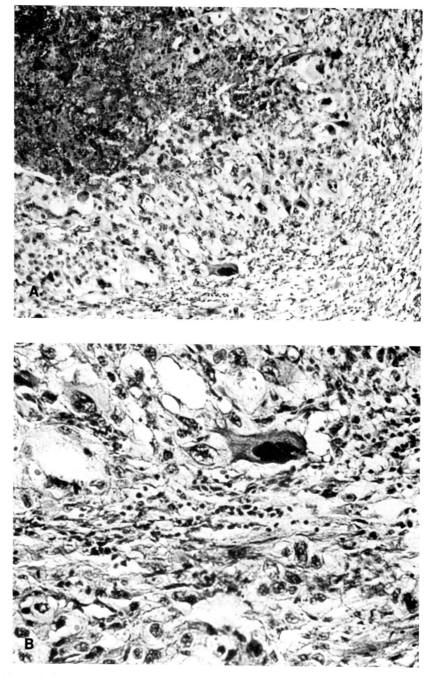

FIG. 7–40. A: Choriocarcinoma with sheets of mononuclear cytotrophoblastic cells, scattered syncytiotrophoblasts, and extensive hemorrhage. (H&E × 100, original) **B:** Higher magnification of syncytiotrophoblast and surrounding cytotrophoblastic cells. (H&E × 400, original)

Pathologic Features

Choriocarcinomas are solid, soft, hemorrhagic, friable, nonencapsulated neoplasms that are frequently combined with other germ cell tumors such as teratomas or embryonal carcinomas.

Histologically, they are composed of solid sheets of large, round cytotrophoblastic cells with clear cytoplasm admixed with multinucleated syncytiotrophoblasts (Fig. 7-40). The tumor cells do not form placental villi and are often arranged in a characteristic plexiform pattern with occasional acinar formation. Immunocytochemical techniques are useful for the demonstration of hCG in multinucleated giant cells, an important diagnostic finding.

Treatment and Prognosis

Choriocarcinomas are highly malignant neoplasms that metastasize rapidly to the lungs, brain, bone, and other organs. Patients are treated with chemotherapy (160–162).

DIFFERENTIAL DIAGNOSIS OF GERM CELL TUMORS OF THE MEDIASTINUM

Germ cell tumors of the mediastinum, in particular embryonal carcinomas, are not infrequently misdiagnosed as metastatic poorly differentiated carcinomas or as adenocarcinomas.

The diagnosis of germ cell tumor should be considered in neoplasms composed of very large pleomorphic cells with prominent nucleoli arranged in the various patterns described. In questionable cases, the histologic sections should be studied with immunocytochemical techniques for the detection of placental alkaline phosphatase, α_1-antitrypsin, AFP, and hCG. The presence of these markers in tumor cells is useful for confirming the diagnosis and for the histologic classification of the neoplasm.

The demonstration of a mediastinal origin of the tumor, however, remains largely the responsibility of our clinical colleagues, as there are no reliable pathologic features that will distinguish a gonadal from an extragonadal germ cell tumor.

As discussed earlier in the chapter, flow cytometry may offer useful information to answer this problem, as mediastinal germ cell tumors are frequently diploid, which is an unusual finding in their testicular counterparts.

The Development of Non–Germ Cell Malignancies within Germ Cell Tumors

Carcinomatous and sarcomatous components have been described within germ cell tumors in the mediastinum and other locations following chemotherapy and/or radiotherapy (142,163). They include adenocarcinoma, adenosquamous carcinoma, rhabdomyosarcoma, angiosarcoma, leiomyosarcoma, cystosarcoma phylloides, and other non–germ cell malignancies. These tumors are thought to arise as a malignant component of a teratoma or from totipotential cells that can differentiate along germ cell and non–germ cell lines (142). The tumors probably do not develop as a result of radiotherapy and chemotherapy, as second malignancies usually arise at an average interval of 13 years following therapy (163). It has been suggested that the treatment with chemotherapy and/or radiotherapy selects tumor elements by eliminating the sensitive germ cell neoplastic components and allowing the proliferation of the more resistant sarcomatous or carcinomatous cell lines (142,163).

Association Between Mediastinal Germ Cell Tumors and Hematologic Malignancies

Myers and associates (164), DeMent and associates (165,166), and Nichols and associates (167) have described the unusual association between germ cell tumors and various hematologic malignancies including erythroleukemia, malignant histiocytosis, subacute myelogenous leukemia, chronic granulocytic leukemia, acute myelomonocytic leukemia, acute undifferentiated leukemia, and acute monocytic leukemia. In most patients the tumors were malignant teratomas, but a few instances of embryonal carcinoma and combined germ cell tumors have also been reported (166). The association between these two dissimilar groups of neoplasms is of particular interest because of the common site of origin of primordial germ cells and hematologic stem cells in the yolk sac during embryogenesis (166). Indeed, Pierce and associates (143) have documented in an experimental model that embryonal carcinoma cells are totipotential and can differentiate into hematopoietic and other cell lines. The regulatory gene control of germ cell growth and differentiation are under current study (143).

LYMPHOMAS OF THE THYMUS

Malignant lymphomas are the most frequent malignant tumors of the anterior mediastinum, where they can involve the regional lymph nodes and/or the thymus (168–171). Indeed, the mediastinum is a frequent site of involvement by malignant lymphoma, as is discussed in detail in Chapter 9 (1).

In a large series of mediastinal malignant lymphomas, 50% to 60% of the patients have Hodgkin's disease (168). The other 40% to 50% have any one of the histologic variants of non-Hodgkin's lymphomas.

About half of the patients with mediastinal Hodgkin's disease have thymic involvement (172). In few individuals, however, does the malignant lymphoma present as a primary thymic neoplasm that exhibits the interesting pathologic features discussed in detail in this chapter.

HODGKIN'S DISEASE OF THE THYMUS (SO-CALLED GRANULOMATOUS THYMOMA)

Hodgkin's disease of the thymus has been a subject of interest and indeed controversy in the pathology literature for many years (173–185).

It was first described as a distinct entity in 1916 by Ewing (186), who considered the lesion as a thymoma of granulomatous type. In his view, the lesion originated from reticulum epithelial cells of the thymus, a concept supported by the presence of collections of epithelial cells and glandular structures within the lesion. This view was supported by other pathologists (173–185).

Thus, for many years, "granulomatous thymoma" was considered as an entity distinct from Hodgkin's disease, although it exhibited all the morphologic features characteristic of the malignant lymphoma.

In 1955, Castleman (188) recognized the error and correctly classified instances of so-called granulomatous thymoma as examples of Hodgkin's disease of the thymus. This is the currently accepted view (1,187,188).

Perhaps influenced by Castleman's concept, Thompson (189) suggested in 1955 that all instances of Hodgkin's disease originate from the thymus. This view has been discarded, however, as autopsy studies have shown that only 26% of patients with Hodgkin's disease have thymic involvement (177).

Clinical Features

Hodgkin's disease of the thymus is more frequent in young, female patients (174). They can be asymptomatic at the time a large mediastinal mass is discovered or present with cough, dyspnea, chest pain, fever, fatigue, anorexia, weight loss, pruritus, anemia, and hoarseness. A few patients present with the superior vena cava syndrome (174). Patients with Hodgkin's disease of the thymus seldom have splenomegaly or peripheral lymphadenopathy at the time of initial diagnosis (174).

Systemic conditions are unusually associated with Hodgkin's disease of the thymus. They include erythroid hypoplasia and myasthenia gravis (1,190). Null and associates (180) reported an interesting patient in whom the symptoms of myasthenia gravis subsided after surgical removal of the thymic lymphoma. Whether the disease was indeed related to the neoplasm or to areas of thymic hyperplasia adjacent to the lymphoma or to both is not known. The authors postulated that the neoplastic T cells of the lymphoma could have elaborated thymopoietin, a thymic hormone that produces neuromuscular block. No measurements of the hormone in serum were available in their patient to prove the hypothesis.

Peck (191) reported a patient with hypertrophic osteoarthropathy and mediastinal Hodgkin's disease.

Radiologic Findings

Hodgkin's disease of the thymus appears as solid, lobulated, noncalcified anterior mediastinal tumors (Fig. 7-41) (174,175). Occasionally, they appear as cystic lesions or as partially cavitated masses (184,185,192).

Cystic degeneration of thymic Hodgkin's disease can follow radiotherapy (185).

Pathologic Features

Hodgkin's disease of the thymus presents as large, partially encapsulated, firm, lobulated neoplasms that are encountered in the thymic region at the time of surgery and not infrequently exhibit the presence of thymic horns attached to the tumor. An important gross observation for establishing the origin of the lesion (Fig. 7-42). The neoplasms can reach a large size and weigh over 1,800 g. They frequently infiltrate into adjacent soft tissues and may extend locally into the lung, mediastinal nerves, and/or blood vessels. Lymph nodes adjacent to the thymus can also be involved by the malignant lymphoma.

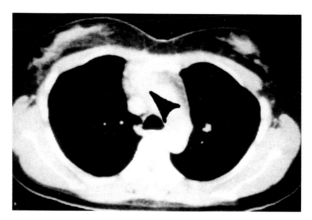

FIG. 7–41. Hodgkin's disease of the thymus presenting as an ill-defined anterior mediastinal mass (*arrowhead*).

On section, the lesions are gray, firm, and nodular with focal areas of necrosis and/or cystic degeneration. The nodules are usually round and pink–gray and are separated by broad white sclerotic fibrous bands that may vary in size and are usually smaller and more irregular than those encountered in thymomas. By contrast, thymomas have larger nodules with angulated borders and of regular size, separated by thin gray septa.

In rare instances, Hodgkin's disease of the thymus becomes predominantly cystic.

Histologically, the lesions exhibit findings characteristic of nodular sclerosis Hodgkin's disease. Other histologic variants of Hodgkin's disease have not been described in the thymus (174). The tumors are composed of nodules of polymorphic infiltrates containing lymphocytes, histiocytes, eosinophils, plasma cells, large malignant mononuclear cells, multinucleated giant cells with prominent nucleoli, and occasional Reed–Sternberg cells (Figs. 7-43 to 7-45). The latter establish the diagnosis of Hodgkin's disease.

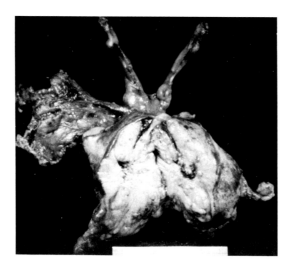

FIG. 7–42. Hodgkin's disease of the thymus. The neoplasm is firm, nodular, poorly circumscribed, and extends into adjacent tissues.

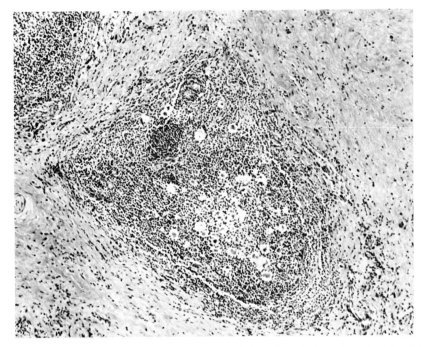

FIG. 7–43. Hodgkin's disease of the thymus, nodular sclerosis type. (H&E × 40, original)

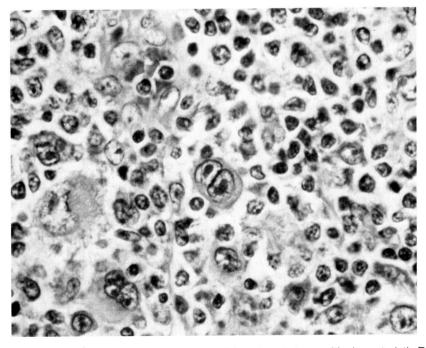

FIG. 7–44. Hodgkin's disease of the thymus, nodular sclerosis type, with characteristic Reed–Sternberg cell. (H&E × 400, original)

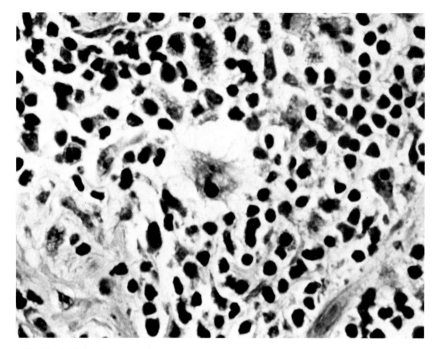

FIG. 7–45. Hodgkin's disease of the thymus, nodular sclerosis type, with characteristic "lacunar" cell. (H&E × 400, original)

In addition, the lesions exhibit at their periphery remnants of thymic tissue that establish the thymic involvement by the tumor.

Hodgkin's disease of the thymus also exhibits histological features that are unique to the neoplasm in this location. There are areas in which the lymphoma is closely admixed with sheets of squamous epithelial cells, Hassall's corpuscles, glands lined by ciliated epithelium, and cystic spaces lined by simple or squamous epithelium (Fig. 7-46). These epithelial elements are usually in close contact with the neoplastic lymphoid cells and can suggest an epithelial origin of the tumor cells (so-called granulomatous thymoma). It has been shown, however, that the neoplastic cells of Hodgkin's disease of the thymus have ultrastructural features of monocytic cells and lack evidence of epithelial differentiation such as the presence of tonofilaments, desmosomes, and basement membrane formation (1).

It is now believed that the epithelial elements of Hodgkin's disease of the thymus represent thymic tissue that remained trapped during the development of the neoplasm and became hyperplastic (181). Whether these cells modulate the growth of the neoplasm through the secretion of thymopoietin or other thymic hormones that are known to be able to induce growth and differentiation of T lymphocytes is not known.

Treatment and Prognosis

The natural history of Hodgkin's disease of the thymus is similar to that of stage I nodular sclerosis Hodgkin's disease in other locations (193). Patients undergo re-

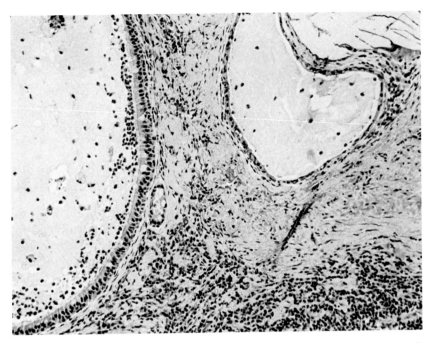

FIG. 7–46. Hodgkin's disease of the thymus with remnant of thymic tissue showing glandular elements. (H&E × 100, original)

section of their lesions combined with postoperative radiotherapy. Seventy-nine percent of patients survive 5 years (181). A few individuals develop recurrences or extrathoracic lesions; others die of complications of treatment.

Bergh and associates (174), in a report of 17 patients with Hodgkin's disease of the thymus, reported better results after aggressive treatment with resection of the tumor, adjacent lymph nodes, and surrounding tissues, radiotherapy, and chemotherapy. Only three of their patients died of complications of treatment. The others survived up to 10 years following therapy. Twenty-one percent of their patients developed local recurrences in the thorax that were controlled with radiotherapy and/or chemotherapy. The authors questioned the value of staging laparotomies in patients with Hodgkin's disease of the thymus, as these patients seldom if ever have involvement of extrathoracic sites by the lymphoma at the time of initial diagnosis.

Poor prognostic signs in patients with Hodgkin's disease of the thymus include the presence of superior vena cava syndrome and pulmonary involvement at the time of initial surgery (181). These patients are at a higher risk of developing recurrences of their disease.

OTHER LYMPHOMAS OF THE THYMUS

Other non-Hodgkin's lymphomas that develop in the anterior mediastinum are discussed in Chapter 9. Szporn and associates (170) reported an interesting patient with true histiocytic lymphoma of the thymus as confirmed by the presence of α_1 antitrypsin and lysozyme in the cytoplasm of the tumor cells. More recently, Isaacson and associates (171) reported two patients with low-grade B-cell lymphomas of mucosa-associated lymphoid tissue arising in the thymus. These tumors exhibited focal lymphoepithelial lesions as seen in myoepithelial sialadenitis.

EXPERIMENTAL MODELS OF THYMIC LYMPHOMAS

Thymic lymphomas have been induced in rats and mice by chemicals such as nitroso-2-hydroxypropylurea, retroviruses, and magnesium deficiency (194,195).

HISTIOCYTOSIS X OF THE THYMUS

A few patients with histiocytosis X (Langerhans' cell granulomatosis) involving the thymus have been described (196–199). Staining with S-100 protein is strongly positive in the tumor cells (198). One of the patients had associated myasthenia gravis (197). The patient reported by Suematsu and associates (199) had a large mediastinal mass with initial features of histiocytosis X in an early biopsy. Additional biopsies showed histopathologic features that were interpreted as consistent with a malignant lymphoma of probable T-cell origin. The thymic gland also is dysplastic and may play a role in patients with systemic histiocytosis X (200–202).

LOCALIZED FIBROUS TUMOR OF THE THYMIC AREA

Localized fibrous tumors (so-called fibrous mesothelioma) can occur in the mediastinum and present as a tumor that is attached to the thymic gland. It may be mistaken for a spindle cell thymoma (Fig. 7-47). The tumor is composed of oval or spindle cells forming interlacing bundles, solid sheets, myxoid areas, perivascular fascicles, and other patterns (Figs. 7-48 and 7-49). Epithelial cells, as seen in thymomas, are not present. The spindle cells exhibit vimentin immunoreactivity (Fig. 7-50), and stains for keratin are negative.

LYMPHANGIOMA OF THE THYMUS

Lymphangiomas arising in the thymus gland are unusual neoplasms (203,205). They can occur as isolated tumors or in patients with generalized lymphangiomatosis (204). They can also be associated with abdominal lymphangiomas (203).

The tumors usually reach a large size and are composed of multiple irregular interconnected vascular spaces lined by flattened endothelial cells. Lymphoid cells are frequently found in their stroma.

Patients are cured by surgical excision. The lesions may recur after incomplete excisions.

METASTATIC TUMORS TO THE THYMUS

The thymus can be involved by metastatic tumors at autopsy in patients with carcinomas of the breast, stomach, larynx, lung, and kidney (206). These findings sel-

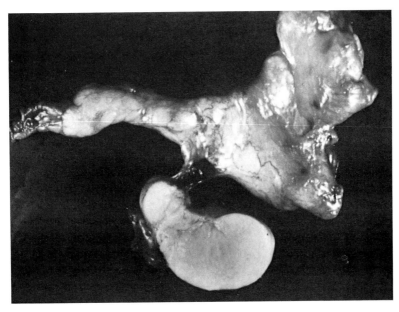

FIG. 7–47. Localized fibrous tumor of the mediastinum. The tumor is attached to the thymus gland.

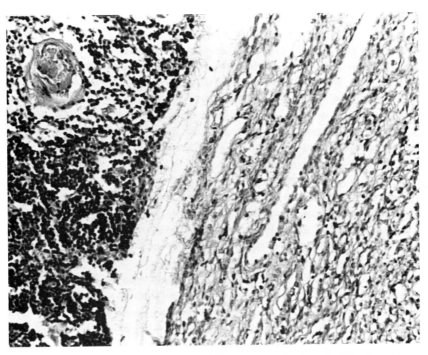

FIG. 7–48. Localized fibrous tumor (so-called fibrous mesothelioma) of the thymic area composed of oval cells in solid sheets. The lesion is attached to the thymus. (H&E × 200, original)

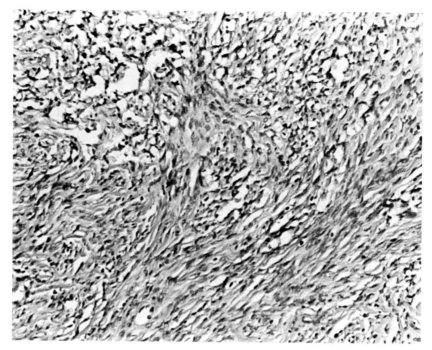

FIG. 7–49. Localized fibrous tumor of the thymic area. The lesion shown in Figs. 7-47 and 7-48 shows dense interlacing bundles of spindle cells. (H&E × 200, original)

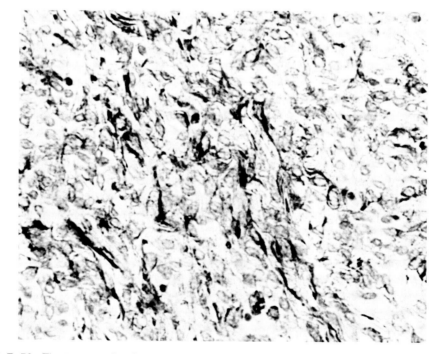

FIG. 7–50. The tumor cells of localized fibrous tumor of the thymic area exhibit vimentin immunoreactivity. (PAP stain × 400, original)

dom have clinical value, as the patients invariably have generalized disease when the thymic metastasis are found.

The thymus can also be involved secondarily by direct extension by mediastinal neoplasms extending into the gland from the lungs, lymph nodes, or adjacent structures (1,206).

REFERENCES

1. Rosai J, Levine GD: Tumors of the thymus, in: *Atlas of Tumor Pathology*, Fasc 13, ser 2. Washington, Armed Forces Institute of Pathology, 1976.
2. Rosai J, Higa E, Davie J: Mediastinal endocrine neoplasms in patients with multiple endocrine adenomatosis. A previously unrecognized association. *Cancer* 1972;29:1075–1083.
3. Fell SC, Sprayregen S, Becker NH: Bilateral carcinoid tumors of the mediastinum. *Ann Thorac Surg* 1966;2:429–434.
4. Lowenthal RM, Gumpel JM, Kreel L, et al: Carcinoid tumour of the thymus with systemic manifestations: a radiological and pathological study. *Thorax* 1974;29:553–558.
5. Judge DM, Changaris DG, Harvey HR, et al: Malignant APUDoma (carcinoid) of the anterior mediastinum: simplified methods of demonstrating biogenic amines in endocrine neoplasms. *Arch Pathol Lab Med* 1976;100:491–494.
6. Manes JL, Taylor HB: Thymic carcinoid in familial multiple endocrine adenomatosis. *Arch Pathol* 1973;95:252–255.
7. Rosai J, Higa E: Mediastinal endocrine neoplasm, of probable thymic origin, related to carcinoid tumor: clinicopathologic study of 8 cases. *Cancer* 1972;29:1061–1074.
8. Rosai J, Levine GD, Weber WR, et al: Carcinoid tumors and oat cell carcinomas of the thymus. *Pathol Annu* 1976;11:201–226.
9. Salyer WR, Salyer DC, Eggleston DC: Carcinoid tumors of the thymus. *Cancer* 1976;37:958–973.
10. Strasberg B, Weinberger I, Kessler E, et al: Thymic carcinoid tumor. *NY State J Med* 1979;79:1755–1757.
11. Levine GD, Rosai J: Thymic hyperplasia and neoplasia: a review of current concepts. *Hum Pathol* 1978;9:495–515.
12. Wick MR, Scott RE, Li CY, et al: Carcinoid tumor of the thymus. A clinicopathologic report of seven cases with a review of the literature. *Mayo Clin Proc* 1980;55:246–254.
13. Kasugai H, Kasai T, Endo Y, et al: A case report of ruptured thymic carcinoid. *Nippon Kyobu Geka Gakkai Zasshi* 1989;37:1602–1607.
14. Jose CC, Varghese CV, Singh AD: Thymic carcinoid in a case of Zollinger–Ellison syndrome. A case report. *Austral Radiol* 1988;32:408–409.
15. Wick MR, Rosai J: Neuroendocrine neoplasms of the thymus. *Pathol Res Pract* 1988;183:188–199.
16. Percopo V, Lorenzo M, Di Prisco B, et al: Thymic carcinoid. Description of 2 cases and review of the international literature. *Minerva Chir* 1988;43:1209–1214.
17. McCaughey ES, Walker V, Rolles CJ, et al: Ectopic ACTH production by a thymic carcinoid tumour. *Eur J Pediatr* 1987;146:590–591.
18. Warren JS, Yum MN: Carcinoid tumor arising in a treated primary germ cell tumor of the mediastinum. *South Med J* 1987;80:259–261.
19. Herbst WM, Kummer W, Hofmann W, et al: Carcinoid tumors of the thymus. An immunohistochemical study. *Cancer* 1987;60:2465–2470.
20. Wick MR, Scheithauer BW: Thymic carcinoid. A histologic, immunohistochemical and ultrastructural study of 12 cases. *Cancer* 1984;53:475–484.
21. Huntrakoon M, Lin F, Heitz PU, et al: Thymic carcinoid with Cushing's syndrome. *Arch Pathol Lab Med* 1984;108:551–554.
22. Kay S, Willson MA: Ultrastructural studies of an ACTH-secreting thymic tumor. *Cancer* 1970;26:445–452.
23. Penman E, Wass JAH, Besser GM, et al: Somatostatin secretion by lung and thymic tumours. *Clin Endocrinol* 1980;13:613–620.
24. Baker J, Holdaway IM, Jagusch M, et al: Ectopic secretion of ACTH and Met-enkephalin from a thymic carcinoid. *J Endocrinol Invest* 1982;5:33–38.
25. Birnberg FA, Webb WR, Selch MT, et al: Thymic carcinoid tumors with hyperparathyroidism. *Am J Roentgenol* 1982;139:1001–1004.
26. Scholz DA, Bahn RC: Thymic tumors associated with Cushing's syndrome. Review of three cases. *Proc Staff Meet Mayo Clin* 1959;34:433–441.

27. Felson B, Castleman B, Levinsohn EM, et al: Cushing's syndrome associated with mediastinal mass. *Am J Roentgenol* 1982;138:815–819.
28. Marchevsky AM, Dikman SH: Mediastinal carcinoid with incomplete Sipple's syndrome. *Cancer* 1979;43:2497–2501.
29. Levine GD, Rosai J: A spindle cell variant of thymic carcinoid. A clinical, histologic and fine structural study with emphasis on its distinction from spindle cell thymoma. *Arch Pathol* 1976;100:293–300.
30. Ho FCS, Ho JCI: Pigmented carcinoid tumor of the thymus. *Histopathology* 1977;1:363–369.
31. Wick MR, Carney JA, Bernatz PE, et al: Primary mediastinal carcinoid tumors. *Am J Surg Pathol* 1982;6:195–205.
32. Fetissof F, Boivin F, Jobard P: Microfilamentous carcinoid of the thymus: correlation of ultrastructural study with Grimelius stain. *Ultrastruct Pathol* 1982;3:9–15.
33. Alvarez-Fernandez E: Intracytoplasmic fibrillary inclusions in bronchial carcinoid. *Cancer* 1980;46:144–151.
34. Carstens PHB, Broghamer WL Jr: Duodenal carcinoid with cytoplasmic whorls of microfilaments. *J Pathol* 1978;124:235–238.
35. Sidhu GS: The endodermal origin of digestive and respiratory tract APUD cells: histopathologic evidence and a review of the literature. *Am J Pathol* 1979;96:5–17.
36. Lange L: Ueber ein Lipom des Thymus. *Zentralbl Allg Pathol* 1916;27:97–101.
37. Hall GFM: A case of thymolipoma with observations on a possible relationship to intrathoracic lipomata. *Br J Surg* 1948;36:321–324.
38. Rubin M, Mishkin S: The relationship between mediastinal lipomas and the thymus. *J Thorac Surg* 1954;27:494–502.
39. Teplick JG, Nedwich A, Haskin ME: Roentgenographic features of thymolipoma. *Am J Roentgenol* 1973;117:873–877.
40. Trites AEW: Thyrolipoma, thymolipoma and pharyngeal lipoma: a syndrome. *Can Med Assoc J* 1966;95:1254–1259.
41. Guilfoil PH, Murray H: Thymolipoma. Report of a case. *Surgery* 1955;38:406–409.
42. Scully NM: Lipothymoma with cystic lymphangioma: case report. *Am Surg* 1960;26:400–404.
43. Ringe B, Dragojevic D, Frank G, et al: Thymolipoma—a rare, benign tumor of the thymus gland. Two case reports and review of the literature. *Thorac Cardiovasc Surg* 1979;27:369–374.
44. Otto HF, Löning TH, Lachenmayer L, et al: Thymolipoma in association with myasthenia gravis. *Cancer* 1982;50:1623–1628.
45. Almog CH, Weissberg D, Herczeg E, et al: Thymolipoma simulating cardiomegaly: a clinico-pathological rarity. *Thorax* 1977;32:116–220.
46. Benton C, Gerard P: Thymolipoma in a patient with Graves' disease: case report and review of the literature. *J Thorac Cardiovasc Surg* 1966;51:428–433.
47. Barnes RDS, O'Gorman P: Two cases of aplastic anaemia associated with tumours of the thymus. *J Clin Pathol* 1962;15:264–268.
48. Bigelow NH, Ehler AA: Lipothymoma: an unusual benign tumor of the thymus gland. *J Thorac Surg* 1952;23:528–538.
49. Boetsch CH, Swoyer GB, Adams A, et al: Lipothymoma: report of two cases. *Dis Chest* 1966;50:539–543.
50. Dunn BH, Frkovich G: Lipomas of the thymus gland with an illustrative case report. *Am J Pathol* 1956;32:41–51.
51. Falor WH, Ferro FE: Lipothymoma. *Surgery* 1956;39:291–296.
52. Homer MJ, Wechsler RJ, Carter BL: Mediastinal lipomatosis. CT confirmation of a normal variant. *Radiology* 1978;128:657–661.
53. Korhonen LK, Laustela E: Thymolipoma. Report of a case. *Scand J Thorac Cardiovasc Surg* 1968;2:147–150.
54. Reintgen D, Fetter BF, Roses A, et al: Thymolipoma in association with myasthenia gravis. *Arch Pathol Lab Med* 1978;102:463–466.
55. Roseff I, Levine B, Gilbert L: Lipothymoma simulating cardiomegaly: case report. *Am Heart J* 1958;56:119–125.
56. Moigneteau C, Cornet E, Gordeef A, et al: Le thymo-lipome. *J Chir* 1967;94:509–520.
57. Pan CH, Chiang CY, Chen SS: Thymolipoma in patients with myasthenia gravis: report of two cases and review. *Acta Neurol Scand* 1988;78:16–21.
58. Iseki M, Tsuda N, Kishikawa M, et al: Thymolipoma with striated myoid cells. *Am J Surg Pathol* 1990;14:395–398.
59. Hirai T, Ito M, Abe R: Small thymolipoma in association with myasthenia gravis. *Nippon Kyobu Geka Gakkai Zasshi* 1989;37:2229–2232.
60. Yamanaka N, Araki S, Sato Y: Thymolipoma in association with myasthenia gravis. *Rinsho Shinkeigaku* 1987;27:663–666.
61. Teilum G: Endodermal sinus tumor of the ovary and testis—comparative morphogenesis of the

so-called mesonephroma ovarii (Schiller) and extraembryonic (yolk sac, allantoic) structures of the rat's placenta. *Cancer* 1959;12:1092–1105.

62. Kurman RJ, Norris HJ: Endodermal sinus tumor of the ovary: a clinical and pathologic analysis of 71 cases. *Cancer* 1976;38:2404–2419.

63. Friedman NB: The comparative morphogenesis of extragenital and gonadal teratoid tumors. *Cancer* 1951;4:265–274.

64. Kiffer JD, Sandeman TF: Primary malignant mediastinal germ cell tumors: a study of eleven cases and a review of the literature. *Int J Radiat Oncol Biol Phys* 1989;17:835–841.

65. Brown K, Collins JD, Batra P, et al: Mediastinal germ cell tumor in a young woman. *Med Pediatr Oncol* 1989;17:164–167.

66. Kawaguchi K, Kishida S, Okeda R, et al: Encephalomyeloneuritis with mediastinal germ cell tumor. A paraneoplastic condition? *Acta Pathol Jpn* 1988;38:351–359.

67. McLeod DG, Taylor HG, Skoog SJ, et al: Extragonadal germ cell tumors. Clinicopathologic findings and treatment experience in 12 patients. *Cancer* 1988;61:1187–1191.

68. Bohle A, Studer UE, Sonntag RW, et al: Primary or secondary extragonadal germ cell tumors? *J Urol* 1986;135:939–943.

69. Kersh CR, Eisert DR, Constable WC, et al: Primary malignant mediastinal germ-cell tumors and the contribution of radiotherapy: a southeastern multi-institutional study. *Am J Clin Oncol* 1987;10:302–306.

70. Aliotta PJ, Castillo J, Englander LS, et al: Primary mediastinal germ cell tumors. Histologic patterns of treatment failures at autopsy. *Cancer* 1988;62:982–984.

71. Kay PH, Wells FC, Goldstraw P: A multidisciplinary approach to primary nonseminomatous germ cell tumors of the mediastinum. *Ann Thorac Surg* 1987;44:578–582.

72. Nichols CR, Saxman S, Williams SO, et al: Primary mediastinal nonseminomatous germ cell tumors. *Cancer* 1990;65:1641–1646.

73. Kersh CR, Constable WC, Hahn SS, et al: Primary malignant extragonadal germ cell tumors. An analysis of the effect of radiotherapy. *Cancer* 1990;65:2681–2685.

74. Wright CD, Kesler KA, Nichols CR, et al: Primary mediastinal nonseminomatous germ cell tumors. Results of a multimodality approach. *J Thorac Cardiov Surg* 1990;99:210–217.

75. Hawkins EP, Finegold MJ, Hawkins HK, et al: Nongerminomatous malignant germ cell tumors in children. *Cancer* 1986;58:2579–2584.

76. Bergh NP, Gatzinsky P, Larsson S, et al: Tumors of the thymus and thymic region: III. Clinicopathological studies on teratomas and tumors of germ cell type. *Ann Thorac Surg* 1978;25:107–111.

77. Cox JD: Primary malignant germinal tumors of the mediastinum: a study of 24 cases. *Cancer* 1975;36:1162–1168.

78. Patcher MR, Lattes R: "Germinal" tumors of the mediastinum: a clinicopathologic study of adult teratomas, teratocarcinomas, choriocarcinomas and seminomas. *Dis Chest* 1964;45:301–310.

79. Richards GJ Jr, Reeves RJ: Mediastinal tumors and cysts of children. *Am J Dis Child* 1958;95:284–291.

80. Ringertz N, Lidholm SO: Mediastinal tumors and cysts. *J Thorac Surg* 1956;31:458–487.

81. Oberman HA, Libcke JH: Malignant germinal tumors of the mediastinum. *Cancer* 1964;17:498–507.

82. Whittaker LD, Lynn HB: Mediastinal tumors and cysts in the pediatric patient. *Surg Clin North Am* 1973;53:893–904.

83. Martini N, Golbey RB, Hajdu SI, et al: Primary mediastinal germ cell tumors. *Cancer* 1974;33:763–769.

84. Recondo J, Libshitz HI: Mediastinal extragonadal germ cell tumors. *Urology* 1978;11:369–375.

85. Vogelzang NJ, Raghavan D, Anderson RW, et al: Mediastinal nonseminomatous germ cell tumors: the role of combined modality therapy. *Ann Thorac Surg* 1982;33:333–339.

86. Irie T, Watanabe H, Kawaoi A, et al: Alpha-fetoprotein (AFP), human chorionic gonadotropin (HCG), and carcinoembryonic antigen (CEA) demonstrated in the immature glands of mediastinal teratocarcinoma. A case report. *Cancer* 1982;50:1160–1165.

87. Lattes R: Thymoma and other tumors of the thymus. *Cancer* 1962;15:1224–1235.

88. Schlumberger HG: Teratoma of the anterior mediastinum in the group of military age: a study of 16 cases and review of theories of genesis. *Arch Pathol* 1946;41:398–404.

89. Scardino PT, Cox HD, Waldmann TA, et al: The value of serum tumor markers in the staging and prognosis of germ cell tumors of the testis. *J Urol* 1977;118:994–999.

90. Oosterhuis JW, Rammeloo RHU, Cornelisse CJ, et al: Ploidy of malignant mediastinal germ-cell tumors. *Hum Pathol* 1990;21:729–732.

91. Lachman MF, Kim K, Koo BC: Mediastinal teratoma associated with Klinefelter's syndrome. *Arch Pathol Lab Med* 1986;110:1067–1071.

92. Nichols CR, Heerema NA, Palmer C, et al: Klinefelter's syndrome associated with mediastinal germ cell neoplasms. *J Clin Oncol* 1987;5:1290–1294.

93. Beasley SW, Tiedemann K, Howat A, et al: Precocious puberty associated with malignant thoracic teratoma and malignant histiocytosis in child with Klinefelter's syndrome. *Med Pediatr Oncol* 1987;15:277–280.

94. Dal Cin P, Drochmans A, Moerman P, et al: Isochromosome 12p in mediastinal germ cell tumor. *Cancer Genet Cytogenet* 1989;42:243–251.

95. Dexeus FH, Logothetis CJ, Chong C, et al: Genetic abnormalities in men with germ cell tumors. *J Urol* 1988;140:80–84.

96. Carter D, Bibro MC, Touloukian RJ: Benign clinical behaviour of immature mediastinal teratoma in infancy and childhood: report of two cases and review of the literature. *Cancer* 1982;49:398–402.

97. Rusby NL: Dermoid cysts and teratomata of the mediastinum. A review. *J Thorac Surg* 1944;13:169–222.

98. Daniel RA Jr, Diveley WL, Edwards WH, et al: Mediastinal tumors. *Ann Surg* 1960;151:783–795.

99. Hodge J, Aponte G, McLaughlin E: Primary mediastinal tumors. *J Thorac Surg* 1959;37:730–744.

100. Mahour GH, Woolley MM, Trivedi SN, et al: Teratomas in infancy and childhood. Experience with 81 cases. *Surgery* 1974;76:309–318.

101. Canty TG, Siemens R: Malignant mediastinal teratoma in a 15-year-old girl. *Cancer* 1978;41:1623–1626.

102. Grimm HW: Mediastinal teratoma. *Radiology* 1927;8:438–439.

103. Pate JW, Buker R, Korones SB: Mediastinal teratoma in the newborn. *Surgery* 1963;54:533–535.

104. Pugsley WS, Carleton RL: Germinal nature of teratoid tumors of the thymus. *Arch Pathol* 1953;56:341–347.

105. Schlumberger HG: Teratoma of the anterior mediastinum in the group of military age. *Arch Pathol* 1946;41:398–444.

106. Robertson JM, Fee HJ, Mulder DG: Mediastinal teratoma causing life-threatening hemoptysis. Its occurrence in an infant. *Am J Dis Child* 1981;135:148–150.

107. Aravanis C, Papasteriades E, Steriotis J: Recurrent pericarditis due to cystic teratoma of the mediastinum: a case report. *Angiology* 1980;31:427–430.

108. Vade A, Nolan J: Posterior mediastinal teratoma involving the esophagus. *Gastrointest Radiol* 1989;14:106–108.

109. Weinraub Z, Gembruch U, Fodisch HJ, et al: Intrauterine mediastinal teratoma associated with non-immune hydrops fetalis. *Prenat Diagn* 1989;9:369–372.

110. Wirtanen GW, Stephenson JA, Wiley AL Jr: Primary anterior mediastinal malignant teratoma. A case report with long-term survival. *Cancer* 1989;63:1823–1825.

111. Saabye J, Elbirk A, Andersen K: Teratomas of the mediastinum. *Scand J Thorac Cardiovasc Surg* 1987;21:271–272.

112. Kreller-Laugwitz G, Kobel HF, Oppermann HC: Mediastinal teratoma in a newborn infant. *Monatsschr Kinderheilkd* 1988;136:270–272.

113. Wilms G, Thijs M: Posterior mediastinal teratoma. *ROFO* 1986;145:112–113.

114. Uyama T, Monden Y, Harada K, et al: Rapidly growing mature teratoma of the mediastinum: do sex hormones affect growth of the tumor? *J Surg Oncol* 1988;38:285–289.

115. Suda K, Mizuguchi K, Hebisawa A, et al: Pancreatic tissue in teratoma. *Arch Pathol Lab Med* 1984;108:835–837.

116. Honicky RE, DePapp EW: Mediastinal teratoma with endocrine function. *Am J Dis Child* 1973;126:650–653.

117. Sales LM, Vontz FK: Teratoma and DiGuglielmo syndrome. *South Med J* 1970;63:448–450.

118. Toyofuku T, Mochizuki I, Kusama S: Mediastinal germ cell tumor in trisomy 8. *Eur J Respir Dis* 1987;70:245–249.

119. Deenadayalu RP, Tuuri D, Dewall RA, et al: Intrapericardial teratoma and bronchogenic cyst. Review of literature and report of successful surgery in infant with intrapericardial teratoma. *J Thorac Cardiovasc Surg* 1974;67:945–951.

120. Thurlbeck WM, Scully R: Solid teratoma of the ovary. A clinicopathological analysis of 9 cases. *Cancer* 1960;13:804–811.

121. Norris HJ, Zirkin HJ, Benson WL: Immature (malignant) teratoma of the ovary: a clinical and pathologic study of 58 cases. *Cancer* 1976;37:2359–2372.

122. Gonzalez-Crussi F, Winkler RF, Mirkin DL: Sacrococcygeal teratomas in infants and children: relationship of histology and prognosis in 40 cases. *Arch Pathol Lab Med* 1978;102:420–425.

123. Levine GD: Primary thymic seminoma—a neoplasm ultrastructurally similar to testicular seminoma and distinct from epithelial thymoma. *Cancer* 1973;31:729–741.

124. Bush SE, Martinez A, Bagshaw MA: Primary mediastinal seminoma. *Cancer* 1981;48:1877–1882.

125. Bagshaw MA, McLaughlin WT, Earle JD: Definitive radiotherapy of primary mediastinal seminoma. *Am J Roentgenol* 1969;105:86–94.

126. Schantz A, Sewall W, Castleman B: Mediastinal germinoma: a study of 21 cases with an excellent prognosis. *Cancer* 1972;30:1189–1194.

127. Sterchi M, Cordell AR: Seminoma of the anterior mediastinum. *Ann Thorac Surg* 1975;19: 371–377.

128. Hurt RD, Bruckman JE, Farrow GM, et al: Primary anterior mediastinal seminoma. *Cancer* 1982;49:1658–1663.

129. Polansky SM, Barwick KW, Ravin CE: Primary mediastinal seminoma. *Am J Roentgenol* 1979;132:17–21.

130. Reynolds TF, Yagoda A, Vugrin D, et al: Chemotherapy of mediastinal germ cell tumors. *Semin Oncol* 1979;6:113–115.

131. Burt ME, Javadpour N: Germ-cell tumors in patients with apparently normal testes. *Cancer* 1981;47:1911–1915.

132. Raghavan D, Barrett A: Mediastinal seminomas. *Cancer* 1980;46:1187–1191.

133. Kindig JR, Tavel ME: Acquired pulmonic stenosis due to mediastinal seminoma. *Chest* 1980;78:493–495.

134. Cefaro GA, Luzi S, Turriziani A, et al: Primary mediastinal seminoma. *Br J Urol* 1988;62: 461–464.

135. Bailey D, Baumal R, Marks A: Use of anti-seminoma monoclonal antibody to confirm the diagnosis of mediastinal seminoma. A case report. *APMIS* 1988;96:206–210.

136. Burns BF, McCaughey WT: Unusual thymic seminomas. *Arch Pathol Lab Med* 1986;110: 539–541.

137. Biester RJ, Lippert MC, Mills SE: Late recurrence of a seminoma. *J Urol* 1987;137:749–750.

138. Lee YM, Jackson SM: Primary seminoma of the mediastinum. *Cancer* 1985;55:450–452.

139. Takahashi N, Chifu S, Matsuo K, et al: Primary mediastinal seminoma—a case report. *Gan No Rinsho* 1988;34:331–341.

140. Mostofi FK, Price EB: Tumors of the male genital system, in: *Atlas of Tumor Pathology,* Fasc 8, ser 2, Washington, Armed Forces Institute of Pathology, 1973.

141. Sangalli G, Livraghi T, Giordano F, et al: Primary mediastinal embryonal carcinoma and choriocarcinoma. A case report. *Acta Cytol* 1986;30:543–546.

142. Ulbright TM, Loehrer PJ, Roth LM, et al: The development of non–germ cell malignancies within germ cell tumors. *Cancer* 1984;54:1825–1833.

143. Pierce GB, Arechaga J, Jones A, et al: The fate of embryonal carcinoma cells in mouse blastocysts. *Differentiation* 1987;33:247–253.

144. Curry WA, McKay CE, Richardson RL, et al: Klinefelter's syndrome and mediastinal germ cell neoplasms. *J Urol* 1981;125:127–129.

145. McNeil MM, Leong AS, Sage RE: Primary mediastinal embryonal carcinoma in association with Klinefelter's syndrome. *Cancer* 1981;47:343–345.

146. Kuzur ME, Cobleigh MA, Greco A, et al: Endodermal sinus tumor of the mediastinum. *Cancer* 1982;50:766–774.

147. Norgaard-Pedersen B, Albrechtsen R, Teilum G: Serum alpha-fetoprotein as a marker for endodermal sinus tumor (yolk sac tumor) or a vitelline component of "teratocarcinoma." *Acta Pathol Microbiol Immunol Scand (A)* 1975;83:573–589.

148. Fox MA, Vix VA: Endodermal sinus (yolk sac) tumors of the anterior mediastinum. *Am J Roentgenol* 1980;135:291–294.

149. Roth LM, Panganiban WG: Gonadal and extragonadal yolk sac carcinomas. A clinicopathologic study of 14 cases. *Cancer* 1976;37:812–820.

150. Huntington RW Jr, Bullock WK: Yolk sac tumors of extragonadal origin. *Cancer* 1970;25: 1368–1376.

151. Teilmann I, Kassis H, Pietra G: Primary germ cell tumor of the anterior mediastinum with features of endodermal sinus tumor (mesoblastoma vitellinum). *Acta Pathol Microbiol Immunol Scand* 1967;70:267–278.

152. Mukai K, Adams WR: Yolk sac tumor of the anterior mediastinum. Case report with light and electron-microscopic examination and immunohistochemical study of alpha-fetoprotein. *Am J Surg Pathol* 1979;3:77–83.

153. Sham JS, Fu KH, Chiu CS, et al: Experience with the management of primary endodermal sinus tumor of the mediastinum. *Cancer* 1989;64:756–761.

154. Truong LD, Harris L, Mattioli C, et al: Endodermal sinus tumor of the mediastinum. A report of seven cases and review of the literature. *Cancer* 1986;58:730–739.

155. Chamsi-Pasha H, Bernstein A: Mediastinal yolk sac tumour mimicking pericardial effusion. *Thorax* 1988;43:339–340.

156. Goo Neratne S, Keh P, Sreekanth S, et al: Anterior mediastinal endodermal sinus (yolk sac) tumor in a female infant. *Cancer* 1985;56:1430–1433.

157. Greenwood SM, Goodman JR, Schneider G, et al: Choriocarcinoma in a man. The relationship of gynecomastia to chorionic somatomammotropin and estrogens. *Am J Med* 1971;51:416–422.

158. Sickels EA, Belliveau RE, Wiernik PH: Primary mediastinal choriocarcinoma in the male. *Cancer* 1974;33:1196–1203.
159. Wenger ME, Dines DE, Ahmann DL, et al: Primary mediastinal choriocarcinoma. *Mayo Clin Proc* 1968;43:570–575.
160. Sandhaus L, Strom RL, Mukai K: Primary embryonal choriocarcinoma of the mediastinum in a woman. A case report with immunohistochemical study. *Am J Clin Pathol* 1981;75:573–578.
161. Candes FP, Ajinkya MS: Primary mediastinal choriocarcinoma (a case report). *J Postgrad Med* 1987;33:219–221.
162. Kathuria S, Jablokow VR: Primary choriocarcinoma of mediastinum with immunohistochemical study and review of the literature. *J Surg Oncol* 1987;34:39–42.
163. Manivel C, Wick MR, Abenoza P, et al: The occurrence of sarcomatous components in primary mediastinal germ cell tumors. *Am J Surg Pathol* 1986;10:711–717.
164. Myers TJ, Kessimian N, Schwartz S: Mediastinal germ cell tumor associated with the hemophagocytic syndrome. *Ann Intern Med* 1988;109:504–505.
165. DeMent SH, Eggleston JC, Spiva KJL: Association between mediastinal germ cell tumors and hematologic malignancies. *Am J Surg Pathol* 1985;9:23–30.
166. DeMent SH: Association between mediastinal germ cell tumors and hematologic malignancies: an update. *Hum Pathol* 1990;21:699–703.
167. Nichols CR, Roth BJ, Heerema N, et al: Hematologic neoplasia associated with primary mediastinal germ cell tumors. *N Engl J Med* 1990;322:1425–1429.
168. Benjamin SP, McCormack LJ, Effler DB, et al: Primary lymphatic tumors of the mediastinum. *Cancer* 1972;30:708–712.
169. van Heerden JA, Harrison EG Jr, Bernatz PE, et al: Mediastinal malignant lymphoma. *Chest* 1970;57:518–529.
170. Szporn AH, Dikman S, Jagirdar J: True histiocytic lymphoma of the thymus. *Am J Clin Pathol* 1984;82:734–737.
171. Isaacson PG, Chan JKC, Tang C, et al: Low-grade B-cell lymphoma of mucosa-associated lymphoid tissue arising in the thymus. A thymic lymphoma mimicking myoepithelial sialadenitis. *Am J Surg Pathol* 1990;14:342–351.
172. Lowenhaupt E, Brown R: Carcinoma of the thymus of granulomatous type; a clinical and pathological study. *Cancer* 1951;4:1193–1209.
173. Nickels J, Franssila K, Hjelt L: Thymoma and Hodgkin's disease of the thymus. *Acta Pathol Microbiol Immunol Scand (A)* 1973;81:1–5.
174. Bergh NP, Gatzinsky P, Larsson S, et al: Tumors of the thymus and thymic region: II. Clinicopathological studies on Hodgkin's disease of the thymus. *Ann Thorac Surg* 1978;25:99–106.
175. Eiser NM, Samarrai AAR: Thymic lymphoma—an unusual presentation. *Thorax* 1975;30:588–591.
176. Klempman S, Leibowitz M: Hodgkin's disease of the thymus. A case report. *S Afr Med J* 1982;62:961–963.
177. Marshall AHE, Wood C: The involvement of the thymus in Hodgkin's disease. *J Pathol Bacteriol* 1957;73:163–166.
178. Katz A, Lattes R: Granulomatous thymoma or Hodgkin's disease of thymus? A clinical and histologic study and a re-evaluation. *Cancer* 1969;23:1–15.
179. Fechner RE: Hodgkin's disease of the thymus. *Cancer* 1969;23:16–23.
180. Null JA, LiVolsi VA, Glenn WWL: Hodgkin's disease of the thymus (granulomatous thymoma) and myasthenia gravis. A unique association. *Am J Clin Pathol* 1977;67:521–525.
181. Keller AR, Castleman B: Hodgkin's disease of the thymus gland. *Cancer* 1974;33:1615–1623.
182. Lattes R: Thymoma and other tumors of the thymus: an analysis of 107 cases. *Cancer* 1962;15:1224–1260.
183. Eisenberg SJ, Sahyoun PF: Mixed tumors of the thymus. Criteria for their differentiation and their radiotherapeutic response. *Arch Pathol* 1950;49:404–417.
184. Lewis CR, Manoharan A: Benign thymic cysts in Hodgkin's disease: report of a case and review of published cases. *Thorax* 1987;42:633–634.
185. Kim HC, Nosher J, Haas A, et al: Cystic degeneration of thymic Hodgkins's disease following radiation therapy. *Cancer* 1985;55:354–356.
186. Ewing J: The thymus and its tumors. Report of three cases of thymoma. *Surg Gynecol Obstet* 1916;22:461–472.
187. Thompson AD, Thackray AC: The histology of tumors of the thymus. *Br J Cancer* 1957;11:348–357.
188. Castleman B: Tumors of the thymus gland, in: *Atlas of Tumor Pathology*, Fasc 19. Washington, D.C., Armed Forces Institute of Pathology, 1955.
189. Thompson AD: The thymic origin of Hodgkin's diseases. *Br J Cancer* 1955;9:37–50.
190. Remigio PA: Granulomatous thymoma associated with erythroid hypoplasia. *Am J Clin Pathol* 1971;55:68–72.

191. Peck B: Hypertrophic osteoarthropathy with Hodgkin's disease in the mediastinum. *JAMA* 1977;238:1400–1401.
192. Federle MP, Callen PW: Cystic Hodgkin's lymphoma of the thymus: computed tomography appearance. *J Comput Assist Tomogr* 1979;3:542–544.
193. Lukes RJ, Butler JJ, Hicks EB: Natural history of Hogdkin's disease as related to its pathologic picture. *Cancer* 1966;19:317–344.
194. Konishi N, Ward JM, Reynolds CW, et al: Thymic T-cell lymphoma with the CD8+ (OX-8), CDH+ (W3125) phenotype, induced in F344/Ncr rats by nitroso-z-hydroxypropylurea. *Thymus* 1988;12:225–237.
195. Mueller RE, Ball JK, Chan FP: Characterization of cell markers in type B retroviral-induced thymic lymphomas—II. Surface antigen phenotype, karyotype and proviral integration pattern in cultured lymphoma cells and cloned lines. *Leuk Res* 1989;13:561–571.
196. Ladanyi M, Roy I, Ladanyi M: Mediastinal germ cell tumors and histiocytosis. *Hum Pathol* 1988;19:586–590.
197. Bramwell NH, Burns BF: Histiocytosis X of the thymus in association with myasthenia gravis. *Am J Clin Pathol* 1986;86:224–227.
198. Siegal GP, Dehner LP, Rosai J: Histiocytosis X (Langerhans' cell granulomatosis) of the thymus. A clinico pathologic study of four childhood cases. *Am J Surg Pathol* 1985;9:117–124.
199. Suematsu N, Watanabe S, Shimosato Y: A case of large "thymic granuloma." Neoplasm of T-zone histiocyte. *Cancer* 1984;54:2480–2486.
200. Abramson SJ, Berdon WE, Reilly BJ, et al: Cavitation of anterior mediastinal masses in children with histiocytosis-X. Report of four cases with radiographic, pathologic findings and clinical follow up. *Pediatr Radiol* 1987;17:10–14.
201. Consolini R, Cini P, Cei B, et al: Thymic dysfunction in histiocytosis-X. *Am J Pediatr Hematol Oncol* 1987;9:146–148.
202. Newton WA Jr, Hamoudi AB, Shannon BT: Role of the thymus in histiocytosis-X. *Hematol Oncol Clin North Am* 1987;1:63–74.
203. Pardes JG, LiPuma JP, Haaga JR, et al: Lymphangioma of the thymus in a child. *J Comput Assist Tomogr* 1982;6:825–827.
204. Case records of the Massachusetts General Hospital: weekly clinicopathological exercises. Case 30, 1980. *N Engl J Med* 1980;303:270–276.
205. Edagawa M, Iwamoto I, Shibata K, et al: A case of giant mediastinal cystic lymphangioma. *Nippon Kyobu Geka Gakkai Zasshi* 1989;37:2241–2244.
206. Middleton G: Involvement of the thymus by metastatic neoplasm. *Br J Cancer* 1966;20:41–46.

8

Endocrine and Salivary Gland Lesions of the Mediastinum

The mediastinum can be the site of origin of thyroid, parathyroid, and paraganglial lesions. They are more frequent in the anterosuperior compartment but can arise from the posterior mediastinum or other compartments.

MEDIASTINAL THYROID LESIONS

In the second half of the 19th century, several reports in the European literature described instances of goiters that extended down into the thoracic cavity (1). In 1858, for example, Malard described cases of "goitre plongeant" (1). Several subsequent reports have described the clinical, radiographic, and pathologic features of mediastinal goiters (1–14).

There has been controversy regarding the nomenclature of mediastinal goiters (1). The lesions have been classified according to whether they were continuous with an enlarged cervical thyroid gland (partially intrathoracic goiters) or completely enclosed within the chest without a palpable cervical goiter (substernal, completely intrathoracic goiter) (1). Other reports utilize the more general terms: mediastinal goiter or intrathoracic thyroid tissue (2–12).

As recently emphasized by Hall and associates (13), there are therapeutic implications of differentiating substernal goiters that are in continuity with the thyroid gland from true ectopic or aberrant intrathoracic thyroid lesions. The latter are unusual, representing less than 1% of surgically removed goiters, and they derive their blood supply from intrathoracic vessels, an important consideration at the time of surgical resection.

Mediastinal goiters are relatively common thoracic lesions. They account for up to 10% of mediastinal masses and are most frequent in the anterior mediastinum (15). They can occur, however, in other mediastinal compartments (16). Indeed, up to 25% of mediastinal goiters occur in the posterior mediastinum (9,12).

Pathogenesis

The thyroid gland is derived embryologically from a central anlage arising from the medial laryngeal fold and two lateral outpouches from the fourth branchial pouches that migrate to the neck during embryogenesis (1). Anomalies of their development can result in the formation of ectopic thyroid tissue at any site between the tip of the tongue to the diaphragm (1,17). Indeed, ectopic thyroid tissue has been encountered in all mediastinal compartments as well as in the wall of the trachea, larynx, esophagus, aorta, pericardium, and myocardium (1,17).

Mediastinal goiters can develop from these ectopic thyroid tissue foci. Most instances of thyroid mediastinal pathology result, however, from extension of cervical goiters from the neck into the thorax because of mechanical factors (1). Indeed, up to 20% of cervical goiters are accompanied by the presence of intrathoracic thyroid tissue (3,4).

The thyroid gland is normally enclosed in the neck within soft tissues and muscles that extend upward to the larynx and hyoid bone. The gland is not surrounded by rigid structures that will prevent its downward migration into areas of least mechanical resistance. Several factors favor the migration of cervical goiters into the thorax, including the weight of the enlarged gland, shortness of the neck, the negative intrathoracic pressure, and the respiratory movements (1). Once goiters are in the mediastinum, they grow preferentially into the right side because the aortic arch and other great vessels offer a mechanical barrier to their growth in the left side of the thorax (1).

Clinical Features

Mediastinal goiters are more frequent in female patients (1). They are found occasionally on routine chest roentgenograms, but patients usually present with various symptoms related to the compression of thoracic structures by the enlarged thyroid gland, including cough, retrosternal pain, feeling of weight in the chest that increases in the supine position, and others (1–17). Patients are usually euthyroid, but they may rarely have thyrotoxicosis. Very rarely, mediastinal goiters result in the superior vena cava syndrome.

On physical examination, the patients frequently have a palpable cervical goiter or a mass that can be detected in the suprasternal notch.

Radiologic Features

Mediastinal goiters appear on chest roentgenograms as large masses with a bosselated border and focal areas of calcification (Fig. 8-1) (8,9). They frequently change in position during swallowing, as seen on fluoroscopy. Mediastinal thyroid lesions also can be detected and characterized on the basis of their location and density utilizing computed tomography (CT) scans (Fig. 8-2) (11,12). Intravenous contrast media facilitate the CT scan diagnosis of mediastinal goiter (11). Thyroid lesions can also be detected with ^{131}I thyroid scans that demonstrate an enlarged gland with multiple nodules and with sonograms and ^{99m}Tc-pertechnetate scans (2,4,5).

Thyroid scans can be very helpful in demonstrating ectopic mediastinal thyroid lesions that have no attachment to a normal cervical thyroid, an important fact in the preoperative assessment of a mediastinal lesion. Indeed, the removal of such a lesion through a standard cervical approach may result in severe bleeding from intrathoracic vessels. However, nonfunctional mediastinal thyroid lesions can present with negative scans (18).

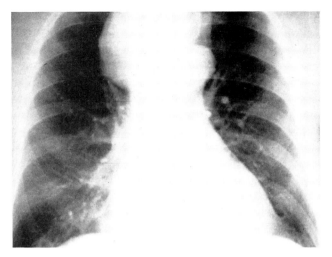

FIG. 8–1. Intrathoracic goiter appearing as a large superior mediastinal mass.

Pathologic Features

Most mediastinal thyroid lesions are diffuse colloid or adenomatous goiters (1). Follicular adenomas of the thyroid occasionally can be encountered in the mediastinum. Other lesions of the gland, such as thyroiditis or malignant neoplasms, are unusual in the thorax.

The pathologic features of thyroid lesions of the mediastinum are identical to those present in the cervical gland. They have been described in detail in other textbooks of surgical pathology (19).

Multinodular or adenomatous goiters, the most frequent form of mediastinal thyroid pathology, are characterized by a gland that is usually markedly enlarged and greatly distorted by multiple nodules surrounded by a fibrous capsule (Fig. 8-3) (1–

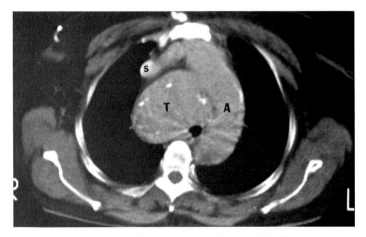

FIG. 8–2. Large mediastinal goiter with areas of calcification (*T*). The lesion is posterior to the superior vena cava (*S*) and displaces the trachea and aortic arch (*A*) to the left side.

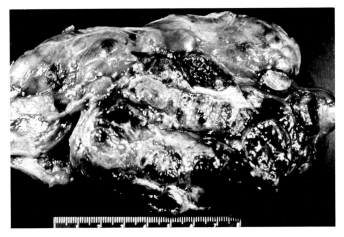

FIG. 8–3. Intrathoracic goiter. The markedly enlarged thyroid has numerous irregular colloid-containing adenomatous nodules with areas of calcification and fibrosis.

12). Areas of hemorrhage, calcification, or cystic degeneration are frequent. Histologically, the nodules are composed of thyroid follicles of various sizes lined by amphophilic or oxyphilic follicular cells (Fig. 8-4). Areas of epithelial hyperplasia that can be mistaken for a follicular carcinoma of the thyroid may also be present.

Diffuse hyperplasia of the thyroid gland is less frequent in the mediastinum (1–12).

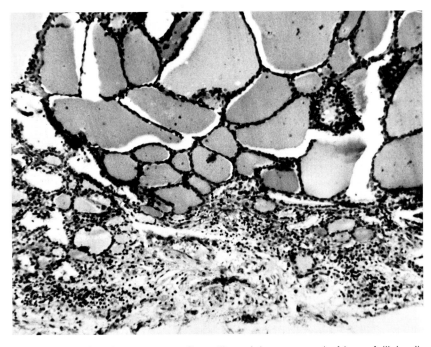

FIG. 8–4. Intrathoracic adenomatous goiter with nodule composed of large follicles lined by low cuboidal cells and containing colloid. (H&E × 40, original)

The gland is uniformly and symmetrically enlarged with preservation of its usual shape. Histologically, the thyroid follicles exhibit marked epithelial hyperplasia with loss of their round shape and presence of papillary infoldings.

Follicular adenomas of the thyroid infrequently arise from the mediastinum. They appear as well-encapsulated nodules composed of thyroid follicles of different sizes (fetal, microfollicular, macrofollicular, trabecular adenomas) (19).

Malignant neoplasms of the thyroid are unusual primary tumors of the mediastinum (20). Waggoner (21) reported an instance of papillary carcinoma of the thyroid arising from ectopic thyroid tissue located in the tracheal wall. We have encountered an instance of primary follicular carcinoma of the thyroid in the anterior mediastinum (Fig. 8-5).

However, in daily practice, most thyroid carcinomas present in the mediastinum should be considered as metastatic tumors until proven otherwise.

MEDIASTINAL PARATHYROID LESIONS

There are normally four parathyroid glands in man, located on the posterior aspects of the thyroid lobes. They can vary in number, however, from two to five (22). Indeed, 2% to 6.5% of adults have supernumerary parathyroid glands (22).

The parathyroids derive embryologically from the third and fourth branchial pouches. The superior glands develop from the fourth branchial pouches (22). The inferior parathyroids derive from the third branchial pouches in close contact with the developing thymic anlage. In about 10% of patients, the parathyroid glands are located in the submaxillary area, thyroid gland, thymus, mediastinum, or pericardium (Fig. 8-6) (23–28).

In the thorax, ectopic parathyroids are present in the anterior mediastinum in ap-

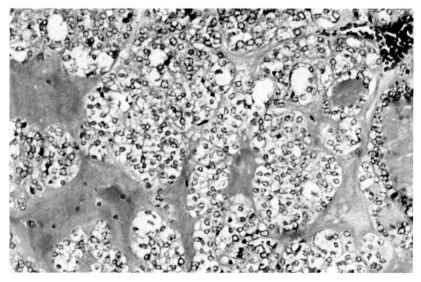

FIG. 8–5. Intrathoracic follicular carcinoma of the thyroid. The tumor is composed of small follicles and solid nests of clear polygonal cells. The lesion exhibited capsular invasion in other areas. (H&E × 100, original)

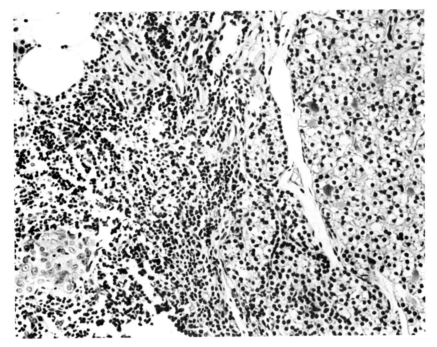

FIG. 8–6. Intrathymic ectopic parathyroid gland. (H&E × 100, original)

proximately 80% of cases, adjacent to or within the thymus, a finding explained by the common embryologic origin of the thymus and the inferior parathyroids.

Ectopic parathyroids have also been described in other compartments such as the posterior mediastinum (23–33).

In a recent review, Clark (27) reported mediastinal parathyroid tumors in 22% of patients undergoing surgery for hyperparathyroidism and in 38% of patients requiring reoperation for persistent or recurrent hyperparathyroidism. In patients where the lower parathyroid glands were not present in the neck, the glands were usually located in the anterior mediastinum within the thymic area. In instances of upper parathyroids missing from the neck at the time of exploration, the glands were usually found in the posterior mediastinum (27).

Parathyroid Adenomas

Patients with mediastinal parathyroid tumors are usually women (3:1) in their fourth through seventh decades of life (23). They present internists, radiologists, and particularly thoracic surgeons with difficult diagnostic problems.

Clinical Features

Patients with mediastinal parathyroid tumors present with symptoms of skeletal abnormalities, renal stones, peptic ulcer, pancreatitis, mental changes, hypercalcemia, and other manifestations of hyperparathyroidism (22,23). However, unusual patients with nonfunctioning parathyroid adenomas have been reported (26). They frequently undergo several surgical procedures until their mediastinal lesions are located and resected (23,30).

The localization of parathyroid tumors in the mediastinum has been greatly facilitated by the use of modern diagnostic techniques such as computerized tomography and selective venous catheterization with parathormone measurements, ultrasonography, thallium-technetium scans, and magnetic resonance imaging (MRI) (27,31–34). Glands located in the posterior mediastinum or the pericardium are particularly difficult to localize (29).

There is controversy as to what diagnostic method is most sensitive and specific for the diagnosis of mediastinal parathyroid lesions. Selective venous catheterization is the most accurate method for the lateralization of these lesions, and MRI scan appears to be the most useful test for localizing parathyroid tumors in patients with persistent or recurrent hyperparathyroidism (27).

Parathyroid adenomas can undergo spontaneous hemorrhage with pain and progressive respiratory symptoms (35).

Parathyroids located in the anterior and superior mediastinum can usually be resected at the time of neck exploration without an additional thoracotomy in instances in which the ectopic glands have been localized preoperatively (23).

Pathologic Features

Most patients with parathyroid abnormalities in the mediastinum present with a single adenoma. Instances of parathyroid hyperplasia or carcinoma are unusual in the mediastinum. For example, in a series of 84 patients with mediastinal parathyroid tumors studied at the Massachusetts General Hospital by Nathaniels and associates (23), there was only one instance of parathyroid hyperplasia and one other of parathyroid carcinoma; all other patients had adenomas of the gland. It is also of interest that 21% of these lesions were located intrathymically.

Parathyroid adenomas have morphologic features in the mediastinum similar to their neck counterparts (22). They are usually single, well-encapsulated nodules composed of trabeculae, solid nests, and microacini lined by chief cells, oncocytic cells, and/or clear cells (Figs. 8-7 and 8-8). A rim of normal parathyroid tissue can usually be seen in adjacent tissues external to the capsule. Occasionally, the epithelial cells exhibit various degrees of pleomorphism, but mitotic figures are absent.

Parathyroid adenomas are difficult to distinguish from hyperplasia on histologic grounds, as there are no pathognomonic diagnostic morphologic features. Indeed, the diagnosis of parathyroid adenoma is established in the presence of an enlarged parathyroid gland and in the absence of enlargement of the other parathyroid, as demonstrated by surgical exploration and biopsy of at least one normal gland (22).

Lipoadenoma

Wolff and Goodman (36) and Hargreaves and Wright (37) described instances of mediastinal functioning lipoadenomas arising from supernumerary parathyroid glands.

Lipoadenomas of the parathyroid can be easily overlooked as instances of normal parathyroids and are well-encapsulated nodules composed of adipose tissue admixed

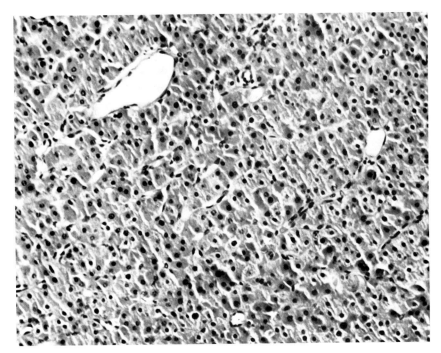

FIG. 8–7. Ectopic intrathoracic parathyroid adenoma composed entirely of oxyphilic cells arranged in a trabecular pattern. (H&E × 100, original)

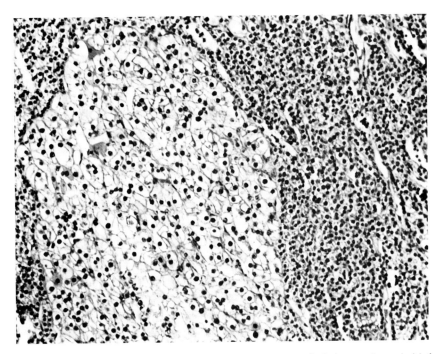

FIG. 8–8. Ectopic intrathoracic parathyroid adenoma composed of clear cells and chief cells. (H&E × 100, original)

with trabeculae and microacini lined by chief cells or oncocytic cells (36). The presence of fat in the lesion presents a diagnostic challenge, as it is absent in parathyroid adenomas and present in a normal gland. On low-power microscopy, however, lipoadenomas are well-encapsulated tumors with a distinct internal architecture that can be distinguished from a normal gland.

Lipoadenomas are usually small and functional and are associated with hyperparathyroidism. It is controversial whether they are benign tumors or parathyroid gland hamartomas (38).

MEDIASTINAL LESIONS OF PARAGANGLIAL ORIGIN

The paraganglia are important structures of the diffuse neuroendocrine system composed of neuroepithelial cells with intracytoplasmic dense-core membrane-bound granules containing catecholamines and are scattered throughout the body (39).

The mediastinum has parasympathetic paraganglia in close contact with the great vessels (aorticopulmonary paraganglia or aortic body) and sympathetic paraganglia located along the paraaortic regions (40).

The aorticopulmonary paraganglia are chemoreceptors able to sense fluctuations in blood oxygen tension, temperature, and pH (40). They become hyperplastic in patients with chronic hypoxemia (40). The paraaortic thoracolumbar paraganglia probably represent small homologs of the adrenal medulla (39,40).

Paragangliomas (Chemodectomas)

Paragangliomas are endocrine tumors that originate from paraganglia such as the carotid body, glomus jugulare, Zuckerkandl's body, and others (39). In the mediastinum, paragangliomas develop most frequently in the superior mediastinum from the supraaortic or aorticopulmonary bodies (40–56). They can also originate from paraaortic sympathetic paraganglia in the posterior mediastinum (47–50). Fernandez and associates (51) reported a chemodectoma arising from the vagus nerve.

Clinical Features

Aorticopulmonary paragangliomas are infrequent tumors. Mediastinal paragangliomas in other locations are even less frequent (40–56). They occur in all age groups (mean age 47 years) and are more frequent in women (1.8:1) (40–56).

Approximately 50% of the patients are asymptomatic at the time of original diagnosis and are found to have a superior mediastinal tumor mass on routine chest roentgenograms. Others present with hoarseness, dysphagia, chest pain or discomfort, cough, hemoptysis, and/or clinical manifestations of the superior vena cava syndrome (39). Mediastinal paragangliomas can be multiple and/or present in familial clusters (52–54). They have also been described in association with gastric leiomyosarcomas and pulmonary chondromas (Carney's triad) (57,58).

Radiologic Features

Mediastinal paragangliomas are round, well-circumscribed masses on chest roentgenograms that vary in size from 1.2 to 17 cm (average diameter 7.5 cm) (39). Aortic body tumors are located in close contact with the great aorticopulmonary vessels and the base of the heart and can be confused radiologically with vascular structures (39). These aorticopulmonary tumors are difficult to locate even with the aid of computerized tomograms and MRI.

Angiography is most useful for the diagnosis and location of these highly vascular, well-circumscribed lesions (59).

Pathologic Features

Paragangliomas are well encapsulated, gray–pink, highly vascular, and frequently exhibit areas of hemorrhage. Histologically, they are composed of characteristic nests of cuboidal cells surrounded by vascularized fibrous septa (cell balls or *Zellballen*) (Fig. 8-9). The tumor cells have a round nucleus and a clear or eosinophilic granular cytoplasm (Fig. 8-10). Nerve trunks may be found at the periphery of the neoplasm.

Cellular pleomorphism with occasional bizarre giant tumor cells, rare mitotic figures, and focal vascular invasion may be seen. These features should not be considered, however, as evidence of malignancy. Indeed, there are no reliable histologic criteria to distinguish benign from malignant paragangliomas (39). Paragangliomas are diagnosed as malignant only after they have metastasized (60,61).

Special Studies

Silver staining techniques such as those described by del Rio Ortega and Grimelius are useful for the detection of argyrophilia in the cytoplasm of tumor cells in paragangliomas (39). They confirm the neuroendocrine nature of the tumor. Tumor cells also exhibit formalin-induced fluorescence in freeze-dried preparations, indicative of the presence of catecholamines in their cytoplasm (39).

Ultrastructurally, paragangliomas exhibit three cell types: endothelial cells, pericytes, and chief cells (39). The latter are the neoplastic cells and are characterized by the presence of numerous intracytoplasmic membrane-bound dense neurosecretory granules ranging from 100 to 300 nm in size. Chief cells are in close proximity to vascular structures and are separated from endothelial cells and pericytes by their basement membranes.

Differential Diagnosis

Paragangliomas may be difficult to distinguish from other endocrine tumors such as thymic carcinoids, metastatic medullary carcinomas of the thyroid, and pheochromocytomas. Carcinoids and other endocrine neoplasms lack the typical pattern with "cell-ball" formation characteristic of paragangliomas. Pheochromocytomas are indistinguishable on morphologic grounds from paragangliomas.

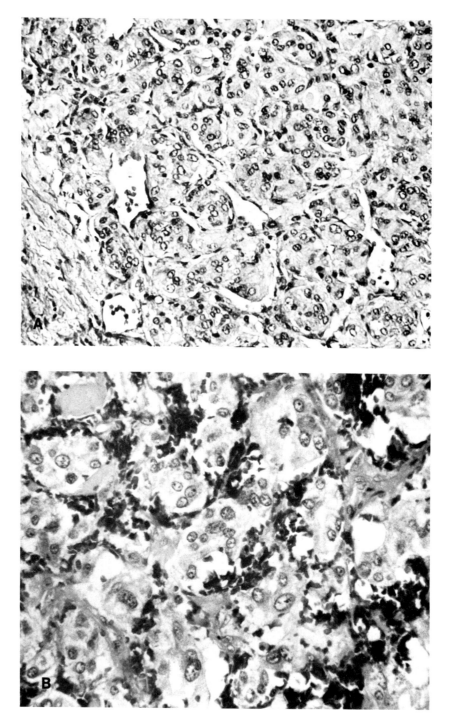

FIG. 8–9. A: Mediastinal paraganglioma composed of "*Zellballen*" of polygonal cells surrounded by capillaries. (H&E × 100, original) **B:** Higher magnification showing polygonal tumor cells with amphophilic or eosinophilic cytoplasm and central round to oval nuclei. (H&E × 400, original)

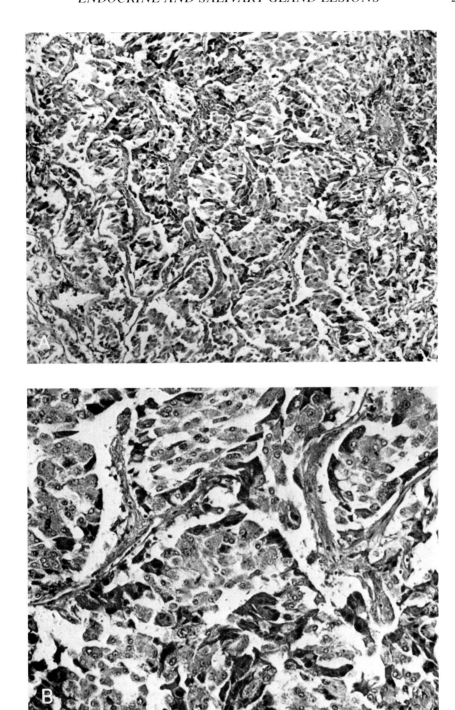

FIG. 8–10. A: Mediastinal pheochromocytoma composed of small nests of polygonal cells surrounded by highly vascularized stroma. (H&E × 100, original) **B:** Higher magnification of polygonal cells with amphophilic or eosinophilic cytoplasm. (H&E × 400, original)

Treatment and Prognosis

Mediastinal paragangliomas are benign tumors in most instances. Only 13% of cases are malignant and metastasize to the skeletal system, lungs, and other organs (39,55).

Paragangliomas can be cured by complete excision (39). Optimal surgical treatment is not always possible, however, because of the location of these tumors in close proximity to the great vessels, heart, and other mediastinal structures. In these instances, radiotherapy is only of limited value.

PHEOCHROMOCYTOMAS

Pheochromocytomas are tumors from the adrenal medulla characterized by the presence of intracytoplasmic epinephrine and/or norepinephrine. Their morphologic features are identical to those of paragangliomas (Fig. 8-10).

Pheochromocytomas have been described in extraabdominal locations including the mediastinum (62).

TUMOR OF SALIVARY GLAND ORIGIN: PLEOMORPHIC ADENOMA

A patient with a benign mixed tumor of salivary gland origin (pleomorphic adenoma) was described in the middle mediastinum (63,64). It was a well-circumscribed, 7.0 × 5.0 × 4.0 cm tumor with a pale–tan, mucoid surface, located adjacent to the carina and the aortic arch. Microscopically, it was composed of a myxoid stroma

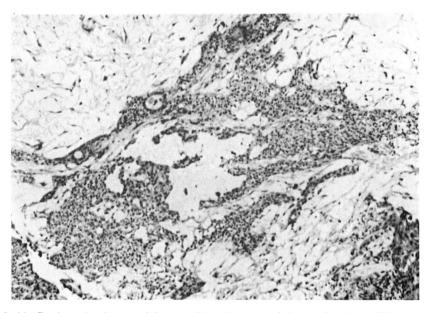

FIG. 8–11. Benign mixed tumor (pleomorphic adenoma) of the mediastinum. The tumor has epithelial cells with focal acinar formation, solid sheets of myoepithelial cells, and a myxoid stroma. (H&E × 100, original)

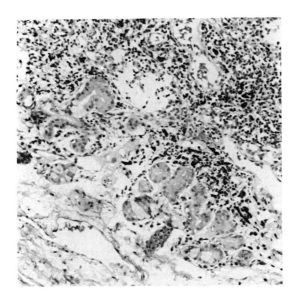

FIG. 8–12. Mediastinal lymph node with inclusions of benign salivary gland tissue. (H&E × 100, original)

with stellate cells admixed with solid nests, trabeculae, and glands lined by epithelial cells and myoepithelial cells (Fig. 8-11) (Color fig. 8*). We encountered an additional patient exhibiting ectopic salivary gland–type glandular inclusions in a mediastinal lymph node, suggesting a possible site of origin for pleomorphic adenomas in this unusual location (Fig. 8-12).

REFERENCES

1. Lindskog BI, Malm A: Diagnostic and surgical considerations on mediastinal (intrathoracic) goiter. *Dis Chest* 1965;47:201–207.
2. Morris UL, Colletti PM, Ralls PW, et al: CT demonstration of intrathoracic thyroid tissue. *J Comput Assist Tomogr* 1982:6:821–824.
3. Gourin A, Garzon AA, Karlson KE: The cervico mediastinal approach to intrathoracic goiter. *Surgery* 1971;69:651–654.
4. Kaplan WD, Watnick M, Holman BL: Scintigraphic identification of complete thoracic goiter with normal appearing cervical thyroid: a case report. *J Can Assoc Radiol* 1974;25:193–195.
5. Salvatore M, Gallo A: Accessory thyroid in the anterior mediastinum. Case report. *J Nucl Med* 1975;16:1135–1136.
6. Shimshak RR, Schoenrock GJ, Taekman HP, et al: Preoperative localization of a parathyroid adenoma using computed tomography and thyroid scanning. *J Comput Assist Tomogr* 1979;3:117–119.
7. Sweet RH: Intrathoracic goiter located in the posterior mediastinum. *Surg Gynecol Obstet* 1949;89:57–66.
8. Ellis FH Jr, Good CA: Intrathoracic goiter. *Ann Surg* 1952;135:79–90.
9. Reitz K-A, Werner B: Intrathoracic goiter. *Acta Chir Scand* 1960;119:379–388.
10. Irwin RS, Braman SS, Arvanitidis AN, et al: [131]I Thyroid scanning preoperative diagnosis of mediastinal goiter. *Ann Int Med* 1978;89:73–74.
11. Glazer GM, Axel L, Moss AA: CT diagnosis of mediastinal thyroid. *Am J Roentgenol* 1982;138:495–498.
12. Binder RE, Pugatch RD, Faling LJ, et al: Diagnosis of posterior mediastinal goiter by computed tomography. *J Comput Assist Tomogr* 1980;4:550–552.

*Color figure 8 appears following page 64.

13. Hall TS, Caslowitz P, Popper C, et al: Substernal goiter versus intrathoracic aberrant thyroid: a critical difference. *Ann Thorac Surg* 1988;46:684–685.
14. Zapatero J, Baamonde C, Gonzalez Aragoneses F, et al: Ectopic goiters of the mediastinum: presentation of two cases and review of the literature. *Jpn J Surg* 1988;18:105–109.
15. Daniel RA Jr, Diveley WL, Edwards WH, et al: Mediastinal tumors. *Ann Surg* 1960;151:783–795.
16. Burkell CC, Cross JM, Kent HP, et al: Mass lesions of the mediastinum. *Curr Probl Surg* 1969;6:2–57.
17. Helidonis E, Dokianakis G. Papazoglou G, et al: Ectopic thyroid gland in the submandibular region. *J Laryngol Otol* 1980;94:219–224.
18. Bashist B, Ellis K, Gold RP: Computed tomography of intrathoracic goiters. *Am J Roentgenol* 1983;140:453–456.
19. Rosai J: *Ackerman's Surgical Pathology*. St. Louis, CV Mosby, pp 330–378, 1981.
20. Fish J, Moore RM: Ectopic thyroid tissue and ectopic thyroid carcinoma: a review of the literature and report of a case. *Ann Surg* 1963;157:212–221.
21. Waggoner LG: Intralaryngeal, intratracheal thyroid. *Ann Otol Rhinol Laryngol* 1958;67:61–71.
22. Castleman B, Roth SI: Tumors of the parathyroid glands, in: *Atlas of Tumor Pathology*, Fasc 14, ser 2. Washington D.C., Armed Forces Institute of Pathology, 1978.
23. Nathaniels EK, Nathaniels AM, Wang C-A: Mediastinal parathyroid tumors: a clinical and pathological study of 84 cases. *Ann Surg* 1970;171:165–170.
24. Wang CA: The anatomic basis of parathyroid surgery. *Ann Surg* 1976;183:271–275.
25. Deleplanque G, Kraimps JL, Coste G, et al: A case of parathyroid adenoma localized in the middle mediastinum. *Ann Chir* 1989;43:393–396.
26. Murphy MN, Glennon PG, Diocee MS, et al: Nonsecretory parathyroid carcinoma of the mediastinum. Light microscopic, immunocytochemical, and ultrastructural features of a case, and review of the literature. *Cancer* 1986;58:2468–2476.
27. Clark OH: Mediastinal parathyroid tumors. *Arch Surg* 1988;123:1096–1100.
28. Nudelman IL, Deutsch AA, Reiss R: Primary hyperparathryoidism due to mediastinal parathyroid adenoma. *Int Surg* 1987;72:104–108.
29. Doppman JL, Krudy AG, Brennan MF, et al: CT appearance of enlarged parathyroid glands in the posterior superior mediastinum. *J Comput Assist Tomogr* 1982;6:1099–1102.
30. Brennan MF, Doppman JL, Marx SJ, et al: Reoperative parathyroid surgery for persistent hyperparathyroidism. *Surgery* 1978;83:669–676.
31. Krudy AG, Doppman JL, Brennan MF, et al: The detection of mediastinal parathyroid glands by computed tomography, selective arteriography and venous sampling: an analysis of 17 cases. *Radiology* 1981;140:739–744.
32. Whitley NO, Bohlman M, Connor TB, et al: Computed tomography for localization of parathyroid adenomas. *J Comput Assist Tomogr* 1981;5:812–817.
33. Massac E Jr, Righini M, Seremetis M: Mediastinal hyperfunctioning parathryoid adenoma. *J Natl Med Assoc* 1982;74:385–387.
34. Wang CA, Gaz RD, Moncure AC: Mediastinal parathyroid exploration: a clinical and pathologic study of 47 cases. *World J Surg* 1986;10:687–695.
35. Hotes LS, Barzilay J, Cloud LP, et al: Spontaneous hematoma of a parathyroid adenoma. *Am J Med Sci* 1989;297:331–333.
36. Wolff M, Goodman EN: Functioning lipoadenoma of a supernumerary parathyroid gland in the mediastinum. *Head Neck Surg* 1980;2:302–307.
37. Hargreaves HK, Wright TC Jr: A large functioning parathyroid lipoadenoma found in the posterior mediastinum. *Am J Clin Pathol* 1981;76:89–93.
38. Le Golvan DP, Moore BP, Nishiyama RH: Parathyroid hamartoma. *Am J Clin Pathol* 1977;67:31–35.
39. Lack EE, Stillinger RA, Colvin DB, et al: Aortico-pulmonary paraganglioma. Report of a case with ultrastructural study and review of the literature. *Cancer* 1979;43:269–278.
40. Dripps RD Jr, Comroe JH Jr: The clinical significance of the carotid and aortic bodies. *Am J Med Sci* 1944;208:681–694.
41. Lack EE: Hyperplasia of vagal and carotid body paraganglia in patients with chronic hypoxemia. *Am J Pathol* 1978;91:497–516.
42. Olson JL, Salyer WR: Mediastinal paragangliomas (aortic body tumor): a report of four cases and a review of the literature. *Cancer* 1978;41:2405–2412.
43. Patcher MR: Mediastinal nonchromaffin paraganglioma. A clinicopathological study based on 8 cases. *J Thorac Cardiovasc Surg* 1963;45:152–160.
44. Arom KV, Nicoloff DM: Intrathoracic paraganglioma arising from aorticosympathetic paraganglion. *Arch Surg* 1976;111:275–279.
45. Ashley DJB, Evans CJ: Intrathoracic carotid-body tumour (chemodectoma). *Thorax* 1966;21:184–185.
46. Barrie JD: Intrathoracic tumours of carotid body type (chemodectoma). *Thorax* 1961;16:78–86.

47. Ogawa J, Inoue H, Koide S, et al: Functioning paraganglioma in the posterior mediastinum. *Ann Thorac Surg* 1982;33:507–510.
48. Routh A, Hickman BT, Hardy JD, et al: Malignant chemodectoma of posterior mediastinum. *South Med J* 1982;75:879–881.
49. Nickels J, Friman CE: Chemodectoma of the lower mediastinum. Report of a case. *Ann Chir Gynaecol Fenn* 1972;61:124–127.
50. Shaw KM, Kennedy JD: Chemodectoma (non-chromaffin paraganglioma) of the ninth intercostal space. *Thorax* 1956;11:57–59.
51. Fernandez BB, Hernandez FJ, Staley CJ: Chemodectoma of the vagus nerve: report of a case with ultrastructural study. *Cancer* 1975;35:263–269.
52. Del Fante FM, Watkins E Jr: Chemodectoma of the heart in a patient with multiple chemodectomas and familial history. Case report and survey of literature. *Lahey Clin Found Bull* 1967;16:224-229.
53. Lacquet LK, Moulijn AC, Jongerius CM, et al: Intrathoracic chemodectoma with multiple localizations. *Thorax* 1977;32:203–209.
54. Haber S: Retroperitoneal and mediastinal chemodectoma. Report of a case and review of the literature. *Am J Roentgenol* 1964;92:1029–1041.
55. Aggarwal P, Wali JP, Venugopal P, et al: Functional, malignant intrathoracic paraganglioma. *Postgrad Med J* 1989;65:177–179.
56. Dunn GD, Brown MJ, Sapsford RN, et al: Functioning middle mediastinal paraganglioma (phaeochromocytoma) associated with intercarotid paragangliomas. *Lancet* 1986;1:1061–1064.
57. Dajee A, Dajee H, Hinrichs S, et al: Pulmonary chondroma, extra-adrenal paraganglioma, and gastric leiomyosarcoma: Carney's triad. *J Thorac Cardiovasc Surg* 1982;84:377–381.
58. Grace MP, Batist G, Grace WR, et al: Aorticopulmonary paraganglioma and gastric leiomyoblastoma in a young woman. *Am J Med* 1981;70:1288–1292.
59. D'Altorio RA, Rishi US, Bhagwanani DG: Arteriographic findings in mediastinal chemodectoma. *J Thorac Cardiovasc Surg* 1974;67:963–965.
60. Victor S, Anand KV, Andappan P, et al: Malignant mediastinal chemodectoma. *Chest* 1975;68:583–584.
61. Enquist RW, Tormey DC, Jenis EH, et al: Malignant chemodectoma of the superior mediastinum with elevated urinary homovanillic acid. *Chest* 1974;66:209–211.
62. Kawai K, Kimura S, Miyamoto J, et al: A case of multiple extra-adrenal pheochromocytomas. *Endocrinol Jpn* 1979;26:693–696.
63. Feigin GA, Robinson B, Marchevsky A: Mixed tumor of the mediastinum. *Arch Pathol Lab Med* 1986;110:80–81.
64. Gale JT, Mendelson DS, Cohen BA, et al: Benign mixed tumor of salivary gland origin presenting as a mediastinal mass. *J Comput Tomogr* 1986;10:23–25.

9

Lymphoid Proliferations and Malignant Lymphoma of the Mediastinum

Jonathan W. Said, M.D. and Alberto M. Marchevsky, M.D.

Both lymph nodes in the mediastinum and the thymus may be involved in a variety of lymphoproliferative disorders ranging from true reactive lymphoid hyperplasias to malignant lymphomas. Lymphoid proliferations are among the most common causes of mediastinal masses, and malignant lymphomas are the most frequent malignant tumors of the mediastinum (1,2).

DISTRIBUTION OF MEDIASTINAL LYMPH NODES

Mediastinal lymph nodes are characterized according to their anatomic location as: (a) anterior mediastinal nodes, including those to the right and front of the superior vena cava and right innominate vein and along the border of the thymus and phrenic nerve, and on the left along the main pulmonary artery and in front of the aortic arch and left carotid artery along the phrenic and vagus nerves; (b) peritracheobronchial nodes, including the right and left paratracheal, subcarinal, retrotracheal, pretracheal, and pulmonary root nodes; (c) posterior mediastinal nodes behind the esophagus and in front of and alongside the aorta; (d) hilar lymph nodes; (e) intrapulmonary lymph nodes; and (f) parietal lymph nodes (3). Although any lymph node group may be affected by lymphoproliferative disorders, the anterosuperior and middle peritracheobronchial and hilar lymph nodes are most commonly involved.

CLASSIFICATION OF MEDIASTINAL LYMPHADENOPATHIES

A spectrum of lymphadenopathies both benign and malignant involve the mediastinum (Table 1). Most commonly encountered are malignant lymphoma and metastatic carcinoma, granulomatous lymphadenitis, and other forms of reactive lymphoid hyperplasia.

MALIGNANT LYMPHOMA OF THE MEDIASTINUM

The mediastinum may be involved in approximately 15% to 20% of patients with malignant lymphoma (1,2,4–7) but is less frequently the site of presentation of primary disease. In a series reported by Lichtenstein and associates (8), patients presenting with symptoms of an enlarging mediastinal mass comprised only 17 of 184

TABLE 1. *Mediastinal lymphadenopathies*

Granulomatous lymphoid proliferations
   Tuberculosis
   Fungal infections (histoplasmosis, coccidiomycosis, etc.)
   Sarcoidosis
   Silicosis
   Wegener's granulomatosis
Reactive lymphoid hyperplasias
   Nonspecific lymphoid hyperplasia
   Systemic lupus erythematosus
   Infectious mononucleosis
Angiofollicular lymphoid hyperplasia (Castleman's disease)
Neoplasms
   Hodgkin's disease
   Non-Hodgkin's lymphomas
   Plasmacytoma
   Leukemic infiltration
   Metastatic carcinoma

adult patients with non-Hodgkin's lymphomas of the thorax. Hodgkin's disease (nodular sclerosis or mixed cellularity type) is the most common form of malignant lymphoma involving the mediastinum in adults. In children, lymphoblastic lymphoma is more common than Hodgkin's disease in terms of primary mediastinal presentation.

Hodgkin's Disease

Hodgkin's disease is the most frequent form of malignant lymphoma involving the mediastinum in adults, where it usually affects the prevascular, tracheobronchial, and/or paratracheal node groups (9). The thymus may also be primarily involved. Other lymph node chains, such as the posterior mediastinal lymph nodes, are affected less frequently.

Etiology

Hodgkin's disease affects both sexes and has a bimodal age distribution with the largest peak in the third to fourth decades and a second lower peak after age 50. Men are affected more often than women, although the subtype of nodular sclerosis is somewhat more common in females. Epidemiologic studies suggest an increased risk among family members but there is no increased risk among physicians and nurses caring for Hodgkin's disease patients, and there is no clear evidence that Hodgkin's is caused by an infectious agent or is the result of viral oncogenesis. Monoclonal integration of Epstein–Barr (EB) virus genomes (10) and detection of EB virus messenger RNA in Reed–Sternberg (RS) cells (11) suggests a direct role for EB virus in the pathogenesis of at least some cases of Hodgkin's disease.

Pathology

Hodgkin's disease usually presents with peripheral lymphadenopathy, and in most cases there is an orderly sequence of disease progression to adjacent node groups.

Cervical, axillary, and, less commonly, inguinal nodes may be the site of presentation. Mediastinal lymph node extension most commonly follows involvement of the right supraclavicular lymph nodes (12). The current classification of Hodgkin's disease was described by Lukes (13) and modified at the Rye symposium.

Nodular sclerosis Hodgkin's disease is the most frequent type involving the mediastinum and is characterized by birefringent collagen bands surrounding nodules with a mixed background of small lymphocytes, plasma cells, histiocytes, eosinophils, and both lacunar and diagnostic RS cells (Fig. 9-1). Lacunar cells are characterized by abundant, clear cytoplasm that retracts leaving an artifactual clear space in formalin-fixed tissues (Fig. 9-2). Classic RS cells are large polyploid cells with bilobed or multilobed nuclei and large inclusion like nucleoli surrounded by a clear halo (Fig. 9-3). With the exception of the RS cells in lymphocyte predominance Hodgkin's disease, which mark as B-lymphocytes (14), RS cells are characteristically negative for common leukocyte antigen and express Leu M1 (CD15) and Kil or Ber H2 (CD30).

Nodular sclerosis can be subclassified into grades 1 and 2 as reported by the British National Lymphoma Investigation (BNLI) (15). Grade 2, which is characterized by a background proliferation in which there are areas of lymphoid depletion or numerous pleomorphic RS cells, is associated with a relatively poor prognosis. In the "syncytial variant" of Hodgkin's disease, which may also involve the mediastinum, RS variants are present in sheets and cohesive clusters (Fig. 9-4) that can simulate

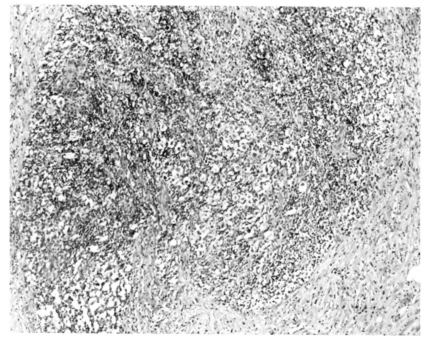

FIG. 9–1. Nodular sclerosis Hodgkin's disease with lymphoid nodules, many lacunar cells, and polymorphic lymphoid infiltrates surrounded by irregular, dense fibrous bands. (H&E × 40, original)

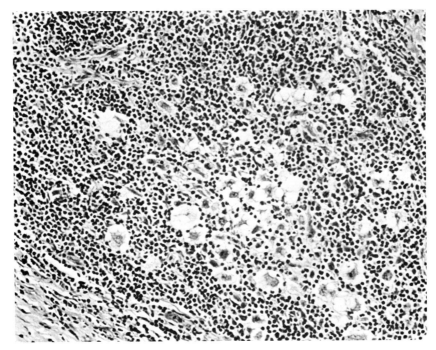

FIG. 9–2. Nodular sclerosis Hodgkin's disease with lacunar cells. (H&E × 100, original)

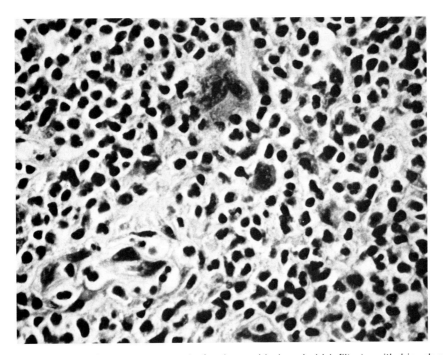

FIG. 9–3. Hodgkin's disease composed of polymorphic lymphoid infiltrate with binucleated Reed–Sternberg cells. (H&E × 400, original)

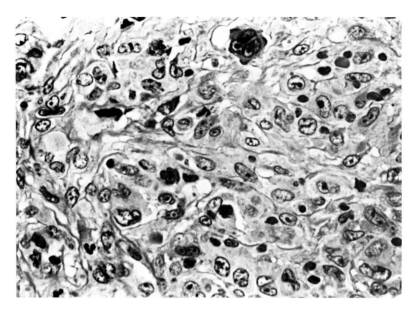

FIG. 9–4. Syncytial variant of nodular sclerosis Hodgkin's disease. Nodule is comprised of sheets of lacunar Reed–Sternberg cells with one diagnostic binucleate cell (top). (H&E × 120, original)

metastatic neoplasms, thymoma, and non-Hodgkin's lymphomas particularly in small biopsy specimens (16).

Lymphocyte predominance Hodgkin's disease (less than 10% of the total cases in most series) occurs in a nodular and diffuse variety (Fig. 9-5) and consists of lymphocytes and histiocytes in variable proportions with numerous lymphocyte and histiocyte (L&H) RS variants but only rare diagnostic RS cells (13). Mixed cellularity Hodgkin's disease has a polymorphous cellular composition in which diagnostic RS cells are readily identified (Fig. 9-6). This accounts for approximately 30% of cases and tends to involve the older age group. Lymphocyte depletion Hodgkin's disease, rare in the mediastinum, occurs in a diffuse fibrosis variant in which there is a disorderly proliferation of nonbirefringent reticulum fibers and a reticular variant with many diagnostic and sarcomatous RS cells (Fig. 9-7).

Staging of Hodgkin's Disease

Hodgkin's disease is staged according to the number of involved sites and their distribution above and below the diaphragm (Table 2). In addition to histologic type and stage of disease, presence of B-symptoms, which include fever, night sweats, and loss of 10% of the body weight in the preceding six months, are of prognostic significance.

Mediastinal Involvement by Hodgkin's Disease

Mediastinal involvement is most common with nodular sclerosis, less frequent in mixed cellularity, and unusual in lymphocyte predominance and lymphocyte de-

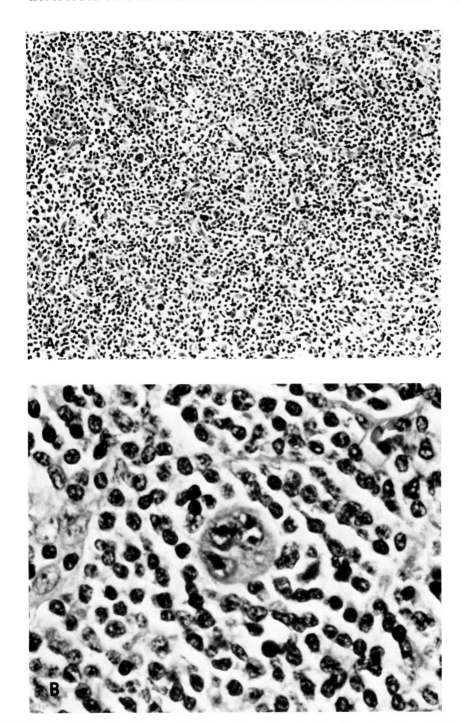

FIG. 9–5. A: LPHD with diffuse proliferation of small lymphoid cells and scattered "L & H" Reed–Sternberg variants. (H&E × 100, original) **B:** Higher magnification reveals a rare diagnostic Reed–Sternberg cell. (H&E × 400, original)

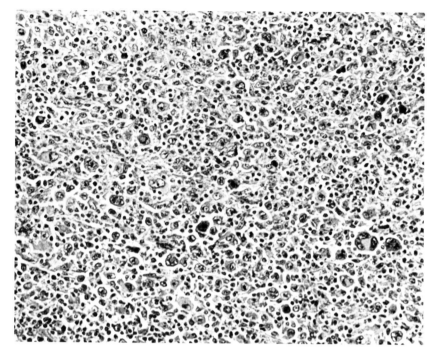

FIG. 9–6. Mixed cellularity Hodgkin's disease showing polymorphic lymphoid infiltrate with many Reed–Sternberg cells. (H&E × 100, original)

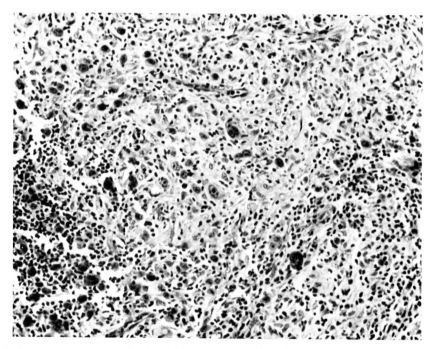

FIG. 9–7. Lymphocyte depletion Hodgkin's disease with multiple pleomorphic giant cells and fibrosis. (H&E × 100, original)

TABLE 2. *Staging classification of Hodgkin's disease*

Stage	Definition
I	Single lymph node region (I) or extralymphatic site (I$_E$)
II	Two or more lymph node regions on the same side of the diaphragm (II), or one or more nodes on the same side of diaphragm and a site of extralymphatic involvement on the same side of the diaphragm (II$_E$)
III	Lymph node regions on both sides of the diaphragm (III), which may include the spleen (III$_S$) or extralymphatic site (III$_E$)
IV	Disseminated disease with involvement of one or more extralymphatic organs including bone marrow, liver, lung, and skin

pleted subtypes. Presence of a large mediastinal mass (Fig. 9-8) is an unfavorable prognostic factor, and treatment with single modality therapy may be unsuccessful (17). Unfortunately, authors have proposed different criteria for bulky mediastinal disease. In most series, results depend on the retrospective review of chest radiographs; the measurement that has been most consistently used is the ratio of maximal mediastinal width to chest diameter (mediastinal mass ratio, or MMR) (18). Large mediastinal masses are usually considered those with an MMR between 33% and 50%.

Treatment and Prognosis of Mediastinal Hodgkin's Disease

Mediastinal Hodgkin's disease generally has a favorable prognosis, and the presenting stage is usually early with stage I or II disease. The adjacent cervical lymph nodes are the nodal site most often involved by direct extension. Patients with stage I and II disease and mediastinal involvement at the time of initial diagnosis have a 88% 5-year survival rate compared with 98% survival rates for individuals in similar stages lacking mediastinal masses (19). Patients with stage III disease have a similar 5-year survival rate regardless of the presence of a mediastinal mass, although those with mediastinal involvement have lower disease-free survivals. Ferrant and associates (20) recommend combined modality therapy consisting of nitrogen mustard,

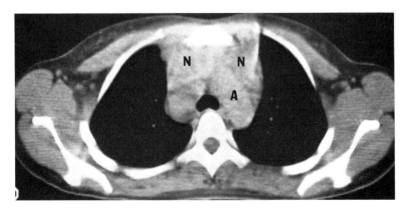

FIG. 9–8. Hodgkin's disease. Computed tomographic scan at the level of the aortic arch (*A*) demonstrates marked anterior and superior mediastinal lymphadenopathy (*N*).

vincristine, procarbazine, and prednisone (MOPP) chemotherapy followed by radiotherapy in patients with mediastinal Hodgkin's disease to increase complete remission rate and survival. Symptomatic patients with large mediastinal masses may respond poorly despite combined modality therapy (20).

Mediastinal Non-Hodgkin's Lymphomas (Other Than Lymphoblastic Lymphoma)

With the exception of lymphoblastic lymphoma, which will be discussed separately and is more common in children, malignant lymphoma localized to the mediastinum and adjacent structures at presentation is unusual and occurs in only about 6% of non-Hodgkin's lymphoma patients (21). Table 3 is a classification of non-Hodgkin's lymphomas according to the working formulation and their equivalents in the Rappaport classification. Many mediastinal lymphomas are not easily classified according to the formulation, however. Primary mediastinal non-Hodgkin's lymphomas are diffuse, and the vast majority are of large cell morphology. Evidence suggests that thymic and mediastinal large cell lymphomas are similar B-lineage neoplasms and originate in resident nonneoplastic thymic B-cells (22). These B-cells are normally present in the medulla and extraparenchymal septae, and phenotypically they express positivity for CD19, CD20, CD22, IgM, and IgD heavy chains (22).

Clinical Findings

Mediastinal lymphomas occur in all age groups, with the highest incidence in the fourth decade of life. There is a female preponderance of greater than 60%. Involvement of visceral organs, such as the kidneys, is relatively common compared with the extent of simultaneous lymph node involvement (22). In one series, malignant lymphomas of the high-grade immunoblastic subtype occurred at an older age (mean 54 years) (23). The majority of patients who present with symptoms of mediastinal enlargement also have contiguous nodal as well as extranodal disease (Fig. 9-9), including infiltration of the pulmonary parenchyma, pericardium, sternum, sternal soft tissues, chest wall, and vena cava (Fig. 9-10) (21). Cough, chest pain, dyspnea, and venous obstruction are common early signs (24).

While regional radiotherapy has been used to treat localized mediastinal non-Hodgkin's lymphoma with variable results, the high incidence of contiguous and extranodal spread has led many authors to recommend combination chemotherapy with or without adjuvant mediastinal irradiation (21). Achievement of complete remission after chemotherapy appears to be a major prognostic factor (25).

Histologic Appearance

Although mediastinal involvement occurs with roughly equal frequency in follicular and diffuse non-Hodgkin's lymphomas, almost all patients with primary mediastinal disease have diffuse histologic types (21), most commonly intermediate-grade diffuse large cell lymphomas. Mediastinal large cell lymphomas are often associated with sclerosis (mediastinal diffuse large cell lymphoma with sclerosis) (Fig. 9-11) (26), but sclerosis may be variable and is not always present. High-grade

TABLE 3. *Working formulation of non-Hodgkin's lymphomas for clinical usage: comparison with the Rappaport classification*

Working formulation	Rappaport classification
Low grade	

A.   Malignant lymphoma
    Small lymphocytic consistent with CLL
      plasmacytoid
	Lymphocytic, well-differentiated

B.   Malignant lymphoma, follicular
    Predominantly small cleaved cell; diffuse
      areas, sclerosis
	Nodular, poorly differentiated
	  lymphocytic

C.   Malignant lymphoma, follicular
    Mixed, small cleaved and large cell; diffuse
      areas, sclerosis
	Nodular, mixed, lymphohistiocytic

Intermediate grade	

D.   Malignant lymphoma, follicular
    Predominantly large cell
      Diffuse areas
      Sclerosis
	Nodular histiocytic

E.   Malignant lymphoma, diffuse
    Small cleaved cell
      Sclerosis
	Diffuse, poorly differentiated
	  lymphocytic

F.   Malignant lymphoma, diffuse
    Mixed, small and large cell
      Sclerosis
      Epithelioid cell component
	Diffuse, mixed, lymphohistiocytic

G.   Malignant lymphoma, diffuse
    Large cell
      Cleaved cell
      Noncleaved cell
      Sclerosis
	Diffuse, histiocytic

High grade	

H.   Malignant lymphoma
    Large cell, immunoblastic
      Plasmacytoid
      Clear cell
      Polymorphous
      Epithelioid cell component
	Diffuse, histiocytic

I.   Malignant lymphoma
    Lymphoblastic
      Convoluted cell
      Nonconvoluted cell
	Lymphoblastic

J.   Malignant lymphoma
    Small noncleaved cell
      Burkitt's
      Follicular areas
	Undifferentiated Burkitt's and
	  undifferentiated non-Burkitt's

Miscellaneous Composite Mycosis fungoides Histiocytic Extramedullary plasmacytoma Unclassifiable Other	

B-cell lymphomas, according to the Working Formulation (immunoblastic and Burkitt-like lymphomas), occur infrequently. Lymphomas may arise from mediastinal lymph nodes or in the thymus. Areas of uninvolved thymic cortex may be evident, and there may be thymic cysts with squamous epithelial lining infiltrated by lymphocytes (22).

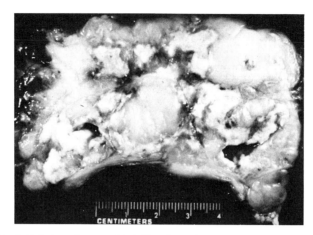

FIG. 9–9. Non-Hodgkin's lymphoma with infiltration of lymph nodes and surrounding soft tissues and with extensive tumor necrosis.

Large B-cell Lymphoma of the Thymus and Mediastinum

Many B-cell malignant lymphomas of the thymus and mediastinum have abundant, clear cytoplasm (22) and have been called *mediastinal clear cell lymphomas* (Fig. 9-12). A relationship to sinusoidal (monocytoid) B-cells has been suggested (27), and, immunophenotypically, cells correspond to a late stage of B-cell differentiation (CD19$^+$, CD20$^+$) with loss of surface immunoglobulins. Although these tumors are difficult to classify histologically, these have a rapid proliferation rate and an aggressive clinical course. These lymphomas may be derived from a unique population of B-cells that is normally present within the thymus.

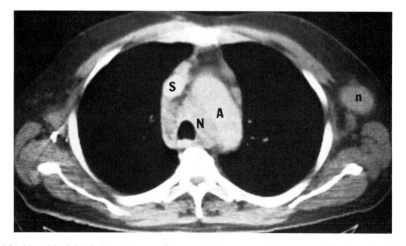

FIG. 9–10. Non-Hodgkin's lymphoma. Computed tomographic scan at the level of the aortic arch demonstrates lymphadenopathy (*N*) surrounding the trachea and displacing the aortic arch (*A*) and superior vena cava (*S*). An enlarged lymph node is also noted in the left axilla (*n*).

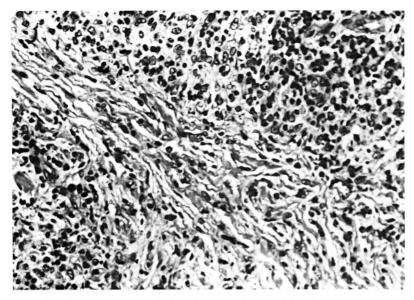

FIG. 9–11. Mediastinal non-Hodgkin's lymphoma with broad band of sclerosis. (H&E × 80, original)

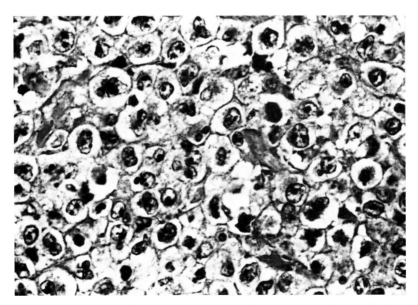

FIG. 9–12. Mediastinal clear cell lymphoma. Large malignant lymphoid cells with B-cell phenotype have irregular nuclei and clear cytoplasm with well-defined cell membranes. (H&E × 250, original)

Histologic subtypes of large B-cell mediastinal lymphoma include *large cleaved* and *large noncleaved* follicular center cell lymphomas. Mixtures of angulated, cleaved, and noncleaved cells may be present (Fig. 9-13), and subtypes are frequently difficult to classify in the working formulation (22). Nuclei show variable but usually mild pleomorphism and are two to four times the size of a small lymphocyte. Nuclear heterochromatin is fine and marginated against the nuclear membrane. In addition to noncleaved nuclei, nuclei with cleaved and angulated nuclear outlines may be present. Multinucleated giant cells, including RS-like forms, may be present, but the uniform proliferation of large lymphoid cells rules out Hodgkin's disease. Variable numbers of small lymphoid cells and histiocytes may be present as part of the reactive lymphoid proliferation and may be intimately admixed with the large lymphoid cells.

In rare cases, mediastinal large cell lymphomas have an immunoblastic appearance and consist of sheets of large, transformed, lymphoid cells with immunoblastic or plasmacytoid features (Fig. 9-14). Nuclei are large with two or three evenly spaced nucleoli frequently aligned along the nuclear membrane, and the cytoplasm is relatively abundant and amphophilic on Giemsa stain.

Immunophenotyping

With rare exceptions mediastinal non-Hodgkin's lymphomas, other than the lymphoblastic type, are B-cell neoplasms. Surface immunoglobulins may be absent in

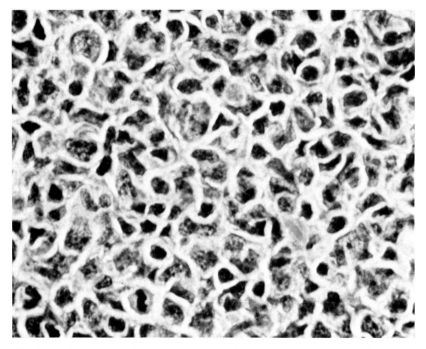

FIG. 9–13. Follicular center cell lymphoma comprised of large lymphoid cells, many with irregular, angulated, and cleaved nuclear outlines.

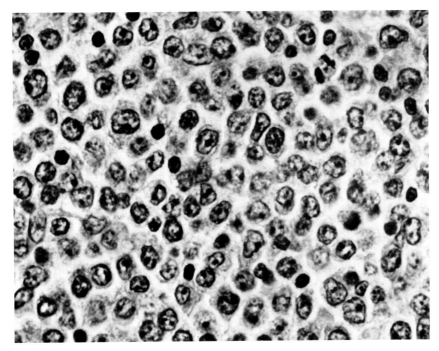

FIG. 9–14. Malignant lymphoma, large cell, immunoblastic, composed of large immunoblasts with open nuclei, prominent nucleoli, and rim of basophilic cytoplasm. Smaller plasmacytoid cells are also present. (H&E × 400, original)

mediastinal large cell lymphomas, but almost all express common leukocyte antigen and B-cell–restricted/associated antigens such as CD20 (23,27). Table 4 summarizes commonly used monoclonal antibodies in the phenotyping of B- and T-cell mediastinal lymphomas.

Rare Mediastinal Non-Hodgkin's Lymphomas

T-cell lymphomas (other than lymphoblastic lymphoma) are rare in the mediastinum and are predominantly T-cell large lymphoid or T-immunoblastic type (28). T-cell non-Hodgkin's lymphomas resemble their B-cell counterparts in terms of age at presentation, male to female ratio, and incidence of concomitant nodal and extranodal disease. T-cell lymphomas on one series responded poorly to therapy compared with large B-cell lymphomas of the mediastinum (28).

Other types of lymphoma, including composite Hodgkin's disease and non-Hodgkin's lymphoma, occur rarely (26). Burkitt-like lymphoma (high-grade malignant lymphoma, small noncleaved cell type) (Fig. 9-15) with a mediastinal presentation is rare but has been described in immunosuppressed individuals following transplantation (29). B-cell immunoblastic lymphomas primary in the mediastinum may be seen in patients with acquired immune deficiency syndrome (J. W. Said, unpublished observation).

TABLE 4. *Monoclonal antibodies useful in phenotyping mediastinal lymphomas*

CD1* (OKT6, Leu6)	Cortical thymocyte marker
	T-lymphoblastic lymphomas (65%)
CD2 (OKT11, Leu5b)	Sheep red blood cell receptor
	T-cell lymphomas (>70%).
CD3 (OKT3, Leu4)	T-cell receptor in the T-cell membrane
	80%–95% peripheral T-cells
	>50% T-lymphoblastic lymphoma
CD4 (OKT4, Leu3a)	T-cells of helper/inducer type
CD5 (OKT1, Leu1)	T1 antigen present on 95% peripheral T-cells
	95% thymocytes
	Some B-cell lymphomas and CLL
CD7 (3A1, Leu9)	FC receptor for IgM
	All thymocytes
	Human natural killer cells
	T-lymphoblastic lymphomas
CD8 (OKT8, Leu2a)	Suppressor cytotoxic T-cells
CD15 (LeuM1)	Reed–Sternberg cells
	Antibody (LeuM1 useful in paraffin sections
CD20 (B1, Leu16)	B-cell antigen
	L26 antibody useful in paraffin sections
CD30 (Ki1, BerH2)	Activated T-cells
	Large cell anaplastic lymphomas
	Reed–Sternberg cells
	BerH2 antibody useful in paraffin sections
CD43 (MT1, Leu22)	T-cells and some B-cell lymphomas
	Antibody Leu22 useful in paraffin sections
CD45 (LCA, 9.4)	Leukocyte common antigen
CD45R (UCHL1)	Antibody UCHL1 (CD45R) stains predominantly
	T-cells in paraffin sections

*CD group with examples of commonly used antibodies in parentheses.

Low-Grade B-Cell Lymphoma of Mucosa-Associated Lymphoid Tissue (MALT) Arising in the Thymus

Rare cases of primary low-grade B-cell lymphoma (Fig. 9-16) have been described with histologic features similar to B-cell lymphomas arising in mucosa-associated lymphoid tissues (30). Lymphoid proliferation is present within residual Hassall's corpuscles, and consists of centrocyte-like, small lymphoid cells with variable but usually mild nuclear irregularity and clear cytoplasm and sharp cell borders. Occasional large, transformed lymphoid cells and scattered plasma cells are also present. With immunophenotyping, these cases show light chain restriction similar to MALT lymphomas at other sites. Although few cases have been described in the thymus, MALT lymphomas tend to be localized at presentation with a low mitotic rate and an indolent clinical course. The interrelationship between rare, low-grade thymic B-cell lymphomas and the more common large cell lymphomas is unclear. Both may be related to the unique B-cell population that is normally present in the thymus.

Differential Diagnosis of Mediastinal Non-Hodgkin's Lymphomas

Presence of pleomorphic RS-like cells in some non-Hodgkin's lymphomas can make differentiation from Hodgkin's disease difficult. Immunohistochemistry may

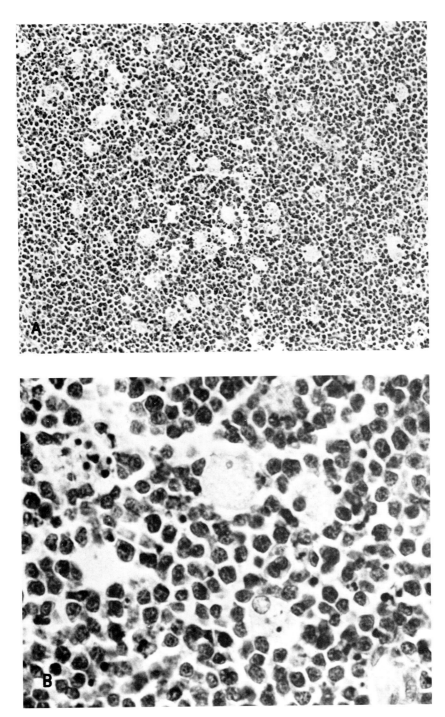

FIG. 9–15. A: Malignant lymphoma, small noncleaved cell, Burkitt's type, showing typical "starry-sky" feature. (H&E × 100) **B:** Higher magnification showing small noncleaved cells and interspersed benign histiocytes with tingible bodies. (H&E × 400, original)

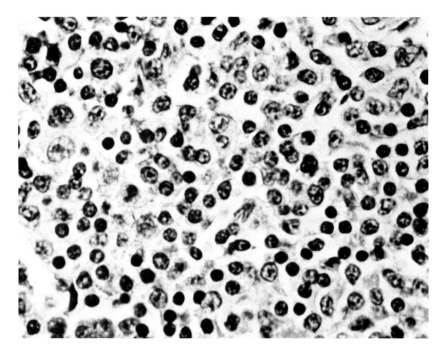

FIG. 9–16. Low-grade B-cell lymphoma comprised of small lymphoid cells. (H&E × 400, original)

be helpful since RS cells are usually common leukocyte antigen negative and CD15 and CD30 positive, while most mediastinal non-Hodgkin's lymphomas are common leukocyte antigen positive and express monoclonal immunoglobulins or B-cell–associated antigens such as CD20. Gene rearrangement studies may be helpful since most B-cell lymphomas have rearrangement of the immunoglobulin genes, rarely present in Hodgkin's disease.

Because of the presence of large, cohesive clusters of malignant cells sometimes with clear cytoplasm and associated sclerosis, malignant lymphoma may be confused with malignant thymoma, germ cell tumors (including seminoma), and metastatic carcinoma. Immunohistochemical staining for keratin in the case of thymoma and carcinoma, and for placental alkaline phosphatase in cases of seminoma, helps avoid this pitfall.

Mediastinal Lymphomas in the Pediatric Age Group

Hodgkin's disease accounts for 25% to 30% of malignant lymphomas in children and is rare under the age of three. Cases with mediastinal involvement are usually of the nodular sclerosis type, and pathology is similar to that described in adults. However, non-Hodgkin's lymphomas in children differ from those in adults in that they are mostly derived from precursor or stem cells. Burkitt's or small noncleaved cell lymphomas only rarely involve the mediastinum in nonimmunosuppressed individuals. Lymphoblastic lymphoma, however, which is biologically closely related to acute lymphoblastic leukemia (ALL) (31), involves the mediastinum in approximately 50% of cases.

Lymphoblastic Lymphoma

In 1975 Barcos and Lukes (32) described a type of non-Hodgkin's lymphoma that tended to affect older children, teenagers, and young adults with a male-female ratio of 2:1. The prognosis was poor, with a median survival of only 10 months. Most of these cases were previously classified as diffuse, poorly differentiated lymphocytic lymphomas, but certain morphologic features distinguish this proliferation from the rest of the group. Lymphoblastic lymphoma comprises about 33% of childhood and 5% of adult non-Hodgkin's lymphomas and involves the mediastinum in approximately 50% of patients.

The lymphoid proliferation in these cases is cytologically identical to that observed in tissues involved with ALL (31). Other findings include peripheral adenopathy, particularly cervical and supraclavicular lymph nodes, and pleural effusions. Bone marrow and peripheral blood involvement may be apparent at diagnosis or occur shortly thereafter. Involvement of the central nervous system is common and requires prophylactic chemotherapy. Recognition of this lymphoma type is of clinical importance, and aggressive chemotherapy regimens modeled after those used in high-risk ALL patients with meningeal prophylaxis, for example, have resulted in an improved prognosis, with up to 80% complete remission rates.

Pathology

Lymph nodes infiltrated by lymphoblastic lymphoma reveal diffuse effacement of the nodal architecture. The cells have fine chromatin, inconspicuous nucleoli, and a rapid proliferative rate with numerous mitoses (Fig. 9-17). In many cases, the cells have distinctive nuclear irregularities or fine convolutions resulting in nuclei with a "hand-in-glove" or "chicken's-foot" morphology. These irregularities may be best appreciated in thin, plastic sections or electron micrographs (Fig. 9-18). In some cases with identical clinical features, cells are round or oval, and nuclear convolutions may not be discerned (33). Although cells are usually intermediate in size, there may be a spectrum of lymphoid cells including small lymphoid or "microlymphoblastic" variants. Nuclear convolutions may be present in cells of all sizes, but nuclear complexity usually is increased in larger cells. In some cases, phagocytic histiocytes or "starry-sky" macrophages may be present, indicative of a rapid cell turnover.

A large cell variant of lymphoblastic lymphoma has also been described (34). In these cases, malignant cells have irregular nuclei and fine chromatin, but nucleoli are prominent in contrast to the small or inconspicuous nucleoli in other morphologic variants. Mediastinal involvement is usually not present with the large cell variant, however.

Immunophenotyping

The majority of mediastinal lymphoblastic lymphomas are T-cell neoplasms, and most reveal markers consistent with a common thymocyte stage of differentiation. Lymphoblastic lymphomas are the only type of non-Hodgkin's lymphomas that express CD1 (T6) and the DNA synthetic enzyme terminal deoxynucleotidyl transferase (TdT) (35). Assessment of intranuclear TdT is of value in classifying and con-

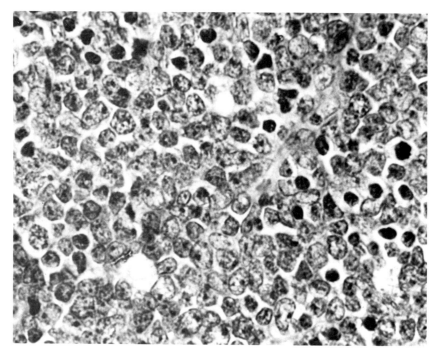

FIG. 9–17. Mediastinal lymphoblastic lymphoma consists of intermediate-sized lymphoid cells with fine chromatin, scant cytoplasm, and inconspicuous nucleoli. (H&E × 400, original)

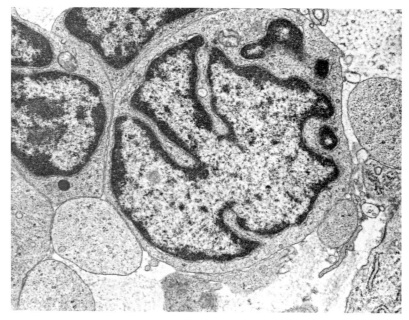

FIG. 9–18. Electron micrograph of mediastinal lymphoblastic lymphoma with a thymic T-cell phenotype (CD1 +, CD2 +, CD5 +, CD7 +, TdT +). The nucleus has characteristic dispersed heterochromatin and convoluted nuclear outline. (Uranyl acetate, lead citrate × 30,000, original)

firming the diagnosis of lymphoblastic lymphoma. Immunohistochemical stains for TdT are best performed on fresh tissue or imprints but can be determined in routinely processed formalin-fixed tissue if the sections are subjected to predigestion with pronase (36).

In some cases of lymphoblastic lymphoma, cells conform to an earlier stage of thymic maturation. T-cell markers most often expressed by lymphoblastic lymphomas include CD2 (T11), CD3 (T3), CD5 (T1), and CD7 (Leu9) (37). The presence of a mediastinal mass is most often seen in T-cell lymphoblastic lymphomas. Other phenotypes include expression of CD10 (CALLA), possibly with T-cell associated antigens. Expression of natural killer (NK) cell antigens has also been described (38,39). If only fixed tissue sections are available, T-cell antigens may be identified with UCHL-1 in a minor proportion of cases (40,41) and with CD43 (Leu22). Polyclonal antibodies to CD3 may also stain lymphoblastic lymphomas in paraffin sections (41).

Most lymphoblastic lymphomas that are not of thymic T-cell phenotype express a pre–B-cell phenotype (37,38,42). Surface immunoglobulins are usually absent, but cells express B-cell differentiation antigens, particularly CD19 (B4). Many also express CD20 (B1) and CD10 (CALLA).

MEDIASTINAL MASS WITH ACUTE LEUKEMIA

Mediastinal masses are frequent in children with lymphoblastic lymphomas and ALL as described previously. Acute monoblastic leukemia and acute myelogenous leukemia (AML) can also be associated with mediastinal masses.

In fewer than 3% of cases of AML, a tumor mass composed of malignant hematopoietic cells is the initial manifestation of the leukemic process (43). These lesions are designated as granulocytic sarcomas or chloromas and can pose difficult diagnostic problems for the surgical pathologist.

Indeed, granulocytic sarcomas are difficult to distinguish from poorly differentiated malignant lymphomas on routine histologic sections. They can be diagnosed, however, with accuracy with the aid of ultrastructural, histochemical, and immunocytochemical techniques. For example, lymphoid cells usually exhibit intracytoplasmic immunoglobulins that are absent in myelogenous cells. Myeloblastic cells exhibit a positive naphthol ASD chloroacetate esterase (NASD-CAE) reaction stainable with the Leder's reaction. Myeloid and monocytic cells have intracytoplasmic lysozyme detectable with immunoperoxidase techniques. All of these reactions can be performed on paraffin sections from lymph node biopsy specimens (44,45).

In addition, touch imprints of biopsy material can be stained with black Sudan B and myeloperoxidase, both of which identify early myeloid cells and blasts.

Ultrastructural studies are more expensive and time consuming but can be useful for demonstration of characteristic electron-dense granules in the cytoplasm of myelogenous cells (43,44).

MEDIASTINAL EXTRAMEDULLARY PLASMACYTOMAS

Extramedullary plasmacytomas are unusual forms of plasma cell dyscrasias in which there is a tumor mass composed of malignant plasma cells in the absence of multiple myeloma. These neoplasms usually occur in the head and neck area of mid-

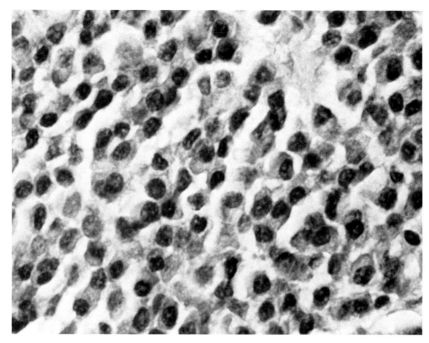

FIG. 9–19. Plasmacytoma composed of sheets of slightly pleomorphic plasma cells. (H&E × 400, original)

dle-aged men, but a few instances have been described in the mediastinum (46–48). The involvement of mediastinal lymph nodes by multiple myeloma also occurs (49). Diagnosis is made by the presence of sheets of plasma cells (Fig. 9-19) effacing normal architecture. Immature forms (plasmablasts), dysplastic, and multinucleate forms may be present but are not essential to the diagnosis.

METASTATIC NEOPLASMS

Numerous thoracic and extrathoracic neoplasms can metastasize to the mediastinal lymph nodes (50–56).

Metastases from thoracic organs usually originate from the esophagus or the lungs and are a poor prognostic sign (Figs. 9–20 and 9–21) (50,54).

Mediastinal metastases from extrathoracic neoplasms originating from the oral cavity, neck, upper respiratory passages, breast, and genitourinary tract (Fig. 9-22) are less frequent causes of mediastinal lymphadenopathy and are frequently accompanied by lymphangitic or hematogenous spread to the lungs (50). For example, 2.3% of 1,071 extrathoracic malignant neoplasms reviewed by McLoud and associates metastasized to the mediastinum; 40% of these patients had associated pulmonary involvement (56).

The mechanisms of extension of these neoplasms into the thorax are still incompletely understood. Head and neck tumors probably metastasize to the mediastinum through the anterior cervical lymph nodes, which communicate with the anterior mediastinal nodal chain (50).

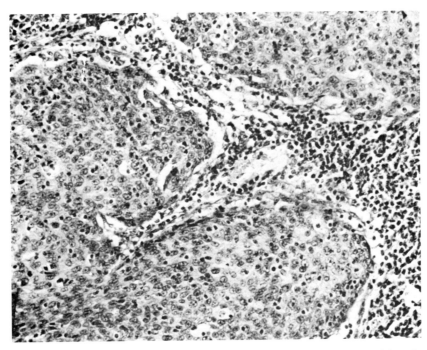

FIG. 9–20. Metastatic squamous cell carcinoma of the lung to mediastinal lymph node. (H&E × 100, original)

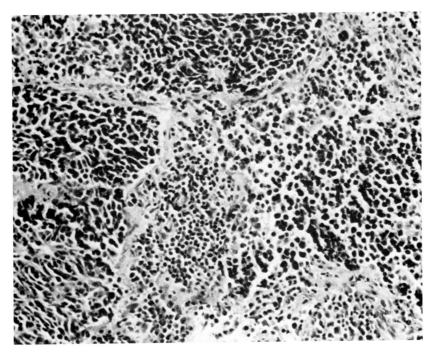

FIG. 9–21. Metastatic small-cell carcinoma of the lung, oat-cell type, to mediastinal lymph node. (H&E × 100, original)

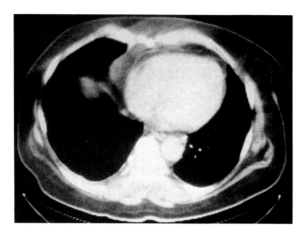

FIG. 9–22. Metastatic breast carcinoma to the anterior mediastinum.

Nasopharyngeal carcinoma (Schmincke's tumor) is a head and neck tumor that is of special interest to surgical pathologists because this neoplasm is frequently misdiagnosed as a large cell lymphoma when its characteristic sheets of large epithelial cells with vesicular nucleus, prominent nucleolus, and indistinct cytoplasm are not recognized (Fig. 9-23). Immunoperoxidase staining for cytokeratin in tumor cells can be helpful for the identification of difficult cases. The malignant cells will also be negative for common leukocyte antigen.

Genitourinary neoplasms such as renal cell carcinomas (Fig. 9-24), prostatic carcinomas (Fig. 9-25), and Wilm's tumors can also metastasize to the mediastinum through tumor emboli that migrate from the abdominal lymphatics into the thoracic duct and reflux into the bronchomediastinal trunks because of the absence or incompetence of the thoracic duct valves (52,53). This reflux mechanism can be demonstrated in 5% to 14% of patients undergoing lymphangiograms (50).

The breast is another source of metastatic tumors to the mediastinum because carcinomas located in the inner quadrants invade lymphatics that drain into the internal mammary and anterior mediastinal lymph nodes (50).

Malignant melanomas can also spread to the mediastinum through various lymphatic routes according to the location of the primary neoplasm (51).

GRANULOMATOUS LYMPHADENITIS AND LYMPHADENOPATHIES

Lymph node enlargement from granulomas is a frequent cause of mediastinal lymphadenopathy (57–59). Granulomas are specialized immune reactions that may be caused by insoluble and/or particulate substances that are phagocytized and mobilized by cells of the mononuclear phagocyte system (60,61). Lymph nodes are a frequent site of granulomas because they drain and filter the lymph, which carries various antigens, and also have all the cells necessary to produce an immunologic reaction (61).

Granulomas are localized compact collections of mature macrophages, which may evolve into epithelioid and giant cells. They can be classified on the basis of morphologic features into epithelioid cell, foreign body type, necrotizing, and nonnecro-

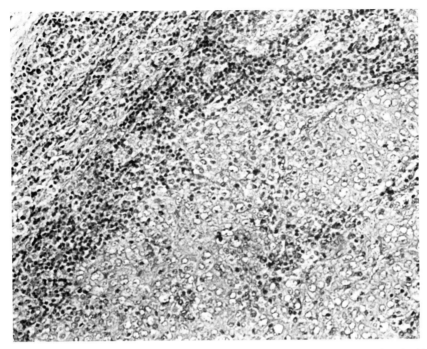

FIG. 9–23. Metastatic nasopharyngeal carcinoma (Schmincke's tumor) to mediastinal lymph node with characteristic sheets of large anaplastic cells with open nuclei and prominent nucleoli. (H&E × 100, original)

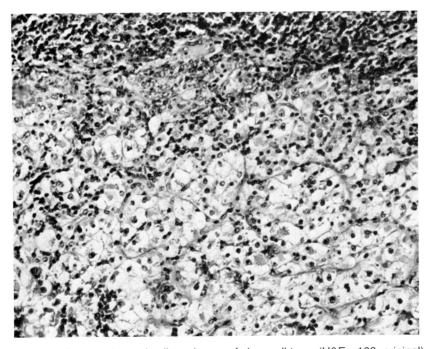

FIG. 9–24. Metastatic renal cell carcinoma of clear cell type. (H&E × 100, original)

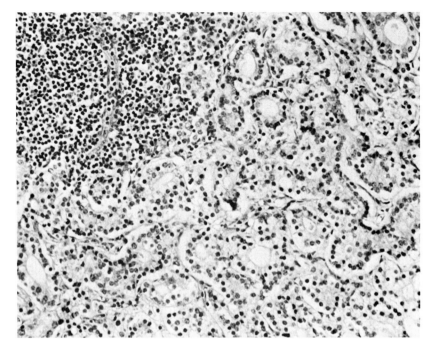

FIG. 9–25. Metastatic prostatic adenocarcinoma with characteristic small, regular glands lined by cuboidal cells with foamy cytoplasm. (H&E × 100, original)

tizing granulomas. Morphologic features such as the presence of necrosis in the granulomas give an indication about the cellular turnover rate of the lesions but do not help surgical pathologists to establish a specific etiologic diagnosis (60,61).

Granulomas result from various infectious and noninfectious causes (62). From a practical standpoint, a surgical pathologist confronted with a granulomatous lymphadenopathy in the mediastinum should culture a portion of the lesion for the detection of mycobacteria and fungi, perform special histochemical stains (Ziehl–Neelsen's, Gomori's methenamine silver) for the detection of infectious organisms, and examine the histologic slides with polarized light for the detection of silica and other refractile materials. However, even after all of these procedures, the etiology of granulomas remains unknown in many instances (62).

The most frequent causes of mediastinal granulomatous lymphadenopathies and lymphadenitides are listed in Table 1.

TUBERCULOUS LYMPHADENITIS

Mediastinal and hilar lymphadenopathy secondary to infections by *Mycobacterium tuberculosis* are common in children with primary tuberculosis (59,63–67). They are an unusual mode of presentation of the disease in adults, encountered in only 5% to 7% of pulmonary cases (59,67). Patients exhibit paratracheal, hilar, and/or anterior mediastinal lymph node enlargement and are often considered to have sarcoidosis or lymphomas on the basis of their roentgenologic findings and the markedly decreased frequency of tuberculosis in the United States.

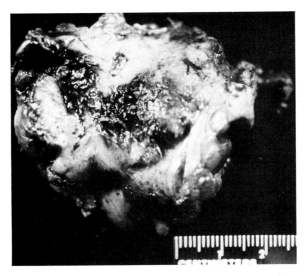

FIG. 9–26. Tuberculous lymphadenitis with matted lymph nodes and extensive necrosis.

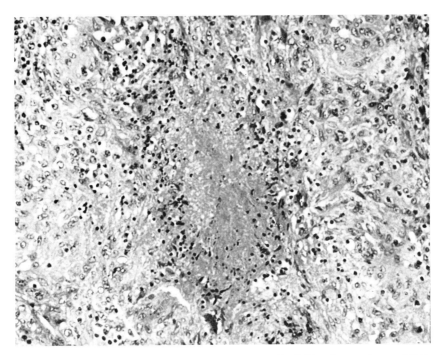

FIG. 9–27. Tuberculous lymphadenitis with caseating epithelioid cell granuloma. (H&E × 100, original)

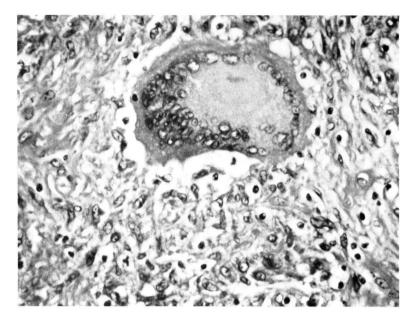

FIG. 9–28. Langerhan's-type giant cell in tuberculous lymphadenitis. (H&E × 400, original)

Tuberculous lymphadenitis presents with enlarged, soft, matted lymph nodes adherent to blood vessels and other mediastinal structures and containing multiple confluent white nodules with a friable "cheesy" material (Fig. 9–26). Smears of this material stained with the Ziehl–Neelsen or the Fite stains exhibit acid-fast bacilli (AFB). Older lesions are firm, gray–white, and calcified.

Histologically, tuberculous lymphadenitis has multiple confluent epithelioid granulomas at different stages of development (Fig. 9-27). Small granulomas are composed of compact collections of epithelioid cells with vesicular nuclei, single nucleoli, and large amphophilic or acidophilic cytoplasm with indistinct cellular borders. Giant cells of the Langhan's type, with multiple nuclei arranged at the periphery of the cells in a C or O shape, are also present (Fig. 9-28). Large granulomas exhibit central caseous, acellular, granular, eosinophilic necrosis. Older lesions have areas of fibrosis and/or calcification. Special stains reveal mycobacteria that are usually found within necrotic areas.

Granulomas caused by atypical mycobacterial infections are infrequent and have similar morphologic features to tuberculosis except in immunosuppressed patients, in whom granulomas may be absent (68,69).

FUNGAL LYMPHADENITIDES

Histoplasma capsulatum, Coccidioides immitis (Fig. 9–29), *Cryptococcus neoformans* (Fig. 9-30), and other fungal infections can cause granulomatous mediastinal lymphadenopathies with areas of central necrosis that are indistinguishable morphologically from tuberculosis, unless the etiologic organisms are identified.

Study of histologic slides stained with periodic acid Schiff reaction (PAS) and/or

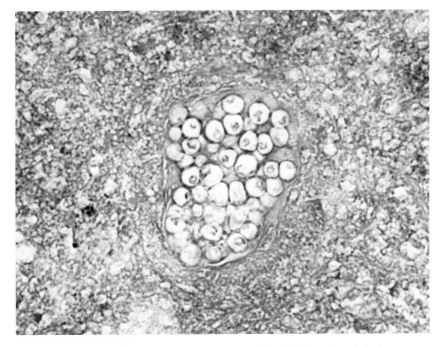

FIG. 9–29. Cyst of *Coccidioides immitis.* (H&E × 400, original)

Gomori's methenamine silver stains, culture of lymph node material, and laboratory tests (i.e., complement fixation test) are needed for a specific diagnosis.

SARCOIDOSIS

Sarcoidosis is a systemic granulomatous disease involving multiple lymph nodes, lung, liver, skin, bones, soft tissues, eyes, and salivary glands (70–75). It has a worldwide distribution and is more frequent in black women in their third through fifth decades of life (black/white 10:1; women/men 2:1).

The etiology of sarcoidosis is unknown. Several immunologic abnormalities have been observed in patients affected by the disease, including circulating immune complexes in serum, hypergammaglobulinemia, cutaneous anergy, and impaired T-cell functions (72). Patients also have elevated serum levels of lysozyme and angiotensin-converting enzyme, enzymes that are thought to be secreted by the epithelioid cells of the granulomas (76). In addition, 78% of sarcoidosis patients react positively with the Kveim–Siltzbach test (72).

The mediastinal lymph nodes are involved in 60% to 90% of patients with sarcoidosis (57). The hilar and paratracheal lymph nodes are the most frequently enlarged (77% of cases), although the anterior and posterior mediastinal nodes can also be involved (57,77,78).

The lymph nodes in sarcoidosis are uniformly enlarged and soft, with small nodules on section. Histologically, they are partially or completely replaced by multiple noncaseating epithelioid cell granulomas that are usually discrete, round, and rela-

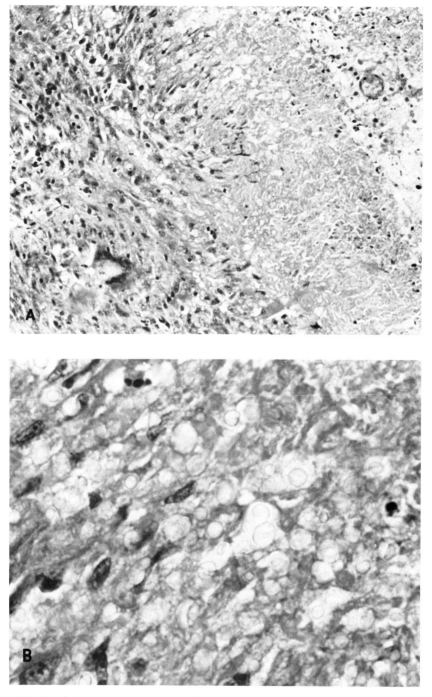

FIG. 9–30. A: Cryptococcal lymphadenitis with necrotizing epithelioid cell granuloma. (H&E × 100, original) **B:** Higher magnification showing numerous yeast forms of *Cryptococcus neoformans.* (H&E × 400, original)

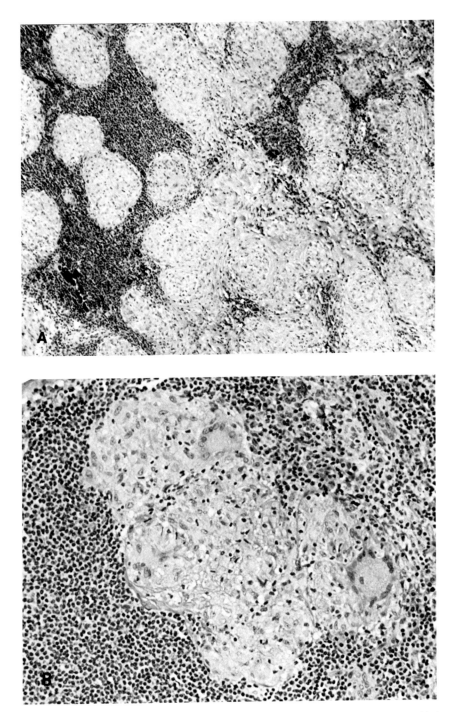

FIG. 9–31. A: Sarcoidosis with almost total replacement of nodal architecture by multiple confluent noncaseating epithelioid cell granulomas. (H&E × 40, original) **B:** Higher magnification of epithelioid cell granuloma with Langhan's-type giant cells. (H&E × 100)

tively uniform in size (Fig. 9-31). These granulomas can exhibit focal central areas of necrosis. Calcification is unusual (75).

Several intracellular and extracellular inclusion bodies have been described in sarcoidosis, such as the asteroid (Fig. 9-32), Schaumann (Fig. 9-33), or Hamazaki–Wesenberg bodies (Fig. 9-34). They are not pathognomonic of sarcoidosis. Asteroid bodies are eosinophilic spider-like intracytoplasmic inclusions composed of lipoproteins (Fig. 9-32). Schaumann bodies are intracellular, round, calcified, concentrically laminated structures (Fig. 9-33). Hamazaki–Wesenberg bodies are giant lysosomes present extracellularly and usually located outside the granulomas (Fig. 9-34). They appear as clusters of yellow–brown, round or spindle-shaped bodies on hematoxylin and eosin (H&E) stained preparations or as "yeasts" on Gomori methenamine-silver–stained preparations and can be confused with fungi (62,63).

SILICOSIS

Silicosis is a form of pneumoconiosis caused by inhalation of silica particles and characterized by silicotic nodules composed of epithelioid cell granulomas containing birefringent particles of silicon dioxide that can be demonstrated with polarized light in the lungs and hilar lymph nodes (79). The nodules become hyalinized in concentric layers, giving the lesion a characteristic "onion skin" appearance (Fig. 9-35).

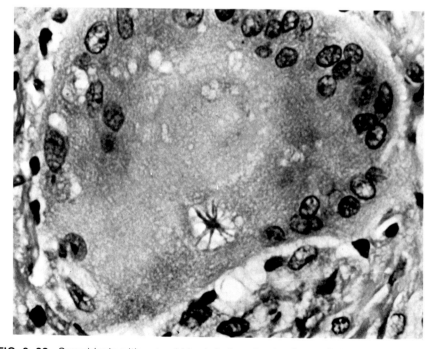

FIG. 9–32. Sarcoidosis with asteroid body in Langhan's giant cell. (H&E × 400, original)

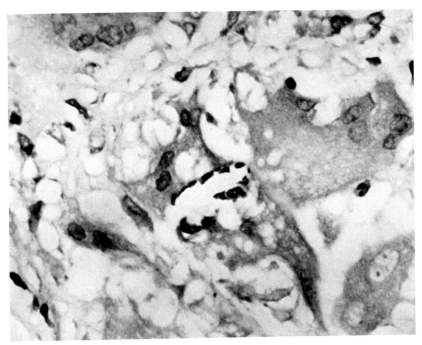

FIG. 9–33. Sarcoidosis. Calcified, laminated Schaumann body. (H&E × 400, original)

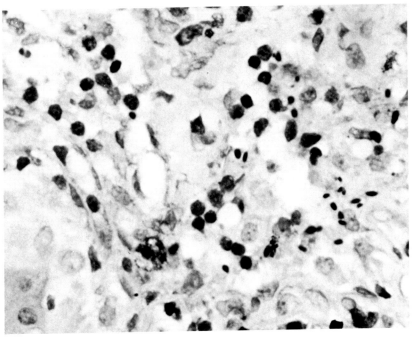

FIG. 9–34. Sarcoidosis. Round to spindle golden–brown extracellular Hamazaki–Wesenberg bodies. (H&E × 400, original)

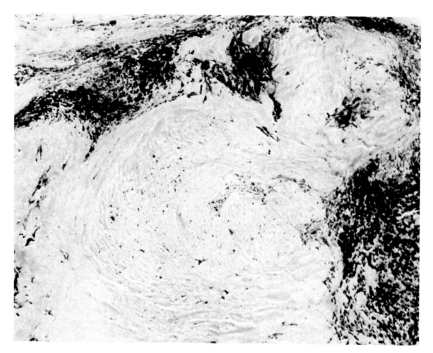

FIG. 9–35. Laminated, densely fibrotic silicotic nodule. (H&E × 40, original)

WEGENER'S GRANULOMATOSIS

Wegener's granulomatosis is a disease of unknown etiology characterized by granulomatous lesions and necrotizing angiitis in the upper respiratory tract, lungs, and kidneys (61). Biopsies of these lesions show fibrinoid necrosis of trabecular, capsular, and perinodal blood vessels, focal infarctions, and epithelioid cell granulomas (Fig. 9-36). Mediastinal lymph node enlargement on chest roentgenograms is frequent in patients with generalized forms of the disease (79).

GRANULOMATOUS LYMPHADENOPATHY ASSOCIATED WITH NEOPLASMS

Epithelial neoplasms, non-Hodgkin's lymphomas, and Hodgkin's disease can be associated with sarcoid-like epithelioid cell granulomas in lymph nodes (60).

The pathogenesis of these granulomas is still unclear. They can be prominent in Hodgkin's disease and obscure the presence of the malignant neoplasm (Fig. 9-37). Indeed, we have seen few cases of Hodgkin's disease misdiagnosed as sarcoidosis on the basis of the presence of abundant granulomas in the lymph nodes infiltrated by the neoplasm. In these cases, however, the epithelioid granulomas were irregularly distributed, did not involve the entire lymph node as is usual in sarcoidosis, and varied considerably in size and shape. In sarcoidosis, granulomas tend to be more uniform and are not admixed with areas of band-like fibrosis and sclerosis as seen in nodular sclerosis Hodgkin's disease. In instances of "sarcoidosis" with unusual histologic features, the pathologist should carefully search for local malignant areas scattered between the granulomas.

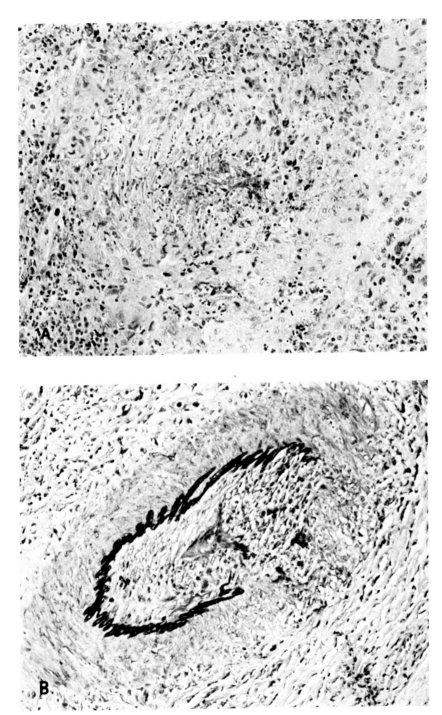

FIG. 9–36. A: Wegener's granulomatosis with characteristic necrotizing granulomas. (H&E × 100, original) **B:** Granulomatous vasculitis in area not adjacent to necrotizing granulomas. (H&E × 100, original)

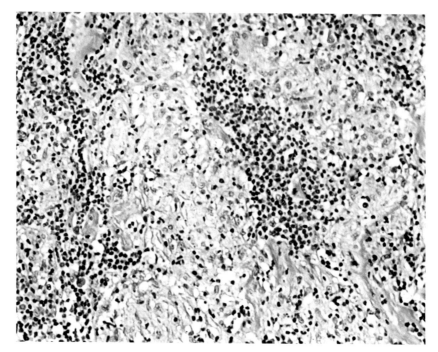

FIG. 9–37. Epithelioid granulomas in Hodgkin's disease. (H&E × 100, original)

ANGIOFOLLICULAR LYMPHOID HYPERPLASIA (CASTLEMAN'S DISEASE)

Angiofollicular hyperplasia was described in 1954 as a form of benign lymph node hyperplasia simulating thymoma (80). The disease appears most commonly as a solitary mass in the mediastinum, although a multicentric variant with systemic manifestations also occurs (81–85).

Clinical Features

Angiofollicular lymph node hyperplasia affects patients of all ages, and there is no sex predominance. Patients with localized disease are often asymptomatic and are found to have a large mediastinal mass on routine chest roentgenograms. Localized symptoms in patients with large mediastinal masses include signs of compression of mediastinal structures (e.g., dyspnea and cough) (86–89).

Systemic symptoms occur most often with multicentric disease and include fever, night sweats, weight loss, anemia, polyclonal hypergammaglobulinemia, elevated sedimentation rates, hypoalbuminemia, peripheral neuropathy, and growth retardation. Multicentric lymphadenopathy may be present as well as hepatosplenomegaly (85).

Radiologic Features

Mediastinal lymphadenopathy is present in about 70% of cases of angiofollicular lymph node hyperplasia. Chest X-ray may reveal large, slightly lobulated masses with smooth margins in the pulmonary hilar areas or in other locations such as the posterior mediastinum (90,91). Angiography demonstrates the vascularity of the lesions (90). Occasionally, angiofollicular lymph node hyperplasia radiologically simulates a pericardial cyst (86).

Pathogenesis

Most authors consider angiofollicular lymphoid hyperplasia to be a form of abnormal immune proliferation. Direct immunofluorescent studies have demonstrated polyclonal immunoglobulins in the lymphoid cells of the lesions, suggesting a reactive lymphoid proliferation (92).

Pathologic Features

Lymph nodes may be markedly enlarged (up to several centimeters in size) (Fig. 9-38), and single or multiple nodes may be involved. Two main histologic subtypes are described, but frequently features of both variants may be present in the same biopsy.

The hyaline-vascular form of angiofollicular hyperplasia is characterized by lymphoid follicles that contain multiple capillaries surrounded by hyaline sheaths. Penetrating postcapillary venules are prominent at the periphery of the follicle leading to the appearance of "lollipop follicles" (Fig. 9-39) (83). Follicles are surrounded by concentric cuffs of lymphocytes arranged in an onion-skin pattern, and there is paracortical vascular hyperplasia (Fig. 9-40).

In the plasma cell variant there are large numbers of plasma cells admixed with immunoblasts, lymphocytes, and macrophages in the interfollicular areas (Fig. 9-41). Follicles are hyperplastic, and may have hyaline vascular germinal centers. Although variable numbers of plasma cells may be present in the interfollicular zone in the hyaline-vascular form of Castleman's disease, the presence of sheets of plasma cells in interfollicular areas is characteristic of the plasma cell variant (93). Most cases of multicentric Castleman's disease are of the plasma cell variant.

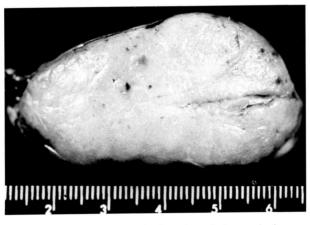

FIG. 9-38. Angiofollicular lymph node hyperplasia.

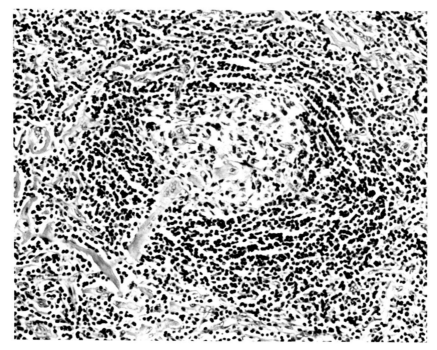

FIG. 9–39. Angiofollicular lymph node hyperplasia showing follicle with multiple capillaries surrounded by hyaline sheaths ("lollipop follicle"). (H&E × 100, original)

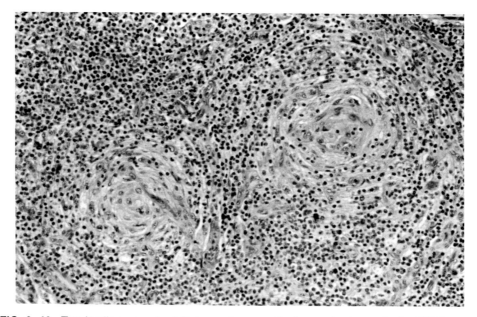

FIG. 9–40. Two hyaline vascular follicles and paracortical vascular hyperplasia. (H&E × 120, original)

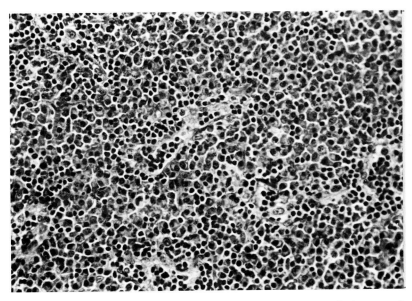

FIG. 9–41. Plasma cell variant of Castleman's disease with sheets of plasma cells in the paracortex. (H&E × 120, original)

Prognosis and Treatment

In localized forms, enlarged lymph nodes may be resected with surgical cure of the disease. Only a few cases of recurrence following surgery have been described (91). Inoperable lesions may benefit from radiotherapy (94,95).

The systemic form of Castleman's disease, however, is associated with significant morbidity and mortality (85). Malignant lymphoma, monoclonal gammopathy and plasmacytoma, Kaposi's sarcoma, peripheral neuropathy, and pseudotumor cerebri have all been reported in patients with the plasma cell variant and generalized disease (93). Multicentric Castleman's disease has also been associated with polyneuropathy, organomegaly, endocrinopathy, monoclonal gammopathy, and skin changes (also known as Takatsuki's syndrome or POEMS) (93).

Development of Vascular Neoplasia in Castleman's Disease

Localized Castleman's disease is associated with vascular hamartoma, histiocytoid hemangioma/angiolymphoid hyperplasia with eosinophilia, and possibly angiomatoid malignant fibrous histiocytoma (96). Cases of vascular neoplasia arising within lesions of Castleman's disease have been described, including one case arising in the mediastinum (96). Histologically, in addition to Castleman's disease of the hyaline vascular type, these masses reveal a mesenchymal spindle cell neoplasm with vascular differentiation. Some of these lesions behave aggressively, resulting in death with metastatic disease (96).

In the general population, systemic Castleman's disease is associated with increased incidence of Kaposi's sarcoma. The relationship between hyaline vascular lymphoid hyperplasia and lymphadenopathic Kaposi's sarcoma is also seen in pa-

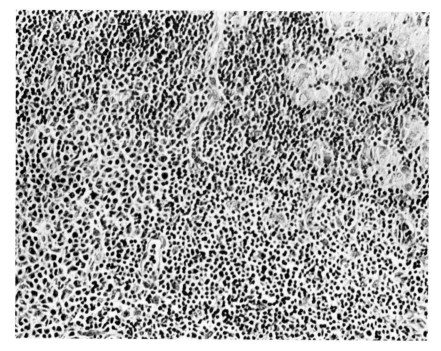

FIG. 9–42. Lymphadenitis in a patient with infectious mononucleosis showing focal proliferation of atypical large immunoblasts and collections of epithelioid cells. (H&E × 100, original)

tients with human immunodeficiency virus (HIV)–related lymphadenopathy. Presence of hyaline vascular lymphoid hyperplasia in HIV-positive individuals suggests that a careful search be made through multiple levels of a lymph node biopsy in order to rule out microscopic infiltration by Kaposi's sarcoma (97). The association between Castleman's disease and vascular neoplasia is unexplained but may possibly be mediated by angiogenic factors produced by activated lymphoid cells (96).

OTHER MEDIASTINAL LYMPHADENOPATHIES

Mediastinal lymphadenopathies have been observed radiologically in other conditions such as angioimmunoblastic lymphadenopathy, infectious mononucleosis (Fig. 9-42), and lupus erythematosus (61,98,99). Patients with these conditions seldom undergo mediastinal biopsies.

REFERENCES

1. Luosto R, Koikkalainen K, Jyrala A, et al: Mediastinal tumours. A follow-up study of 208 patients. *Scand J Thorac Cardiovasc Surg* 1978;12:253–259.
2. Ovrum E, Birkeland S: Mediastinal tumours and cysts. A review of 91 cases. *Scand J Thorac Cardiovasc Surg* 1979;13:161–168.
3. Rouviere H: in Tobias MJ (ed): *Anatomy of the Human Lymphatic System.* Ann Arbor, Edwards Brothers, 1938.
4. Bergh NP, Gatzinsky P, Larsson S, et al: Tumors of the thymus and thymic region. II. Clinicopathologic studies on Hodgkin's disease of the thymus. *Ann Thorac Surg* 1978;25:99–106.

5. Jones SE, Fuks Z, Bull M, et al: Non-Hodgkin's lymphomas. IV. Clinicopathologic correlation in 405 cases. *Cancer* 1973;31:806–823.

6. Chabner BA, Johnson RE, Young RC, et al: Sequential non-surgical and surgical staging of non-Hodgkin's lymphoma. *Ann Intern Med* 1976;85:149–154.

7. Patchefsky AS, Brodovsky HS, Menduke H, et al: Non-Hodgkin's lymphomas: a clinicopathologic study of 293 cases. *Cancer* 1974;34:1173–1186.

8. Lichtenstein AK, Levine A, Taylor CR, et al: Primary mediastinal lymphoma in adults. *Am J Med* 1980;68:509–514.

9. Doll R, Muir C, Waterhouse J (eds): *Cancer Incidence in Five Continents*, vol 2. Berlin, Springer-Verlag, 1970.

10. Weiss LM, Movahed LA, Warnke RA, et al: Detection of Epstein-Barr viral genomes in Reed–Sternberg cells of Hodgkin's disease. *N Engl J Med* 1989;320:502–506.

11. Brousset P, Chittal S, Schlaifer D, et al: Detection of Epstein-Barr virus messenger RNA in Reed–Sternberg cells of Hodgkin's disease by *in situ* hybridization with biotinylated probes on specially processed modified acetone methyl benzoate xylene (ModAMeX) sections. *Blood* 1991;77:1781–1786.

12. Kaplan HS: *Hodgkin's Disease*. Cambridge, Harvard University Press, 1972.

13. Lukes RJ: Criteria for involvement of lymph node, bone marrow, spleen, and liver in Hodgkin's disease. *Cancer Res* 1971;31:1755–1767.

14. Pinkus GS, Said JW: Hodgkin's disease, lymphocyte predominance type, nodular—further evidence for a B-cell derivation. L&H variants of Reed–Sternberg cells express L26, a pan B cell marker. *Am J Pathol* 1988;133:211–217.

15. Haybittle JL, Hayhoe FGJ, Bennett MH: Review of British national lymphoma investigation studies of Hodgkin's disease and development of prognostic index. *Lancet* 1985;1:967–972.

16. Strickler JG, Michie SA, Warnke RA, et al: The "syncytial variant" of nodular sclerosing Hodgkin's disease. *Am J Surg Pathol* 1986;10:470–477.

17. Mauch P, Goodman R, Hellman S: The significance of mediastinal involvement in early stage Hodgkin's disease. *Cancer* 1978;42:1039–1045.

18. Behar RA, Hoppe RT: Radiation therapy in the management of bulky mediastinal Hodgkin's disease. *Cancer* 1990;66:75–79.

19. North LB, Fuller LM, Hagemeister FB, et al: Importance of initial mediastinal adenopathy in Hodgkin's disease. *Am J Roentgenol* 1982;138:229–235.

20. Ferrant A, Hamoir V, Binon J, et al: Combined modality therapy for mediastinal Hodgkin's disease. Prognostic significance of constitutional symptoms and size of disease. *Cancer* 1985;55:317–322.

21. Levitt LJ, Aisenberg AC, Harris NL: Primary non-Hodgkin's lymphoma of the mediastinum. *Cancer* 1982;50:2486–2492.

22. Davis RE, Dorfman RF, Warnke RA: Primary large-cell lymphoma of the thymus. A diffuse B-cell neoplasm presenting as primary mediastinal lymphoma. *Hum Pathol* 1990;21:1262–1268.

23. Lamarre L, Jacobson JO, Aisenberg AC, et al: Primary large cell lymphoma of the mediastinum. A histologic and immunophenotypic study of 29 cases. *Am J Surg Pathol* 1989;13:730–739.

24. Moller P, Moldenhauer G, Momburg F, et al: Mediastinal lymphoma of clear cell type is a tumor corresponding to terminal steps of B cell differentiation. *Blood* 1987;69:1087–1095.

25. Haioun C, Gaulard P, Roudot-Thoravel F, et al: Mediastinal diffuse large cell lymphoma with sclerosis: a condition with poor prognosis. *Am J Clin Oncol* 1989;12:425–429.

26. Perrone T, Frizzera G, Rosai J: Mediastinal diffuse large-cell lymphoma with sclerosis. A clinicopathologic study of 60 cases. *Am J Surg Pathol* 1986;10:176–191.

27. Moller P, Matthaei-Maurer DU, Hoffman WJ, et al: Immunophenotypic similarities of mediastinal clear-cell lymphoma and sinusoidal (monocytoid) B cells. *Int J Cancer* 1989;43:10–16.

28. Treseler PA, O'Hara CJ, Stoll PN, et al: Peripheral T cell lymphoma of the mediastinum: comparison with its B cell counterpart. *Lab Invest* 1989;60:97A.

29. Wolford JH, Krause JR: Posttransplant mediastinal Burkitt-like lymphoma. Diagnosis by cytologic and flow cytometric analysis of pleural fluid. *Acta Cytologica* 1990;34:261–264.

30. Isaacson PG, Chan JKC, Tang C, et al: Low-grade B-cell lymphoma of mucosa-associated lymphoid tissue arising in the thymus. A thymic lymphoma mimicking myoepithelial sialadenitis. *Am J Surg Pathol* 1990;14:342–351.

31. Borowitz MJ, Croker BP, Metzgar RS: Lymphoblastic lymphoma with the phenotype of common acute lymphoblastic leukemia. *Am J Clin Pathol* 1983;79:387–391.

32. Barcos MP, Lukes RJ: Malignant lymphoma of convoluted lymphocytes: a new entity of possible T-cell type, in Sinks LF, Godden JO (eds): *Conflicts in childhood cancer. Proceedings of the symposium* Rockwell Institute, Buffalo, September 1974. Progress in clinical and biological research. New York, Alan R Liss, 1975, pp 147–177.

33. Nathwani BN, Kim H, Rappaport H: Malignant lymphoma, lymphoblastic. *Cancer* 1976;38:9964–9983.

34. Griffith RC, Kelly DR, Nathwani BN, et al: A morphologic study of childhood lymphoma of the lymphoblastic type. *Cancer* 1987;59:1126–1131.

35. Bollum FJ: Terminal deoxynucleotidyl transferase as a hematopoietic marker. *Blood* 1979; 54:1203–1215.
36. Said JW, Shintaku IP, Pinkus GS: Immunohistochemical staining for terminal deoxynucleotidyl transferase (TdT)—an enhanced method in routinely processed formalin-fixed tissue sections. *Am J Clin Pathol* 1988;89:649–652.
37. Weiss LM, Bindl JM, Picozzi VJ, et al: Lymphoblastic lymphoma: an immunophenotype study of 26 cases with comparison to T cell acute lymphoblastic leukemia. *Blood* 1986;67:474–478.
38. Sheibani K, Nathwani BN, Winberg CD, et al: Antigenically defined subgroups of lymphoblastic lymphoma. *Cancer* 1987; 60:183–190.
39. Swerdlow SH, Habeshaw JA, Richards MA, et al: T lymphoblastic lymphoma with leu-7 positive phenotype and unusual clinical course. A multiparameter study. *Leuk Res* 1985;9:167–173.
40. Linder J, Ye Y, Harrington DS, et al: Monoclonal antibodies marking T lymphocytes in paraffin-embedded tissue. *Am J Pathol* 1987;127:1–8.
41. Davey FR, Gatter KC, Ralfkiaer E, et al: Immunophenotyping of non-Hodgkin's lymphomas using a panel of antibodies on paraffin-embedded tissues. *Am J Pathol* 1987;129:54–63.
42. Jaffe ES, Braylan RC, Green FMM, et al: Heterogeneity of immunologic markers and surface morphology in childhood lymphoblastic lymphoma. *Blood* 1976;48:213–222.
43. Krause JR: Granulocytic sarcoma preceding acute leukemia. A report of six cases. *Cancer* 1979;44:1017–1021.
44. Banerjee D, Silva E: Mediastinal mass with acute leukemia. Myeloblastoma masquerading as lymphoblastic lymphoma. *Arch Pathol Lab Med* 1981;105:126–129.
45. Pinkus GS, Said JW: Profile of intracytoplasmic lysozyme in normal tissues, myeloproliferative disorders, hairy cell leukemia, and other pathologic processes. An immunoperoxidase study of paraffin sections and smears. *Am J Pathol* 1977;89:351–366.
46. Arbona GL, Lloyd TV, Lucas J: Mediastinal extramedullary plasmacytoma. *South Med J* 1980;73:670–671.
47. Tokumitsu S, Tokumitsu K, Kohnoe K, et al: Extramedullary hematopoiesis presenting as mediastinal tumor. *Acta Pathol Jpn* 1980;30:315–322.
48. Gupta RM, Roy DC, Gupta IM, et al: Extramedullary plasmacytoma IgG type I presenting as mediastinal syndrome. *Br J Dis Chest* 1974;68:65–70.
49. Kintzer JS, Rosenow EC, Kyle RA: Thoracic and pulmonary abnormalities in multiple myeloma. A review of 958 cases. *Arch Intern Med* 1978;138:727–730.
50. McLoud TC, Meyer JE: Mediastinal metastases. *Radiol Clin North Am* 1982;20:453–468.
51. Webb WR: Hilar and mediastinal lymph node metastases in malignant melanoma. *Am J Roentgenol* 1979;133:805–810.
52. Magill HL, Sackler JP, Parvey LS: Wilm's tumor metastatic to the mediastinum. *Pediatr Radiol* 1982;12:62–64.
53. Lindell MM, Doubleday LC, von Eschenbach AC, et al: Mediastinal metastases from prostatic carcinoma. *J Urol* 1982;128:331–334.
54. Kirsh MM, Sloan H: Mediastinal metastases in bronchogenic carcinoma: influence of postoperative irradiation, cell type and location. *Ann Thorac Surg* 1982;33:459–463.
55. Feldman L, Kricun ME: Malignant melanoma presenting as a mediastinal mass. *JAMA* 1979;241:396–397.
56. McLoud TC, Kalisher L, Stark P, et al: Intrathoracic lymph node metastases from extrathoracic neoplasms. *Am J Roentgenol* 1978;131:403–407.
57. Bein ME, Putman CE, McLoud TC, et al: A reevaluation of intrathoracic lymphadenopathy in sarcoidosis. *Am J Roentgenol* 1978;131:409–415.
58. Sieracki JC, Fisher ER: The ceroid nature of the so-called "Hamazaki-Wesenberg bodies." *Am J Clin Pathol* 1973;59:248–253.
59. Adams DO: The granulomatous response. A review. *Am J Pathol* 1976;84:164–191.
60. Epstein WL: Granuloma formation in man. *Pathobiol Annu* 1977;7:1–31.
61. Ioachim HL: Granulomatous lesions of lymph nodes, in Ioachim HL (ed): *Pathology of Granulomas.* New York, Raven Press, 1983, pp 151–187.
62. Rizzoli PB, Passero MA: Tuberculous mediastinal lymphadenitis presenting as chest wall mass. *Postgrad Med* 1980;68:97–99.
63. Dhand S, Fisher M, Fewell JW: Intrathoracic tuberculous lymphadenopathy in adults. *JAMA* 1979;241:505–507.
64. Morgan H, Ellis K: Superior mediastinal masses: secondary to tuberculous lymphadenitis in the adult. *Am J Roentgenol Radium Ther Nucl Med* 1974;120:893–897.
65. Weber AL, Bird KT, Janower ML: Primary tuberculosis in childhood with partial emphasis on changes affecting the tracheobronchial tree. *Am J Roentgenol Radium Ther Nucl Med* 1968;103:123–132.
66. Kittredge RD, Finby N: Bilateral tuberculous mediastinal lymphadenopathy in the adult. *Am J Roentgenol Radium Ther Nucl Med* 1966;96:1022–1026.
67. Nussbaum E, Hanson GR, Galant S: Nontuberculous mycobacterial infection in an infant with a mediastinal mass. *Clin Pediatr* 1982;21:246–247.

68. Marchevsky AM, Damsker B, Gribetz A, et al: The spectrum of pathology of nontuberculous mycobacterial infections in open-lung biopsy specimens. *Am J Clin Pathol* 1982;78:695–700.

69. Lincoln EM, Gilbert LA: Disease in children due to Mycobacteria other than *Mycobacterium tuberculosis. Am Rev Respir Dis* 1972;105:683–714.

70. Cunningham JA: Sarcoidosis. *Pathol Annu* 1967;2:31–47.

71. James DG, Neville E: Pathobiology of sarcoidosis. *Pathobiol Annu* 1977;7:31–61.

72. Welsh LW, Welsh JJ: Problems of diagnosis in the evaluation of mediastinal sarcoidosis. *Laryngoscope* 1977;87:1635–1644.

73. Munkgaard S, Neukirch F: Comparison of biopsy procedures in intrathoracic sarcoidosis. *Acta Med Scand* 1979;205:179–184.

74. Israel HL, Lenchner G, Steiner RM: Late development of mediastinal calcification in sarcoidosis. *Am Rev Respir Dis* 1981;124:302–305.

75. Rosen Y, Vuletin JC. Pertschuk LP, et al: Sarcoidosis from the pathologist's vantage point. *Pathol Annu* 1979;14:405–439.

76. Kirks DR. Greenspan RH: Sarcoid. *Radiol Clin North Am* 1973;11:279–294.

77. Berkmen YM, Javors BR: Anterior mediastinal lymphadenopathy in sarcoidosis. *Am J Roentgenol* 1976;127:983–987.

78. Seaton A: Silicosis, in Morgan WKC, Seaton A (eds): *Occupational Lung Diseases.* Philadelphia, WB Saunders, 1975, pp 80–123.

79. Symmers WStC (ed): The lymphoreticular system in: *Systemic Pathology.* New York, Churchill Livingstone, 1978.

80. Castleman B, Iverson L, Menendez V: Localized mediastinal lymph node hyperplasia resembling thymoma. *Cancer* 1956;9:822–830.

81. Tuttle RJ, Shier KJ: Angiography of angiomatous lymphoid hamartoma (Castleman tumor) and a suggested pathogenesis. *Radiology* 1979;130:311–315.

82. Gaba AR, Stein RS, Sweet DL, et al: Multicentric giant lymph node hyperplasia. *Am J Clin Pathol* 1978;69:86–90.

83. Keller AR. Hochholzer L, Castleman B: Hyaline-vascular and plasma-cell types of giant lymph node hyperplasia of the mediastinum and other locations. *Cancer* 1972;29:670–683.

84. Bartoli E, Massarelli G, Soggia G, et al: Multicentric giant lymph node hyperplasia: a hyperimmune entity with a rapidly progressive course. *Am J Clin Pathol* 1980;73:423–426.

85. Weisenberger DD, Nathwani BN, Winberg CD, et al: Multicentric angiofollicular lymph node hyperplasia: a clinicopathologic study of 16 cases. *Hum Pathol* 1985;16:162–172.

86. Gibbons JA, Rosencrantz H, Posey DJ, et al: Angiofollicular lymphoid hyperplasia (Castleman's tumor) resembling a pericardial cyst: differentiation by computerized tomography. *Ann Thorac Surg* 1981;32:193–196.

87. Yu GSM, Carson JW: Giant lymph-node hyperplasia, plasma-cell type of the mediastinum, with peripheral neuropathy. *Am J Clin Pathol* 1976;66:46–53.

88. Rosenthal T, Hertz M: Mediastinal lymphadenopathy in infectious mononucleosis. Report of two cases. *JAMA* 1975;233:1300–1301.

89. Scully RE: Case records of the Massachusetts General Hospital. *N Engl J Med* 1984;311:388–398.

90. Olscamp G, Weisbrod G, Sanders D, et al: Castleman's disease: unusual manifestations of an unusual disorder. *Radiology* 1980;135:43–48.

91. Hammond DI: Giant lymph node hyperplasia of the posterior mediastinum. *J Can Assoc Radiol* 1979;30:256–258.

92. Martin JME, Bell B, Ruether BA: Giant lymph node hyperplasia (Castleman's disease) of hyaline vascular type. Clinical heterogeneity with immunohistologic uniformity. *Am J Clin Pathol* 1985;84:439–446.

93. Scully, RE (ed): Case records of the Massachusetts General Hospital. *N Engl J Med* 1987;316:606–618.

94. Nordstrom DG, Twefik HH, Latourette HB: Plasma cell giant lymph node hyperplasia responding to radiation therapy. *Am J Roentgenol* 1978;130:169–171.

95. Weisenburger DD, De Gowin RL, Gibson DP, et al: Remission of giant lymph node hyperplasia with anemia after radiotherapy. *Cancer* 1979;44:457–462.

96. Gerald W, Kostinovsky M, Rosai J: Development of vascular neoplasia in Castleman's disease. *Am J Surg Pathol* 1990;14:603–614.

97. Harris NL: Hypervascular follicular hyperplasia and Kaposi's sarcoma in patients at risk for AIDS. *N Engl J Med* 1984;310:462–463.

98. Kassan SS, Moss ML, Reddick RL: Progressive hilar and mediastinal lymphadenopathy in systemic lupus erythematosus on corticosteroid therapy. *N Engl J Med* 1976;294:1382–1383.

99. Ballow M, Park BH, Dupont B, et al: Benign giant lymphoid hyperplasia of the mediastinum with associated abnormalities of the immune system. *J Pediatr* 1974;84:418–420.

10

Mediastinal Cysts

Mediastinal cysts are uncommon lesions. They comprise 10% to 27% of all mediastinal masses and result, in most instances, from developmental anomalies of the foregut or related embryonal structures (1–6). They also can be acquired as a result of cystic degeneration of mediastinal neoplasms or hematomas, parasitic infections, and/or intrathoracic extension of pancreatic pseudocysts.

A large variety of cysts (listed in Table 1) have been described in the mediastinum (1–6).

The classification of mediastinal cysts into congenital and acquired lesions proposed in Table 1 is convenient but does not apply to all lesions. Indeed, mediastinal cysts may develop as a result of various congenital or acquired mechanisms and present with similar clinicopathologic features. For example, most instances of pericardial cysts are thought to be congenital in origin, but a few cases with identical features have been described following pericarditis (7).

DIAGNOSIS OF MEDIASTINAL CYSTS: ROLE OF FINE-NEEDLE ASPIRATION

Mediastinal cysts often present in adult patients as asymptomatic, incidental lesions on chest roentgenograms. They cannot be reliably distinguished from solid tumors on conventional roentgenograms, and thoracotomy and biopsy were required to establish the diagnosis (1–7). More recent studies with computerized tomography (CT) and contrasted CT demonstrated that most mediastinal cysts have CT densities in the water range that distinguish them from solid tumors (8). However, the distinction between solid tumors and cysts cannot be made reliably in all patients, as cystic mediastinal lesions can exhibit CT densities that approach those of soft tissues (8).

Percutaneous and transbronchial fine-needle aspiration (FNA) under fluoroscopic or CT guidance has been used successfully for the diagnosis and treatment of mediastinal cysts (8,9). With this method the diagnosis of a cyst often can be established with certainty, although the precise diagnosis of the lesion can remain elusive without its resection (8). However, as malignant transformation of a mediastinal cyst is very unusual and cystic neoplasms of the mediastinum are infrequent, the FNA diagnosis of a cyst can be used to preclude a thoracotomy (8). The nature of the cyst's fluid can be helpful for the diagnosis. For example, chylous fluid is aspirated from lymphangiomas or thoracic duct cysts; turbid, mucinous fluid is aspirated from bronchogenic cysts; and clear fluid is aspirated from pericardial or mesothelial cysts. The cytologic examination of the cyst's contents can help to determine the predominant cell type (i.e., bronchial type cells, mucinous cells, mesothelial cells) and to rule out the presence of malignant cells (8,9).

TABLE 1. *Mediastinal cysts*

Congenital
Bronchogenic
Esophageal
Tracheoesophageal
Gastroenteric
Pericardial
Mesothelial
Thymic
Meningocele
Acquired
Thoracic duct
Neoplastic
Teratoma
Thymoma
Lymphangioma
Others
Parasitic
Taenia echinococcus
Cystic hematoma
Pancreatic pseudocyst
Lymphoepithelial cyst

BRONCHOGENIC CYSTS

Bronchogenic (tracheobronchogenous) cysts are the most frequent congenital cystic lesions of the mediastinum (1,2). They account for approximately 40% to 50% of congenital mediastinal cysts (9–24).

Bronchogenic cysts occur in all age groups but are most frequent in adult patients in their third and fourth decades of life. They are slightly more frequent in men (1.5:1) (9–24).

Patients are usually asymptomatic at the time of initial diagnosis and are found to have a mediastinal mass on chest roentgenograms (4). They also can present with symptoms caused by the compression of airways, the esophagus, or other mediastinal structures by a gradually enlarging cyst, such as cough, dyspnea, recurrent respiratory infections, dysphagia, paroxysmal atrial fibrillation, and others (4–20). Rarely, bronchogenic cysts located in the carina cause death in early life by compression of the trachea or a major bronchus (4).

Pathogenesis

Bronchogenic cysts result from abnormal branching of the bronchopulmonary foregut during intrauterine development (4).

The respiratory tree and the esophagus derive from the primitive foregut. The primitive trachea develops from a medial ventral outgrowth from the foregut, the laryngotracheal groove, during the third and fourth weeks of intrauterine life. The laryngotracheal groove develops into a tube that parallels the esophagus and becomes enlarged caudally. The primitive tracheal tube bifurcates during the sixth intrauterine week of life, giving rise to the primitive lung buds. These buds continue to bifurcate dichotomously, resulting in the formation of the bronchi and smaller airways (4).

The tracheobronchial mucosa and glands arise from the endoderm, whereas the surrounding connective tissues, smooth muscle, and cartilage are of mesodermal origin.

It has been postulated that bronchogenic cysts result from supernumerary lung buds that arise after the separation of the trachea from the esophagus by the esophagotracheal septum has taken place (2,4). Bronchogenic cysts develop after the fourth intrauterine week of life according to this theory. The absence of esophageal tissues in bronchogenic cysts and the known occurrence of tracheal diverticula in areas of the airways where these cysts are most frequent support this concept (20).

Bronchogenic cysts can be intrapulmonary or extrapulmonary (4). Intrapulmonary cysts result from abnormal branches of the bronchial tree that remain attached to the bronchial wall during embryogenesis and become enveloped by the developing lung parenchyma. Extrapulmonary cysts result from abnormal buds that lose contact with the airways during embryogenesis, remain in the mediastinum, and gradually increase in size as a result of the secretion of the cyst epithelium into the closed cavity.

Roentgenologic Features

Bronchogenic cysts are round or oval masses located most frequently in the middle anterior mediastinum, in close association with airways (Fig. 10-1). They can be present however, in other mediastinal areas and within the pericardial cavity (Fig. 10-2) (10,18).

Bronchogenic cysts have a sharp border and usually move and change in shape

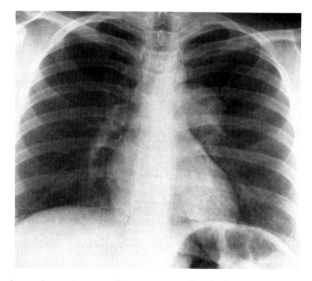

FIG. 10–1. Bronchogenic cyst presenting as a round soft tissue density superimposed over the left hilum (*arrow*).

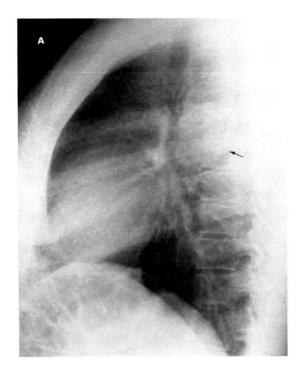

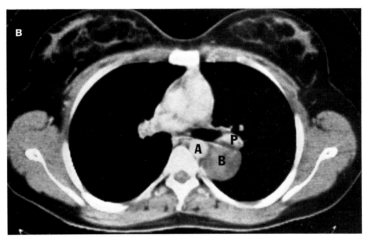

FIG. 10–2. **A:** Bronchogenic cyst extending into the posterior mediastinum (*arrow*). **B:** The bronchogenic cyst (*B*) is posterior to the aorta (*A*) and pulmonary artery (*P*).

with respiration, indicating a close association with the tracheobronchial tree (17). They may also exhibit focal areas of calcification.

These features are useful for differential diagnosis. For example, soft tissue masses such as mediastinal goiters usually have borders that are less sharp, and dermoid cysts usually have a more rigid wall and do not change in shape with respiration (18).

Pathologic Features

Bronchogenic cysts are spherical, cystic, unilocular mediastinal or, less frequently, intrapulmonary masses (Fig. 10-3) (2,4). They can be lobulated, multiloculated, and/or multiple (25). They usually measure only a few centimeters in diameter but may become as large as 15 cm in greatest dimensions.

Bronchogenic cysts have a thin wall with a smooth gray outer surface. Their inner surface is trabeculated because of the presence of smooth muscle and cartilage in

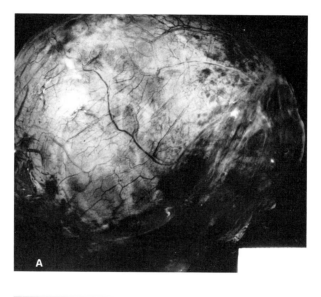

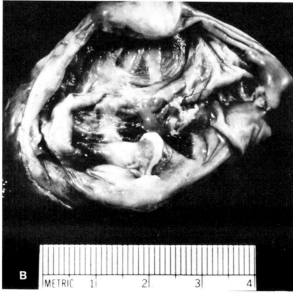

FIG. 10–3. A: Bronchogenic cyst. **B:** Inner aspect of bronchogenic cyst showing thin wall with characteristic trabeculated pattern.

the wall (Fig. 10-3B). The cavity is usually filled with a white–gray, mucinous material, but it can contain, instead, brown inspissated contents that resemble pus.

Recent studies have demonstrated the presence of a high level of carbohydrate antigen (CA) 19-9 and carcinoembryonic antigen (CEA) in the cyst fluid and in the serum of patients with bronchogenic cysts (26).

Histologically, bronchogenic cysts are lined by respiratory epithelium with a lamina propria containing bronchial glands, connective tissue, smooth muscle, and cartilage (Fig. 10-4). The surface epithelium and bronchial type glands of bronchogenic cysts can exhibit immunoreactivity with antibodies to CA 19-9 and CEA (26). Focal areas of calcification may be present. In many instances, the epithelium exhibits focal or extensive squamous metaplasia; it can also become attenuated into a simple flattened epithelial layer. The cyst stroma can have focal chronic inflammation.

Topographic Classification of Bronchogenic Cysts

Bronchogenic cysts can be present in many different areas of the mediastinum.

Maier (14) has divided them according to their location into five groups: paratracheal, carinal, hilar, paraesophageal, and miscellaneous. The latter group includes unusual instances of bronchogenic cysts encountered in the pericardial cavity, on the anterior aspect of the thoracic spine and extending into the vertebral bodies, in the presternal area extending into soft tissues located outside the thoracic cavity, or growing through the diaphragm in a "dumbbell" fashion (4,14,16). This topographic classification of bronchogenic cysts has clinical value, as they usually present with different clinical symptoms according to their location. For example, paratracheal cysts are usually asymptomatic. Carinal cysts are symptomatic early in life as they compress the airways and are detected in childhood. Paraesophageal cysts present with dysphagia because of compression of the esophagus.

A few instances of perforation of a bronchogenic cyst into the lung, airways, or esophagus also have been described (4,14). In this situation, secondary infection is frequent. In most locations, bronchogenic cysts are attached to the airways by fibrous strands. In some instances, however, the cyst is found at surgery to be lying free in the mediastinum, and a bronchogenic origin is more difficult to establish (4,14).

Prognosis and Treatment

Bronchogenic cysts are cured by surgical excision (1,6). Lesions that can only be incompletely excised because of their location or technical problems during surgery can recur and develop bronchial obstruction, compression of the superior vena cava and pulmonary artery, and/or other severe complications (27). However, it is controversial whether all suspected bronchogenic cysts should be resected (23). Some physicians advise older children and adult patients with asymptomatic mediastinal cysts against surgical excision, as the lesions usually grow slowly over many years, frequently remain asymptomatic, and seldom become malignant. This approach has been questioned, however, as bronchogenic cysts can become progressively symptomatic (22). Percutaneous or transbronchial FNA has been utilized successfully for the treatment and diagnosis of these lesions and can be offered as a therapeutic alternative to surgical resection (10).

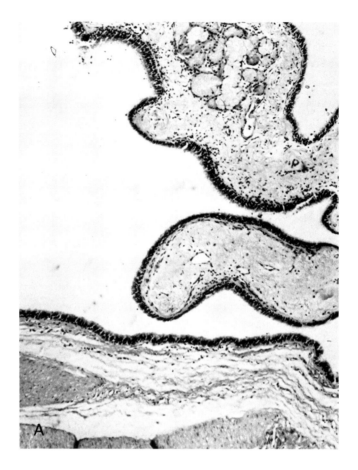

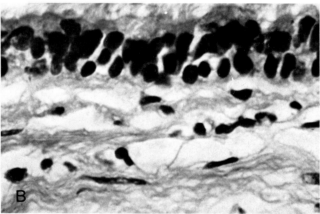

FIG. 10–4. A: Bronchogenic cyst lined by pseudostratified ciliated epithelium with bronchial glands. The cyst wall has smooth muscle and cartilage not shown in the photograph. (H&E × 40, original) **B:** Higher magnification of respiratory epithelium lining the cyst wall. (H&E × 400, original).

Malignant transformation of the epithelial components of a bronchogenic cyst has not been described, to our knowledge. Bernheim and associates (28) reported an instance of leiomyosarcoma in the wall of a bronchial cyst.

ESOPHAGEAL CYST

Esophageal cysts are less common than bronchogenic lesions and are characterized by the presence of a double layer of smooth muscle in their walls (4,29).

These cysts are more frequent in children or young patients in their second decade of life and are more frequent in men. They can be associated with other congenital anomalies such as tracheoesophageal fistulas (2,4).

Patients present with similar symptoms to those with bronchogenic cysts.

Pathogenesis

Esophageal cysts arise from persistent vacuoles in the wall of the foregut that develop during the solid tube stage of development (2,4). Vacuoles that normally would coalesce to form the lumen of the esophagus remain isolated and grow in size to form a cyst in the esophageal wall. The cysts can thereafter grow outside the esophagus.

The theory that esophageal cysts result from abnormal budding from the early foregut is not accepted in most publications (2,4). Both theories are probably correct, however, and can explain the development of two distinct types of esophageal cysts: (a) a type lined by squamous epithelium that resembles adult esophagus, which results from persistent vacuoles in the wall of the foregut, and (b) a type lined by ciliated epithelium, which resembles the fetal esophagus and probably develops from abnormal budding from the foregut (2,4).

Pathologic Features

Esophageal cysts are unilocular, round, and contain mucinous material in their lumina (2,4). They are present in the esophageal wall or in the mediastinum in intimate relation with the esophagus. The cyst wall is lined mostly by nonkeratinized stratified squamous epithelium but can have focal or extensive areas of ciliated columnar epithelium. The cyst wall also has a lamina propria with esophageal-type glands and a muscularis propria composed of two well-defined layers of smooth muscle. Indeed, esophageal cysts have morphologic features that closely resemble those of the esophagus. Focal calcification of the cyst wall can be present.

DIFFERENTIAL DIAGNOSIS BETWEEN BRONCHOGENIC AND ESOPHAGEAL CYSTS

The distinction between bronchogenic and esophageal cysts may be difficult because of their similar topographic distribution and morphology and close embryologic origin.

Bronchogenic cysts can become attached to the esophageal wall during development and, in rare instances, are found within the esophageal wall (2). They can be recognized, however, by the presence of cartilage in the cyst wall and the absence of a well-defined muscularis propria composed of two layers of smooth muscle.

Esophageal cysts can be entirely lined by ciliated columnar epithelium but lack cartilage in their walls and have a well-developed muscularis propria. However, the origin of developmental mediastinal cysts cannot be established in all instances, and there are rare lesions that lack a clear relationship with the airways and the esophagus, have a thin wall lined by ciliated columnar epithelium and connective tissues, lack cartilage and a muscularis propria with two layers of smooth muscle, and cannot be classified into a definite category. These cysts probably form during early embryogenesis at a time when they do not acquire characteristics of the esophagus or the airways.

TRACHEOESOPHAGEAL CYSTS

Tracheoesophageal cysts are rare mediastinal lesions with mixed features of bronchogenic and esophageal cysts (4). They are lined by squamous epithelium in some areas and by ciliated columnar epithelium in others and have esophageal glands, focal areas of cartilage, and a muscularis with two layers of smooth muscle. These cysts probably result from tracheoesophageal fistulas that close off during early embryogenesis and grow slowly in size to become a cystic mass (4).

Prognosis and Treatment

Esophageal cysts are resected surgically with good prognosis. Malignant transformation has not been reported, to our knowledge.

GASTROENTERIC CYSTS

Gastroenteric cysts are unusual developmental cysts of the mediastinum encountered in the posterior mediastinum of patients who usually have vertebral abnormalities (30–43).

They have been reported under various names, such as gastric cysts, enterogenous cysts, foregut duplications, esophageal duplications, gastrogenous cysts, enterocystoma, and others (33–45).

Gastroenteric cysts are more frequent in males and in infants younger than 1 year of life (60% of patients). They can be encountered, however, in adult patients (2,4).

Patients are almost invariably symptomatic at the time of original diagnosis and present with pain and/or signs of compression of paraspinal nerves or other mediastinal structures (2,4,36–43). They include dyspnea, cough, vomiting, poor weight gain, and others. Gastroenteric cysts also can present with massive lethal hemoptysis resulting from ulceration of the cyst wall secondary to the acid secretions of the gastric mucosa lining the lesion rupturing into an airway.

Pathogenesis

Several theories have been proposed to explain the origin of gastroenteric cysts. Fallon and associates (40) and other authors (41) have proposed the currently accepted theory that gastroenteric cysts result from traction diverticula that develop from the primitive gastrointestinal tract as a result of adhesions between the foregut and the primitive vertebrae. This theory is based on the frequent association between gastroenteric cysts and malformations of the cervical and thoracic vertebrae and the fact that the foregut grows in close contact with the notochord during early embryonal life. A traction diverticulum resulting from adhesions between these two structures becomes cut off from the intestinal lumen and grows to develop a cystic mass.

Occasionally, patients with gastroenteric cysts have other associated malformations including intraabdominal cysts or duplications, meningoceles, esophageal atresia, malrotation of the intestines, congenital heart disease, and others (4). The mechanism of these other developmental abnormalities is not known.

Other theories have been proposed to explain the origin of gastroenteric cysts (2–4). They postulate that the cysts result from vestiges of the ductus omphalomesentericus, duplication of the intestine, sequestration of epithelial nodules, diverticula from the foregut, or persistent vacuoles in the wall of the gastrointestinal tract that fail to coalesce with the intestinal lumen (2,4). These theories do not explain the association of gastroenteric cysts with vertebral malformations.

Roentgenologic Features

Gastroenteric cysts appear as round posterior mediastinal masses with sharp borders and focal areas of calcification on chest roentgenograms (31). The thoracic and/or cervical vertebrae exhibit malformations, including hemivertebrae, posterior spina bifida, and scoliosis (2,4,31,33–35). Intrathoracic gastric cysts can be demonstrated by ^{99m}Tc-pertechnetate scintigraphy (42,43).

Pathologic Features

Gastroenteric cysts are spherical, unilocular, and measure up to 9 cm in diameter. They are seldom multiloculated and are frequently attached to the vertebral column by fibrous strands. The cyst wall is pink–gray and usually measures only a few millimeters in thickness. The lumen contains a clear, bloody, or yellow–green fluid that may contain hydrochloric acid, renin, and pepsin. Histologically, gastroenteric cysts have a mucosa, submucosa, and muscularis.

The mucosa of gastroenteric cysts can have a variety of epithelial types including gastric, ciliated, squamous, small intestinal, large intestinal, and/or duodenal epithelium (Figs. 10-5 and 10-6). Gastric mucosa with glands containing chief cells and parietal cells is the most constant component (4). In focal areas, the cyst wall may be lined only by a single layer of mucin-secreting cells.

The mucosa also has a lamina propria and is separated from the submucosa by a muscularis mucosae. The latter may not be present in all histologic sections taken from the cyst wall.

The muscularis propria is composed of two or three distinct layers of smooth muscle. Sympathetic ganglion cells and nerves similar to those seen in the myenteric plexus are frequently found in the muscularis.

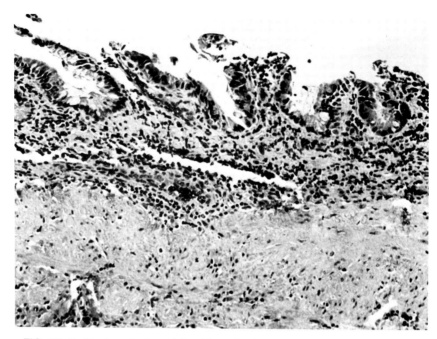

FIG. 10–5. Gastroenteric cyst lined by colonic mucosa. (H&E × 100, original)

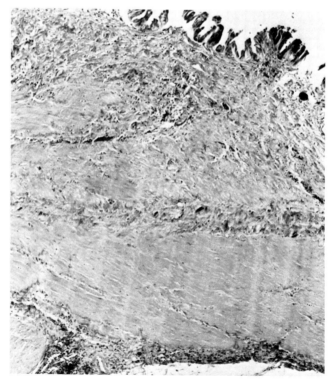

FIG. 10–6. Gastroenteric cyst lined by colonic mucosa, submucosa, and double muscular layer. (H&E × 40, original)

The wall of gastroenteric cysts can be focally calcified and may exhibit areas of ossification.

Prognosis and Treatment

Gastroenteric cysts lined predominantly by intestinal, squamous, or ciliated epithelium have a good prognosis and are cured by surgical excision (1,6). Percutaneous aspiration and cystography have also been utilized for their diagnosis and treatment (44). They seldom undergo malignant transformation. Chuang and associates (46) reported a patient with an adenocarcinoma arising from an "intrathoracic duplication cyst of foregut origin" (Fig. 10-7). The tumor had morphologic features identical to those seen in colonic adenocarcinomas, and a transitional zone between the benign epithelium lining the cyst and the neoplasm was found. This patient has been followed for 14 years after resection without evidence of recurrent disease.

Cysts lined by gastric mucosa have a poorer prognosis and may lead to fatal complications in early life if left undetected (37). These complications arise from the effects of the acid secretions of the cyst epithelium and include development of draining sinuses into the chest wall and neck, erosion of upper thoracic vertebral bodies, and perforation and communication with the pulmonary parenchyma, tracheobronchial tree, or esophagus (32–37).

The prognosis of gastric cysts is excellent, however, if the lesions are discovered and resected early in life.

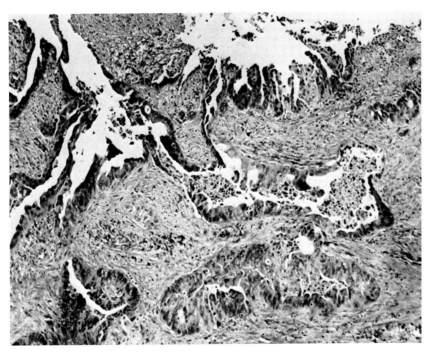

FIG. 10–7. Adenocarcinoma of colonic type developing in gastroenteric cyst. (H&E × 100, original)

MEDIASTINAL CYSTS CONTAINING INTRAMURAL PANCREATIC TISSUE

Shillitoe and Wilson (47) and Carr and associates (48) reported unusual mediastinal cysts containing intramural pancreatic tissue with ducts, acini, and islets of Langerhans.

The lesions lacked other tissue components of mesodermal or ectodermal origin seen in mediastinal teratomas containing pancreatic tissue.

PERICARDIAL AND MESOTHELIAL CYSTS

Pericardial and mesothelial cysts are relatively common developmental lesions of the mediastinum and have been described under various names such as spring water cysts, hydrocele of the mediastinum, mesothelial cyst, pericardial celomic cyst of Lambert, cardiophrenic angle cyst, and pleural cyst of the mediastinum (49–54). Currently, they can be best classified as pericardial cysts when they are attached to the pericardium and as mesothelial cysts when they are encountered in other mediastinal locations.

These cysts are present most frequently in adult patients in their fourth to fifth decades of life and have no sex predilection in some reports, although they can predominate in women (2,4).

Half of the patients with pericardial or mesothelial cysts of the mediastinum are asymptomatic at the time of initial diagnosis and are found to have a mediastinal mass on chest roentgenograms (Fig. 10-8). The other patients present with cough, dyspnea, and other signs of compression of mediastinal structures (4).

Pathogenesis

The pericardium develops during early embryogenesis from discontinued lacunae that appear in the mesenchyme lateral and ventral to the primitive ectodermic plate

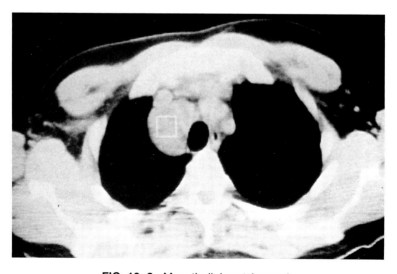

FIG. 10–8. Mesothelial cyst (*cursor*).

or primitive streak (49). These irregularly situated lacunae appear before the formation of the pleuroperitoneal coelom, enlarge, coalesce into one another, and form the pericardial coelom, a horseshoe-shaped space lying on both sides of the primitive streak. The pericardial coelom has ventral and dorsal parietal recesses and persists as an independent cavity until the pleuroperitoneal coelom develops from the pericardial dorsal recess.

A communication persists during embryonic life between the two coelomic cavities until it is closed by the ligamentum transversum and ducts of Cuvier. The latter two structures also separate the pleural cavities from the peritoneal cavity.

Pericardial cysts probably develop from persistent segments of the pericardial coelom ventral parietal recesses that do not establish contact with the pericardial cavity (49). This theory explains the preferential location of these cysts in the cardiophrenic angles and the anterior mediastinum, but it does not explain the predominance of pericardial cysts in the right cardiophrenic angle.

Pericardial cysts also can be acquired. Peterson and associates (7) reported an instance of pericardial cyst developing 10 years after an episode of pericarditis, suggesting a postinflammatory origin.

Mesothelial cysts develop as a result of developmental abnormalities of the pleuroperitoneal coelom or the dorsal recesses of the pericardial coelom through a mechanism similar to that described for pericardial cysts (4).

Pathologic Features

Pericardial cysts are spherical, unilocular, and measure up to 30 cm in diameter (Fig. 10-9). They seldom are multilocular. Their walls are thin and semitranslucent, and their lumina contain clear, watery fluid that has chemical characteristics of a transudate. Histologically, pericardial cysts are lined by a single layer of cuboidal or flattened epithelial cells with an underlying connective tissue stroma that can contain smooth muscle fibers (Fig. 10-10). Inflammation is usually absent.

The morphologic features of mesothelial cysts are identical to those of the pericardial lesions.

Prognosis and Treatment

Pericardial and mesothelial cysts have an excellent prognosis after surgical resection or FNA aspiration (8,49–52). No instances of malignant transformation have been described, to our knowledge.

THORACIC DUCT CYSTS

Thoracic duct cysts of the mediastinum are unusual lesions that are usually recognized only at the time of surgery or are found as an incidental autopsy finding (55–60). They have been described in patients in their third through sixth decades of life and are slightly more frequent in women.

Patients can be asymptomatic at the time a mediastinal mass is encountered on routine chest roentgenograms or present with chest discomfort, substernal soreness, cough, dyspnea, or dysphagia (60). They also can report postprandial chest pain or

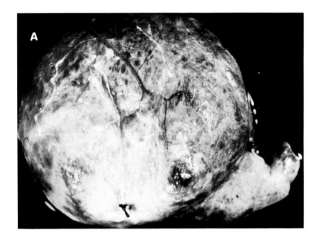

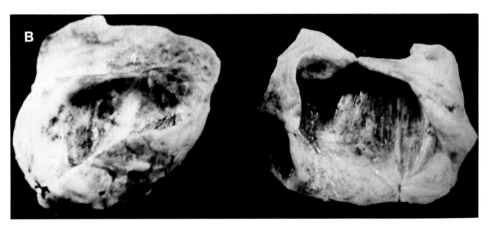

FIG. 10–9. A: Mesothelial cyst with smooth, gray outer surface. **B:** Inner surface of mesothelial cyst lined by thin, semitranslucent gray wall.

develop episodes of acute respiratory obstruction that require emergency surgery following a fatty meal (56,60).

Pathogenesis

Ross (61) described two varieties of thoracic duct cysts: the degenerative and the lymphangiomatous.

Cysts of the degenerative variety are usually encountered as an incidental autopsy finding in elderly patients and are characterized by fibrosis, atherosclerotic plaques, areas of calcification, and other degenerative changes in the cyst wall and the thoracic duct wall (61,62). Sambrook Gowar (59) described an instance of thoracic duct cyst in a patient with a previous episode of neck actinomycosis and speculated on whether the infectious process played a role in the pathogenesis of the lesion.

Lymphangiomatous cysts occur in younger individuals in their fourth or fifth decade of life as single or multiple spaces filled with chyle (63). They are smaller than mediastinal hygromas and have a clear connection with the thoracic duct (64). Lymphangiomatous thoracic duct cysts are probably caused by congenital weakness of

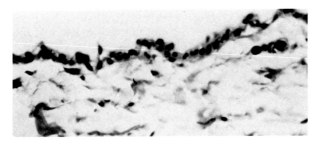

FIG. 10–10. Mesothelial cyst lined by simple cuboidal epithelium. (H&E × 100, original)

the thoracic duct wall with progressive dilatation of the lumen and aneurysm formation.

Radiologic Features

Thoracic duct cysts appear as round or oval sharply circumscribed cystic masses in the posterior mediastinum (63). They have been also described in the hilar and supraaortic areas and exhibit no radiologic features that allow distinction from other mediastinal cysts.

Tsuchiya and associates (63) reported a patient in whom the diagnosis was suspected preoperatively on the basis of postprandial pain and location of the lesion. Lymphangiogram of this patient revealed filling of the cyst with iodized oil 24 hr following injection of the radiopaque material into the patient's foot, establishing the diagnosis of thoracic duct cyst.

Pathologic Features

Thoracic duct cysts are round or oval, single or multiple, and exhibit a clear communication with the thoracic duct (55–63). Indeed, a probe should be passed along the thoracic duct to demonstrate the communication of this structure with the cyst's lumen and confirm the diagnosis.

Thoracic duct cysts have a thin wall, are usually unilocular, and are filled with chyle. Histologically, the cyst wall is lined by a layer of flattened endothelial cells with a connective tissue stroma that contains focal lymphoid infiltrates.

Prognosis and Treatment

Thoracic duct cysts are cured by surgical excision (63). Cervantez-Perez and Fuentes-Maldonado (56) reported an instance in which the pedicle from the thoracic duct was not identified at surgery (54). This patient developed postoperative chylothorax.

PARASITIC CYSTS

Hydatid cysts have been described in the mediastinum. They are caused by the larval stage of the dog tapeworm (*Echinococcus granulosus*) (64,65). They appear as unilocular or multilocular cysts with focal areas of calcification of the wall. They are composed histologically of an outer chitinous layer and an inner germinal layer (Fig. 10-11). The cyst is filled with colorless fluid that contains daughter cysts and scoleces of the parasite with characteristic hooklets (Fig. 10-12).

Marti-Bonmati and associates (65) recently described a primary mediastinal hydatid cyst that ruptured into the aorta.

MEDIASTINAL PANCREATIC PSEUDOCYST

A few cases of pancreatic pseudocysts extending into the mediastinum have been described (66–72). Patients have a history of previous pancreatitis and are found to have a posterior mediastinal mass on chest roentgenograms.

Pancreatic pseudocysts gain access to the thorax through the esophageal or aortic hiati or by eroding through the diaphragm and appear as ill-defined masses in the posterior mediastinum, usually accompanied by pleural effusions (70). Biopsy material from the mass shows only inflamed connective tissue.

Patients with mediastinal pancreatic pseudocysts are now seldom operated on, as the lesions can be diagnosed preoperatively with endoscopic retrograde pancreatography and ultrasonographic studies (68,73,74). Indeed, medical management of mediastinal pancreatic pseudocysts is now recommended (68,73).

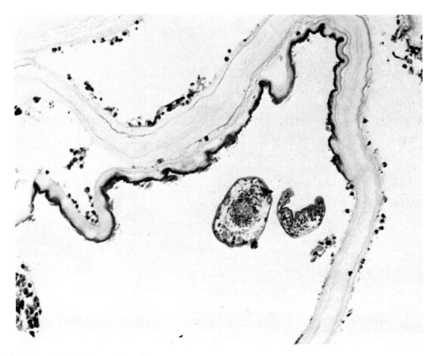

FIG. 10–11. Hydatid cyst lined by germinal layer and containing scoleces of *Echinococcus granulosus.* (H&E × 100, original)

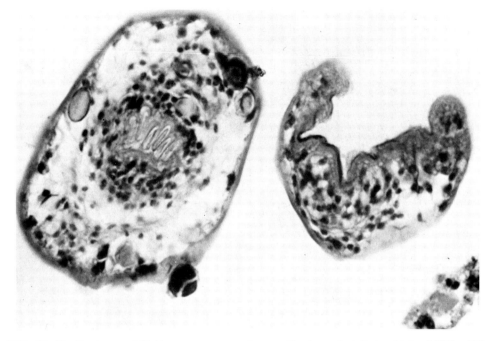

FIG. 10–12. Scoleces of *Echinococcus granulosus* with characteristic hooklets. (H&E × 400, original)

OTHER MEDIASTINAL CYSTS

Thymic cysts and mediastinal neoplasms with cystic formation have been described in other chapters dealing with thymic and soft tissue pathology.

Meningoceles are not true mediastinal cysts, as they do not arise within the area but can appear on chest roentgenograms as posterior mediastinal masses and should be included in the differential diagnosis of cystic lesions of the mediastinum (4). They usually have nerve tissue, nerve roots, and/or neuroglial tissue in their walls.

Ishimaru and associates (75) recently reported a patient with a lymphoepithelial cystic lesion of the mediastinum with a large, solid area of signet-ring adenocarcinoma.

REFERENCES

1. Ovrum E, Birkeland S: Mediastinal tumors and cysts. A review of 91 cases. *Scand J Thorac Cardiovasc Surg* 1979;13:161–168.
2. Salyer DC, Salyer WR, Eggleston JC: Benign developmental cysts of the mediastinum. *Arch Pathol Lab Med* 1977;101:136–139.
3. Bower RJ, Kiesewetter WB: Mediastinal masses in infants and children. *Arch Surg* 1977; 112:1003–1009.
4. Abel MR: Mediastinal cysts. *Arch Pathol* 1956;61:360–379.
5. Laipply TC: Cysts and cystic tumors of the mediastinum. *Arch Pathol* 1945;39:153–161.
6. Luosto R, Koikkalainen K, Jyrälä A, et al: Mediastinal tumours. A follow-up study of 208 patients. *Scand J Thorac Cardiovasc Surg* 1978;12:253–259.
7. Peterson DT, Zatz LM, Popp RL: Pericardial cyst ten years after acute pericarditis. *Chest* 1975;67:719–721.

8. Nath PH, Sanders C, Holley HC, et al: Percutaneous fine needle aspiration in the diagnosis and management of mediastinal cysts in adults. *South Med J* 1988;81:1225–1228.

9. Schwartz AR, Fishman EK, Wang KP: Diagnosis and treatment of a bronchogenic cyst using transbronchial needle aspiration. *Thorax* 1986;41:326–327.

10. Gomes MN, Hufnagel CA: Intrapericardial bronchogenic cysts. *Am J Cardiol* 1975;36:817–822.

11. Burke DW, Folger GM Jr, Magilligan DJ Jr: Pulmonary artery compression caused by bronchogenic cyst. *Angiology* 1979;30:780–783.

12. Agha FP, Master K, Kaplan S, et al: Multiple bronchogenic cysts in the mediastinum. *Br J Radiol* 1975;48:54–57.

13. Eraklis AJ, Griscom NT, McGovern JB: Bronchogenic cysts of the mediastinum in infancy. *N Engl J Med* 1969;281:1150–1155.

14. Maier HC: Bronchogenic cysts of the mediastinum. *Ann Surg* 1948;127:476–502.

15. Mindelzun R, Long P: Mediastinal bronchogenic cyst with esophageal communication. *Radiology* 1978;126:28.

16. Amendola MA, Shirazi KK, Brooks J, et al: Transdiaphragmatic bronchopulmonary foregut anomaly: "dumbbell" bronchogenic cyst. *Am J Roentgenol* 1982;138:1165–1167.

17. Ramenofsky ML, Leape LL, McCauley RGK: Bronchogenic cyst. *J Pediatr Surg* 1979;14:219–224.

18. Robbins LL: The roentgenologic appearance of "bronchogenic" cysts. *Am J Roentgenol* 1943;50:321–333.

19. Mixter CG, Clifford SH: Congenital mediastinal cysts of gastrogenic and bronchogenic origin. *Ann Surg* 1929;90:714–729.

20. Arce J: Diverticulum of the right primary bronchus. *J Thorac Surg* 1943;12:638–641.

21. Jeffries JM III: Asymptomatic bronchogenic cyst of the mediastinum. *Postgrad Med* 1987;81:235–237.

22. Volpi A, Cavalli A, Maggioni AP, et al: Left atrial compression by a mediastinal bronchogenic cyst presenting with a paroxysmal atrial fibrillation. *Thorax* 1988;43:216–217.

23. Estrera AS, Landay MJ, Pass LJ: Mediastinal carinal bronchogenic cyst: is its mere presence an indication for surgical excision? *South Med J* 1987;80:1523–1526.

24. Black TL, Fernandes ET, Wrenn EL Jr, et al: Extralobular pulmonary sequestration and mediastinal bronchogenic chest. *J Pediatr Surg* 1988;23:999–1001.

25. Woodring JH, Vandiviere HM, Dillon ML: Air-filled, multilocular, bronchopulmonary foregut duplication cyst of the mediastinum. Unusual computed tomography appearance. *Clin Imaging* 1989;13:44–47.

26. Uyama T, Monden Y, Sumitomo M, et al: CEA and CA 19-9 in benign pulmonary or mediastinal cystic lesions. *J Surg Oncol* 1989;41:103–108.

27. Miller DC, Walter JP, Guthaner DF, et al: Recurrent mediastinal bronchogenic cyst. Cause of bronchial obstruction and compression of superior vena cava and pulmonary artery. *Chest* 1978;74:218–220.

28. Bernheim J, Griffel B, Versano S, et al: Mediastinal leiomyosarcoma in the wall of a bronchial cyst (letter). *Arch Pathol Lab Med* 1980;104:221.

29. Kassner EG, Rosen Y, Klotz DH Jr: Mediastinal esophageal duplication cyst associated with a partial pericardial defect. *Pediatr Radiol* 1975;4:53–56.

30. Chitale AR: Gastric cyst of the mediastinum: A distinct clinicopathologic entity. *J Pediatr* 1969;75:104–110.

31. Reed JC, Sobonya RE: Morphologic analysis of foregut cysts in the thorax. *Am J Roentgenol Radium Ther Nucl Med* 1974;120:851–860.

32. Piramoon AM, Abbassioun K: Mediastinal enterogenic cyst with spinal cord compression. *J Pediatr Surg* 1974;9:543–545.

33. Laha RK, Huestis WS: Intraspinal enterogenous cyst: delayed appearance following mediastinal cyst resection. *Surg Neurol* 1975;3:67–70.

34. Gimeno A, Lopez F, Figueroa D, et al: Neuroentheric cyst. *Neuroradiology* 1972;3:167–172.

35. Black RA, Benjamin EL: Enterogenous abnormalities: cysts and diverticula. *Am J Dis Child* 1936;51:1126–1137.

36. Schwartz H, Williams CS: Thoracic gastric cysts. Report of two cases with a review of the literature. *J Thorac Surg* 1942;12:117–130.

37. Kirwan WO, Walbaum PR, McCormack RJM: Cystic intrathoracic derivatives of the foregut and their complications. *Thorax* 1973;28:424–428.

38. Poncher HG, Milles G: Cysts and diverticula of intestinal origin. *Am J Dis Child* 1933;45:1064–1078.

39. Ladd WE, Scott HW Jr: Esophageal duplications or mediastinal cysts of enteric origin. *Surgery* 1944;16:815–835.

40. Fallon M, Gordon ARG, Lendrum AC: Mediastinal cysts of foregut origin associated with vertebral abnormalities. *Br J Surg* 1954;41:520–533.

41. Veeneklaas GMH: Pathogenesis of intrathoracic gastrogenic cysts. *Am J Dis Child* 1952;83:500–507.
42. Mark R, Young L, Ferguson C, et al: Diagnosis of an intrathoracic gastrogenic cyst using 99m Tc-pertechnetate. *Radiology* 1973;109:137–138.
43. Kamoi I, Nishitani H, Oshiumi Y, et al: Intrathoracic gastric cyst demonstrated by 99m Tc pertechnetate scintigraphy. *Am J Roentgenol* 1980;134:1080–1081.
44. Zimmer WD, Kamida CB, McGough PF, et al: Mediastinal duplication cyst. Percutaneous aspiration and cystography for diagnosis and treatment. *Chest* 1986;90:772–773.
45. Bortolani EM, Ghilardi G: Endodermal and coelomic mediastinal cysts. *Minerva Chir* 1989;44:1275–1278.
46. Chuang MT, Barba FA, Kaneko M, et al: Adenocarcinoma arising in an intrathoracic duplication cyst of foregut origin: a case report with review of the literature. *Cancer* 1981;47:1887–1890.
47. Shillitoe AJ, Wilson JE: Enterogenous cysts of the thorax with pancreatic tissue as a constituent. *J Thorac Surg* 1957;34:810–814.
48. Carr MJT, Deiraniya AK, Judd PA: Mediastinal cyst containing mural pancreatic tissue. *Thorax* 1977;32:512–516.
49. Lambert AVS: Etiology of thin-walled thoracic cysts. *J Thorac Surg* 1940;10:1–7.
50. Lillie WI, McDonald JR, Clagett OT: Pericardial celomic cysts and pericardial diverticula. A concept of etiology and report of cases. *J Thorac Surg* 1950;20:494–504.
51. Kaimal KP: Computed tomography in the diagnosis of pericardial cyst. *Am Heart J* 1982;103:566–567.
52. Klein DL: Pleural cyst of the mediastinum. *Br J Radiol* 1978;51:548–549.
53. Williamson BR, Spotnitz WD, Gay SB, et al: Pericardial cyst. A rare mass abutting the aorta. *J Comput Tomogr* 1988;12:264–266.
54. Boisserie-Lacroix M, Martigne C, Laurent F, et al: A pleuropericardial cyst in an unusual location: the value of magnetic resonance. *Comput Med Imaging Graph* 1988;12:277–280.
55. Carbone T: Cisti del dotto toracico. *G R Accad Med Torino* 1892;40:136–144.
56. Cervantes-Perez P, Fuentes-Maldonado R: Thoracic duct cyst of the mediastinum (letter). *Chest* 1976;70:411.
57. Emerson GL: Supradiaphragmatic thoracic duct cyst. An unusual mediastinal tumor. *N Engl J Med* 1950;242:575–578.
58. Luosto R, Koikkalainen K, Jyrälä A, et al: Thoracic duct cyst of the mediastinum. A case report. *Scand J Thorac Cardiovasc Surg* 1978;12:261–263.
59. Sambrook Gowar FJ: Mediastinal thoracic duct cyst. *Thorax* 1978;33:800–802.
60. Fromang DR, Seltzer MB, Tobias JA: Thoracic duct cyst causing mediastinal compression and acute respiratory insufficiency. *Chest* 1975;67:725–727.
61. Ross JK: A review of the surgery of the thoracic duct. *Thorax* 1961;16:12–21.
62. Kausel HW, Reeve TS, Stein AA, et al: Anatomic and pathologic studies of the thoracic duct. *J Thorac Cardiovasc Surg* 1957;34:631–642.
63. Tsuchiya R, Sugiura Y, Ogata T, et al: Thoracic duct cyst of the mediastinum. *J Thorac Cardiovasc Surg* 1980;79:856–859.
64. Curley SA, Ablin DS, Kosloske AM: Giant cystic hygroma of the posterior mediastinum. *J Pediatr Surg* 1989;24:398–400.
65. Marti-Bonmati L, Touza R, Montes H: CT diagnosis of primary mediastinal hydatid cyst rupture into the aorta: a case report. *Cardiovasc Intervent Radiol* 1988;11:296–299.
66. Jaffe BM, Ferguson TB, Holtz S, et al: Mediastinal pancreatic pseudocysts. *Am J Surg* 1972;124:600–606.
67. Gooding GAW: Pseudocyst of the pancreas with mediastinal extension: an ultrasonographic demonstration. *J Clin Ultrasound* 1977;5:121–123.
68. Leechawengwong M, Berger HW, Romeu J: Spontaneous resolution of mediastinal pancreatic pseudocyst. *Chest* 1979;75:632–633.
69. Mallard RE, Stilwell CA, O'Neill JA, Jr, et al: Mediastinal pancreatic pseudocyst in infancy. *J Pediatr* 1977;91:445–447.
70. Heiss FW, Shea JA, Cady B, et al: Pancreatic pseudocyst with mediastinal extension and pleural effusion. Demonstration of pathologic anatomy by endoscopic pancreatography. *Dig Dis Sci* 1979;24:649–651.
71. Kirchner SG, Heller RM, Smith CW: Pancreatic pseudocyst of the mediastinum. *Radiology* 1977;123:37–42.
72. Weinfeld A, Kaplan JO: Mediastinal pancreatic pseudocyst. *Gastrointest Radiol* 1979;4:343–347.
73. Johnston RH Jr, Owensby LC, Vargas GM, et al: Pancreatic pseudocyst of the mediastinum. *Ann Thorac Surg* 1986;41:210–212.
74. Gaa J, Deininger HK: Mediastinal pancreas pseudocyst. *Rontgenblatter* 1988;41:406–410.
75. Ishimaru Y, Shibata Y, Ohkawara S, et al: Lymphoepithelial cystic lesion related to adenocarcinoma in the mediastinum. *Am J Clin Pathol* 1989;92:808–813.

11

Mesenchymal Tumors of the Mediastinum

Mesenchymal tumors are unusual in the thorax and account for fewer than 10% of all mediastinal masses (1–8). Approximately half of these neoplasms are of lymphatic or vascular origin, whereas other mesenchymal tumors (Table 1) are less frequent.

We review briefly in this chapter only the basic clinicopathologic aspects of the most frequent mediastinal mesenchymal tumors. The reader should refer to other specialized publications for more detailed information regarding the pathology of each individual pathologic entity (9).

LYMPHANGIOMA

Lymphangiomas are benign lesions characterized by proliferating lymph vessels. It is controversial whether they are neoplastic or hamartomatous in origin (9).

Fewer than 1% of all lymphangiomas are located in the mediastinum only, and these are usually detected in asymptomatic adult patients (10,11).

Mediastinal extensions of cervical lymphangiomas are more frequent. Indeed, as many as 10% of cervical cystic hygromas have mediastinal extensions (10,11). These cervicomediastinal lesions occur almost exclusively in children and are frequently symptomatic. Patients present with large cervical masses accompanied by cough, chest pain, and/or early and potentially severe respiratory distress secondary to airway compression by an enlarging lesion (12,13). These symptoms are age related and occur almost invariably in children younger than 2 years of age. They are infrequent in older patients (11,12).

Pathogenesis

Lymphangiomas result from the proliferation of lymph vessels that remain sequestrated from the lymphatic system early during development. They become cystic as a result of fluid accumulation within their lumina and failure to communicate with the lymphatic tree. This theory is supported by the fact that most lymphangiomas are detected in children and appear in areas such as the neck and axilla where the primitive lymph sacs develop normally during embryogenesis (9). Lymphangiomas can also arise, however, from the mediastinal or cervical mesenchyme itself (13).

TABLE 1. *Mesenchymal tumors of the mediastinum*

Tumors of lymph vessels	Tumors of muscle origin
Lymphangioma	Rhabdomyoma
Lymphangiomatosis	Rhabdomyosarcoma
Lymphangiomyoma	Leiomyoma
Tumors of blood vessel origin	Leiomyosarcoma
Hemangioma	Tumors of pluripotential
Hemangioendothelioma	mesenchyme
Hemangiomatosis	Benign mesenchymoma
Epithelioid hemangioendothelioma	Malignant mesenchymoma
Malignant hemangioendothelioma	Synovial sarcoma
(angiosarcoma)	Tumors of skeletal tissues
Tumors of pericyte origin	Chondroma
Hemangiopericytoma	Osteogenic sarcoma
Tumors and tumor-like fibrohistiocytic	Chondrosarcoma
lesions	Other tumors and tumor-like
Fibromatosis	conditions
Fibrosarcoma	Solitary fibrous tumor (fibrous
Malignant fibrous histiocytoma	mesothelioma)
Tumors of adipose tissue	Myxoma
Lipoma	Meningioma
Lipomatosis	Chordoma
Lipoblastomatosis	Granular cell tumor
Liposarcoma	Extramedullary hematopoiesis
	Histiocytosis X
	Amyloid tumor

Roentgenologic Features

Lymphangiomas occur most frequently in the anterosuperior mediastinum but have also been described in the middle and posterior compartments and other locations (10,14–17). They are round, oval, or lobulated masses with smooth, sharp contours and uniform density and, on chest roentgenograms, can indent and/or displace the trachea and compress other mediastinal structures (15–18). They seldom become calcified.

Computed tomographic (CT) scans, echocardiography, sonograms, thoracic aortography, superior venocavography, lymphangiograms, and magnetic resonance imaging (MRI) are useful for the diagnosis and localization of these lesions.

Pathologic Features

Lymphangiomas can be well or ill circumscribed and vary in size from small to giant lesions that fill a great portion of the thoracic cavity (10,19). They are soft, gray, and exhibit a sponge-like appearance with variably sized spaces filled with white chyle. They can become cystic (cystic hygroma) (Fig. 11-1).

Histologically, lymphangiomas are composed of irregular interconnecting lymphatic vessels of different sizes lined by flattened endothelial cells (Fig. 11-2). In focal areas, the endothelial cells can adopt an epithelioid appearance with a cuboidal, eosinophilic cytoplasm (9). The stroma frequently has lymphoid infiltrates and focal smooth muscle bundles. Areas of hemorrhage caused by operative trauma can also be found. Indeed, red blood cells can be encountered within the lymphatic spaces,

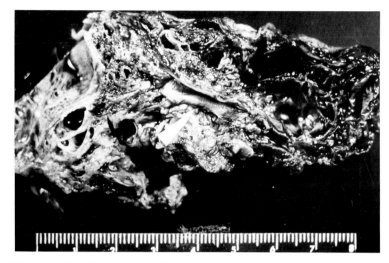

FIG. 11–1. Cystic hygroma with numerous interconnecting lymph vessels.

a feature that should not mislead the surgical pathologist into the diagnosis of a hemangioma.

Lymphangiomas can be classified morphologically according to the size of their lymphatic spaces into cystic hygromas, composed of large cystic spaces, and cavernous lymphangiomas, with smaller spaces forming a sponge-like mass.

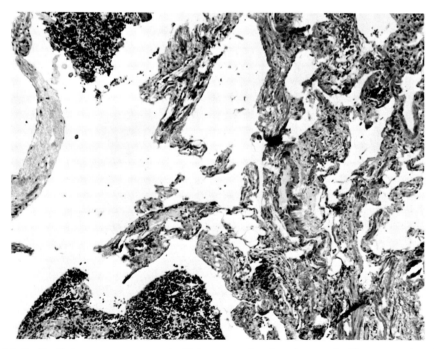

FIG. 11–2. Cystic hygroma composed of interconnecting lymph vessels. The stroma has lymphoid tissue. (H&E × 40, original)

Differential Diagnosis Between Lymphangiomas and Hemangiomas

Hemangiomas exhibit almost identical morphologic features to lymphangiomas. The lymphatic lesions are distinguished from their vascular counterparts, however, by the presence of chyle within their spaces and the frequent finding of microscopic lymphoid infiltrates in their stroma. The presence of chyle within the lesion can be best observed by the surgeon at the time of resection before operative trauma induces secondary hemorrhage. Immunocytochemical techniques also can be useful for the distinction between vascular and lymphatic lesions. The endothelial cells lining lymphatic spaces usually lack intracytoplasmic factor VIII immunoreactivity, which is a finding characteristic of vascular lesions.

Prognosis and Treatment

Lymphangiomas are benign lesions that can nevertheless cause significant clinical problems because of their large size and location. They also can become secondarily infected (9). Complicated lesions frequently develop areas of sclerosis and fibrosis.

Lymphangiomas are cured by surgical excision. Radiotherapy rarely induces regression of the lesions and can result in their malignant transformation (20). However, low-dose radiation can be effective to control chylothorax in lesions refractory to surgical treatment (21). Therapy with sclerosing agents is ineffective.

The complete resection of lymphangiomas can be feasible technically in lesions that invade the pericardium and/or mediastinal vessels and nerves. In these instances, where only incomplete resection is feasible, unroofing of the lesions with resection of as much cyst wall as possible is recommended to decrease the probability of postoperative recurrence (22,23).

LYMPHANGIOMATOSIS

Lymphangiomatosis is an uncommon disorder of children characterized by multiple lymphangiomas in soft tissues, bone, liver, spleen, mediastinum, and/or lungs. It seldom affects patients older than 20 years of age (9,24,25).

Lymphangiomatosis involving the mediastinum is usually accompanied by chylothorax. The mediastinal involvement is a poor prognostic sign in patients with lymphangiomatosis, as the lesions usually infiltrate the area diffusely and cannot be readily resected. Pulmonary lesions also carry a poor prognosis.

LYMPHANGIOMYOMATOSIS

Lymphangiomyomatosis is a rare condition characterized by the proliferation of lymphatics and smooth muscle in mediastinal lymph nodes, lung parenchyma, and retroperitoneum (9). It occurs only in females in their reproductive age and probably results from the development of multiple hamartomas (26–30). Valensi (31) and other authors consider pulmonary lymphangiomyomas as a probable *form fruste* of tuberous sclerosis.

Patients with lymphangiomyomatosis have progressive dyspnea, hemoptysis, chylous bilateral pleural and/or peritoneal effusions, pneumothorax, chyluria, and coarse reticulonodular pulmonary infiltrates with cyst formation distributed irregularly throughout both lungs (29). Pulmonary involvement by lymphangiomyomatosis results in severe impairment in air exchange and respiratory insufficiency with normal pulmonary volumes (26–31).

The diagnosis of lymphangiomyomatosis is suspected after lymphangiograms reveal the presence of obstruction of the major lymphatic ducts, ectasia of lymph vessels distal to the obstruction, and loss of lymph node architecture. It is established by pathologic examination of open lung biopsy specimens or of mediastinal lymph nodes.

Pathologic Features

Lymphangiomyomas appear as red–gray spongy lesions composed of irregularly interconnected endothelial-lined spaces surrounded by short fascicles of smooth muscle cells (9).

The smooth muscle character of the spindle cells surrounding the lymphatic spaces has been the subject of controversy (9). It has been confirmed, however, in immunohistochemical studies demonstrating smooth muscle antigens in the cytoplasm of these cells. Moreover, ultrastructural studies demonstrate myofilaments with dense bodies, pinocytotic vesicles on the cell membrane, and basal lamina formation, all features consistent with a smooth muscle differentiation (26–32).

The diagnosis of lymphangiomyomas can be difficult to establish in mediastinal lymph nodes, where the lesions can be misdiagnosed as metastatic leiomyosarcomas. This error can be avoided, however, if the consistent finding of dilated, interconnecting lymph vessels located central to the smooth muscle fascicles is noted.

Prognosis and Treatment

The prognosis of patients with lymphangiomyomatosis is variable (9). Women with localized lymphangiomyomas usually survive for many years, whereas those with ill-defined lesions and pulmonary involvement develop progressive pulmonary insufficiency and die within 10 years of the initial diagnosis (25–28).

Patients are treated symptomatically to control their recurrent pleural and peritoneal effusions. Radiotherapy in low doses to the lung and mediastinum can result in prolonged survivals (32). McCarty and associates (26) reported the radiographic resolution of pulmonary lesions after progesterone therapy.

Recently, single and double lung transplantation has become an effective therapeutic option for patients with lymphangiomyomatosis and severe respiratory insufficiency (33).

TUMORS OF BLOOD VESSEL ORIGIN

Vascular tumors are unusual in the thorax and represent less than 1% of all mediastinal masses (34). Indeed, fewer than 100 instances of benign and malignant primary mediastinal vascular tumors have been reported (2,34–43). This low incidence is difficult to explain, as the mediastinum is an area containing multiple vascular structures.

Vascular tumors should be distinguished from aneurysms of various mediastinal arteries and/or veins (vascular pseudotumors) (39). They are diagnosed more specifically as mediastinal masses of vascular origin with angiograms and venograms (44,45).

Mediastinal vascular tumors are benign in 75% of instances and include hemangiomas, hemangioendotheliomas, and hemangiopericytomas (2,9,34,46–49). The latter tumors are of pericytic origin but are included together with neoplasms of blood vessel origin in most reports (2,9,34).

Mediastinal vascular tumors affect males and females with equal frequency and can be present in patients of all ages. Cavernous hemangiomas are more frequent in children (38).

Patients with vascular tumors are asymptomatic in about one-third of instances and are found to have a mediastinal mass on routine chest roentgenograms or present, more frequently, with cough, stridor, dyspnea, hoarseness, chest pain, dysphagia, superior vena cava or Horner's syndrome, and/or neurological symptoms resulting from tumor compression of the spinal cord (37–45).

Patients also can have multiple hemangiomas at other sites (angiomatosis) that occur isolated or in association with other abnormalities (e.g., Osler–Weber–Rendu's syndrome) (34,35).

Radiologic Features

Vascular tumors are round or lobulated masses on chest roentgenograms and occur most frequently in the anterosuperior mediastinum (2,41). They also can be present in the posterior mediastinum (40).

Approximately 10% of mediastinal hemangiomas exhibit phlebitis, which appears on chest roentgenograms as areas of ring-like calcifications (37). Mediastinal malignant vascular tumors have ill-defined borders, infiltrate adjacent structures, and can erode the chest wall.

Pathologic Features

Hemangiomas

The vast majority (90%) of benign mediastinal vascular tumors are cavernous or capillary hemangiomas (41). They appear as encapsulated or, less frequently, illcircumscribed, soft, red masses with a spongy appearance that shrink and collapse on section and exude blood. The latter feature is important to distinguish hemangiomas from lymphangiomas, which contain chyle in their lumina instead of blood.

Histologically, hemangiomas are classified according to the size of their vascular spaces into capillary, cavernous, and venous variants (9).

The vast majority of mediastinal hemangiomas are cavernous and are composed of large interconnecting vascular spaces with thick smooth muscle walls and edematous stroma that has focal myxomatous areas containing stellate cells (Fig. 11-3) (38). The latter exhibit ultrastructural features of smooth muscle cells (34).

Occasionally, cavernous hemangiomas have a prominent smooth muscle component and are classified as angiomyomas or hamartomatous hemangiomas (2). These lesions should be distinguished histologically from mesenchymomas. The latter are

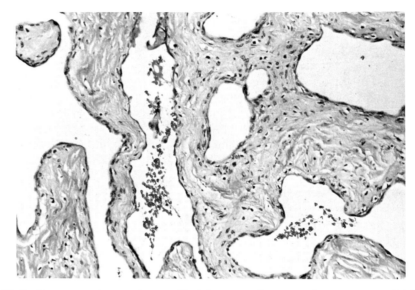

FIG. 11–3. Cavernous hemangioma with interconnecting vascular spaces containing red blood cells and lined by flattened endothelial cells. (H&E × 100, original)

tumors composed of at least two different mesenchymal components other than fibrous tissue. Although hamartomatous hemangiomas are composed of blood vessels and smooth muscle, they are not true mesenchymomas because their muscular component probably represents a nonneoplastic proliferation of the smooth muscle that is normally present in the wall of large vascular spaces. Indeed, it is controversial whether hamartomatous and other hemangiomas are true neoplasms or malformations (9).

Approximately 15% of mediastinal hemangiomas are of the capillary variant and are composed of interconnecting, irregularly dilated, thin-walled, blood-filled vessels (9,37).

Other Vascular Tumors

Benign and malignant hemangiopericytomas and hemangioendotheliomas have been encountered in the mediastinum (2).

Hemangiopericytomas are solitary, well-circumscribed, soft, gray–white masses with focal areas of hemorrhage, cystic degeneration, and/or necrosis composed of densely packed oval, round, or spindle cells arranged in a characteristic perivascular pattern (Fig. 11-4). The lesions are highly vascularized and have multiple anastomosing thin-walled endothelial-lined spaces ranging in size from capillaries to dilated sinusoidal channels with focal "staghorn" configuration (Fig. 11-5). The tumor cells also can form solid areas and focal palisading but are not arranged in fascicles as in other spindle cell mesenchymal tumors (Fig. 11-6). Reticulin stains are useful for the diagnosis of hemangiopericytomas and demonstrate that the tumor cells are located outside the wall of the anastomosing vascular channels.

It is difficult to predict the biologic behavior of hemangiopericytomas on histologic grounds (9). Lesions with four or more mitoses per 10 high-power fields (HPF),

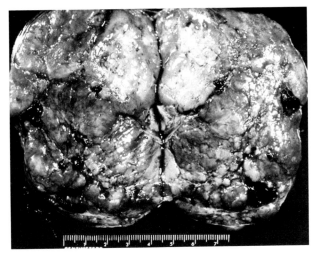

FIG. 11–4. Hemangiopericytoma. The tumor is well-circumscribed, soft, gray, with focal hemorrhages.

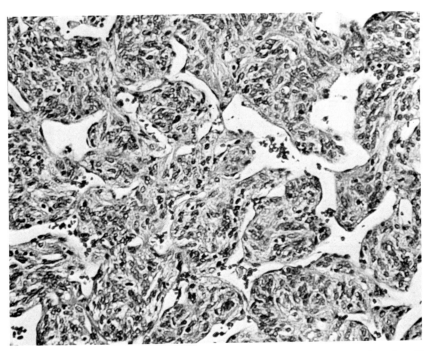

FIG. 11–5. Hemangiopericytoma composed of spindle cells in perivascular location. The lesion is highly vascularized and has multiple interconnecting endothelial-lined spaces with a staghorn configuration. (H&E × 100, original)

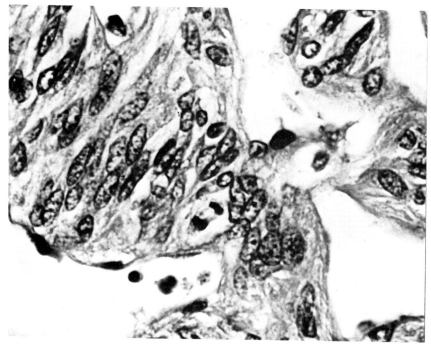

FIG. 11–6. Spindle cells of hemangiopericytoma in typical perivascular location exhibit palisading. Endothelial cells are smaller and flattened. (H&E × 400, original)

prominent cellular pleomorphism and cellularity, and areas of hemorrhage and necrosis are malignant and can metastasize (9).

Hemangioendotheliomas are well-circumscribed but not encapsulated white masses that usually lack hemorrhagic areas and are composed of round to oval endothelial cells arranged in small nests and cords forming inconspicuous vascular channels (Fig. 11-7). Reticulin stains demonstrate that the tumor cells are present within the wall of the vascular spaces and, indeed, line their lumina. Immunocytochemical stains demonstrate the presence of factor-VIII-associated antigen in the cytoplasm of tumor cells. Ultrastructural studies demonstrate Weibel–Palade bodies in their cytoplasm. The latter two findings are characteristic of endothelial cells (9,50).

It is difficult to predict the biologic behavior of hemangioendotheliomas on histologic grounds (9). Features that suggest malignancy in these tumors include mitotic activity greater than one mitosis per 10 HPF, prominent cellular pleomorphism and cellularity, and presence of necrosis.

Toursarkissian and associates (51) recently described a patient with a mediastinal epithelioid hemangioendothelioma, characterized by an intermediate malignant potential.

Prognosis and Treatment

The prognosis of mediastinal vascular tumors is determined by the biologic potential of each individual lesion and its location. Hemangiomas can be suspected clinically in patients with angiomatosis presenting with a round or lobulated, well-circum-

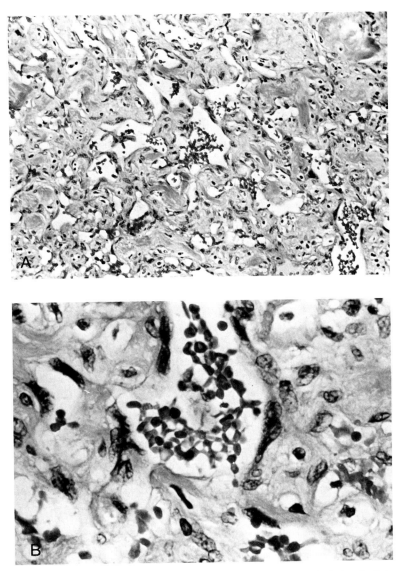

FIG. 11–7. A: Malignant hemangioendothelioma with atypical endothelial cells lining anastomosing irregular vascular channels. (H&E × 100, original) **B:** Higher power showing markedly atypical endothelial cells. (H&E × 400, original)

scribed mediastinal mass detected on chest roentgenograms. These lesions should not be biopsied, however, because of the risk of severe hemorrhage.

Hemangiomas are cured by complete excision, but this optimal therapy is not feasible in all instances, as the lesions may be very large, have local extensions, and be firmly adherent to vital structures. Patients in whom total surgical excision of their lesions is hazardous can be treated with partial resection with a low probability of recurrence (41). There are, to our knowledge, no instances of mediastinal hemangiomas undergoing malignant transformation. Radiation therapy is of little value for the control of incompletely excised hemangiomas.

Benign and malignant hemangioendotheliomas and hemangiopericytomas can also be treated surgically. Recurrent and/or metastatic lesions receive radiotherapy and/or chemotherapy (9,51).

TUMORS AND TUMOR-LIKE CONDITIONS OF FIBROHISTIOCYTIC ORIGIN

Fibromatosis

Fibromatoses are unusual tumor-like conditions characterized by the presence of ill-circumscribed infiltrating masses composed of dense infiltrates by fibroblasts. They are very rare in the mediastinum, where they may be difficult to distinguish from sclerosing mediastinitis. Pachter and Lattes reported three cases (1). We have encountered an additional patient with a thoracic fibromatosis presenting as a retrosternal mass in the anterior mediastinum.

Fibrosarcomas

Fibrosarcomas are very unusual in the mediastinum. Indeed, Barua and associates (52) reviewed the literature in 1979 and encountered only 36 cases, including three of their own.

The lesions occur in patients of both sexes and ranging from 19 to 73 years old. Most patients are in the third through fifth decades of life and have signs and symptoms related to the size and location of their mediastinal lesions. They also may have associated hypoglycemia (53,54).

Fibrosarcomas are well-circumscribed lobulated masses with ill-defined borders on chest roentgenograms that frequently compress and/or infiltrate adjacent mediastinal and thoracic structures such as the ribs and vertebral bodies (53).

They are lobulated, ill-circumscribed white–gray firm masses composed of cellular, pleomorphic spindle cell infiltrates. Mitotic figures and focal areas of necrosis are frequent.

Fibrosarcomas should be distinguished on biopsy material from fibrosing mediastinitis. The latter is more frequent and exhibits fewer cellular spindle cell infiltrates that lack cytologic evidence of malignancy and are admixed with inflammatory cells and/or focal granulomas.

Fibrosarcomas are malignant neoplasms that grow locally in the mediastinum, infiltrate vital structures, and tend to recur following surgical excision (53). They seldom metastasize, however, beyond the thorax (55,56). Most patients die, however, within a few years of initial diagnosis as a result of extensive mediastinal invasion.

Fibrosarcomas are treated by surgical excision and may also respond to radiotherapy (52). Thorbjarnarson (56) reported a patient surviving 13 years after surgery, the longest survivor on record.

Malignant Fibrous Histiocytoma

Malignant fibrous histiocytoma is the most frequent soft tissue sarcoma of late adult life, yet it seldom occurs as a primary mediastinal tumor (9,57–59). The majority of fibrous histiocytomas in the mediastinum are metastatic.

We have observed an additional primary malignant fibrous histiocytoma of the

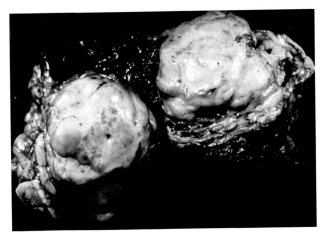

FIG. 11–8. Fibrous histiocytoma. The tumor is poorly circumscribed, firm, tan, and invades the lung parenchyma.

anterior mediastinum in a 35-year-old patient (Fig. 11-8). The tumor was a soft, ill-circumscribed, yellow–gray mass with multiple areas of hemorrhage and necrosis. It weighed 1,350 g. Histologically, this neoplasm was composed of pleomorphic spindle cells arranged in a characteristic storiform pattern (Fig. 11-9). Multinucleated giant cells were also present. Mitotic figures and areas of necrosis were frequent.

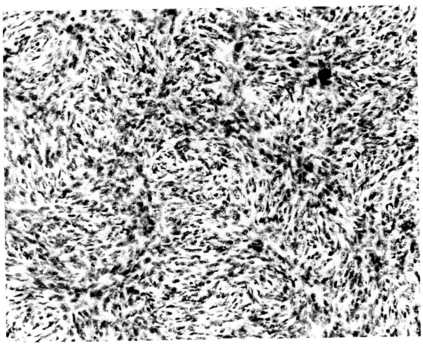

FIG. 11–9. Malignant fibrous histiocytoma with atypical spindle cells arranged in storiform pattern. (H&E × 100, original)

TUMORS OF ADIPOSE TISSUE

Lipoma

Lipomas are rare primary mediastinal tumors (60–62). For example, they accounted for only 1% of the 1,064 mediastinal neoplasms reviewed by Benjamin and associates (47).

Patients may be asymptomatic or present with dyspnea and other symptoms caused by compression of mediastinal structures.

Lipomas are single or multiple, round or oval in the mediastinum and can simulate cardiomegaly or pleural effusions on chest roentgenograms. They have, however, a characteristic coefficient of density on CT scans that allows their identification.

Pathologically, they are well-circumscribed, encapsulated, soft yellow masses that can reach a giant size. Sections of the lesions float in formalin or other aqueous media, a useful gross diagnostic sign. Histologically, lipomas are composed of lobules of mature fat.

Lipomas are benign neoplasms that are cured by complete surgical excision.

Lipomatosis

Lipomatosis is a relatively common cause of mediastinal widening characterized by the accumulation of unencapsulated fat in the area (63–66). It is usually associated with exogenous obesity, steroid ingestion, Cushing's syndrome, or ectopic adrenocorticotropic hormone (ACTH) production by pulmonary neoplasms (65).

Shukla and associates (66) recently reported children with mediastinal lipomatosis secondary to high-dose steroid therapy.

Lipomatosis can simulate on chest roentgenograms various space-occupying lesions of the anterior, middle, or posterior compartments of the mediastinum. It can be diagnosed, however, with CT scans that demonstrate the fatty nature of the lesions (64). Patients with lipomatosis seldom undergo biopsy of their lesions.

Lipoblastomas and Lipoblastomatosis

Lipoblastomatosis is a rare condition first described by Vellios (67) in 1958 and characterized by the development of diffuse, infiltrating benign lipoblastomas in the chest wall, mediastinum, axilla, neck, and prevertebral soft tissues (68). It is a disease of infants younger than 1 year of age.

Lipoblastomas also can appear as isolated, well-encapsulated tumors in the extremities of children that are usually younger than 3 years of age (9).

The lesions of lipoblastomatosis are histologically benign but may infiltrate and compress adjacent structures such as the trachea, causing respiratory distress and even asphyxia.

Histologically, lipoblastomas are composed of irregular lobules of immature fat with lipoblasts at various stages of development that appear as stellate spindle and/or round cells with unilocular intracytoplasmic single vacuoles. The stroma has abundant mucoid material.

The isolated or multiple diffuse lesions are cured by surgical excision. The diffuse lesions of lipoblastomatosis can recur, however, in cases of incomplete resection.

Liposarcoma

Liposarcomas are unusual in the mediastinum. To our knowledge, less than 60 cases have been described (69–76).

Mediastinal liposarcomas occur in patients ranging in age from 5 to 77 years and presenting with dyspnea, chest pain, cough, wheezing, or weight loss (71). Asymptomatic lesions have also been described (70).

Grieger and associates (77) recently reported a mediastinal liposarcoma in a patient infected with the human immunodeficiency virus.

Liposarcomas are large, lobulated masses with ill-defined borders on chest roentgenograms that infiltrate and compress adjacent mediastinal structures. The tumors exhibit on CT scans an EMI density intermediate between those of water and fat. This finding is useful to distinguish lipomas from liposarcomas (72).

Liposarcomas are large, well-circumscribed (but not encapsulated), soft, yellow–gray tumors with areas of hemorrhage and/or necrosis (Fig. 11-10). They also can exhibit a characteristic mucoid appearance and occasionally can reach a large size in the mediastinum, weighing up to 7 kg (71).

Histologically, these tumors can be divided into four types: myxoid, round-cell, well-differentiated, and pleomorphic (73). All of these histologic variants contain various amounts of malignant lipoblasts with large, irregular, round or oval hyperchromatic nuclei and foamy cytoplasm (Fig. 11-11). Identification of these cells is needed to establish the diagnoses.

Myxoid liposarcomas are characterized by the presence of a loose mucoid stroma containing scattered stellate cells and occasional malignant lipoblasts. Round-cell lesions have dense infiltrates of round cells with acidophilic cytoplasm interspersed with lipoblasts. Pleomorphic liposarcomas have abundant lipoblasts with prominent cellular atypia, giant tumor cells, and frequent mitotic figures (Fig. 11-12). All of these variants of liposarcoma have, in addition, areas of necrosis.

Well-differentiated liposarcomas are most difficult to diagnose. They are large, well-circumscribed masses composed of mature fat with only a few scattered atypical lipoblasts and rare mitoses (Fig. 11-13).

Mediastinal liposarcomas are malignant neoplasms that infiltrate adjacent structures and can recur locally and metastasize to the lungs, bones, and other organs

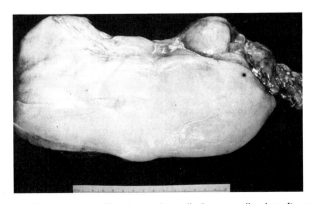

FIG. 11–10. Liposarcoma. The tumor is well-circumscribed, soft, and yellow.

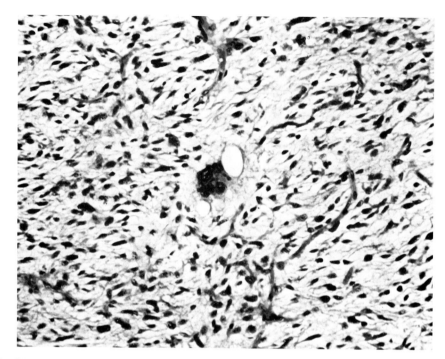

FIG. 11–11. Myxoid liposarcoma with characteristic malignant, multinucleated lipoblast. (H&E × 100, original)

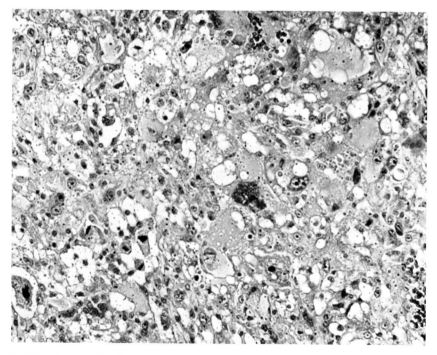

FIG. 11–12. Pleomorphic liposarcoma with markedly atypical lipoblasts with eosinophilic, foamy cytoplasm. (H&E × 100, original)

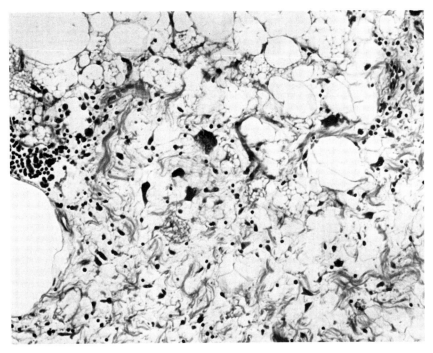

FIG. 11–13. Well-differentiated liposarcoma with occasional malignant lipoblasts. (H&E × 100, original)

(70,71). Their prognosis in the mediastinum appears to be related to the presence or absence of pseudoencapsulation. The few well-circumscribed lesions reviewed by Standerfer and associates (70) had survivals of 3 to 17 years following initial resection, whereas nonencapsulated lesions were more pleomorphic histologically and had a worse prognosis, with death of the patients within 2 years of initial diagnoses.

TUMORS OF MUSCLE ORIGIN

Rhabdomyoma

Rhabdomyomas are unusual benign tumors of striated muscle origin that occur in cardiac and extracardiac locations. The cardiac lesions are probably hamartomatous and usually occur in patients with tuberous sclerosis. Extracardiac rhabdomyomas usually involve the head and neck areas or the female genital tract (9,78).

Miller and associates (78) reported an instance of mediastinal rhabdomyoma and postulated an origin from thymic myoid cells (78). The lesion was a well-encapsulated mass present in the anterosuperior mediastinum of an 80-year-old patient, composed of sheets of large polyhedral cells with acidophilic granular cytoplasm admixed with clear cells. Occasional tumor cells had cross striations on PTAH-stained sections. Ultrastructural studies demonstrated the presence of clusters of intracytoplasmic myofilaments with Z and I bands.

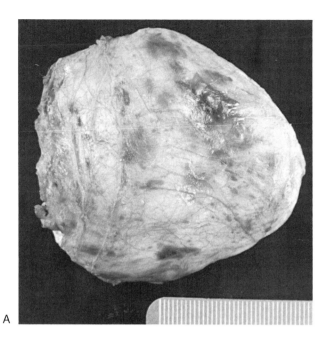

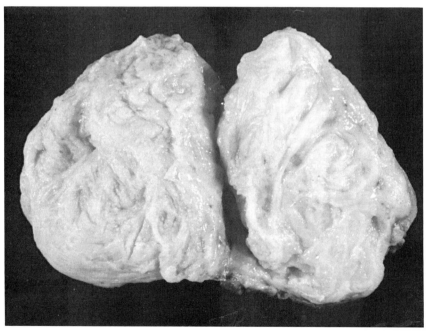

FIG. 11–14. A: Leiomyoma of the mediastinum. The tumor is well encapsulated, firm, and pink–gray. **B:** The cut surface of the leiomyoma of the mediastinum has a typical whorled appearance, similar to that seen in smooth muscle tumors arising at other locations.

Rhabdomyosarcoma

Rhabdomyosarcomas are malignant tumors of striated muscle origin. They are the most frequent soft tissue sarcomas in children, yet they are seldom encountered as primary mediastinal neoplasms (9).

Pachter and Lattes (1) reported three instances of primary mediastinal rhabdomyosarcoma composed of cellular and myxoid areas with small round cells with scanty cytoplasm admixed with larger, elongated tumor cells with abundant eosinophilic cytoplasm. The lesions had characteristic rhabdomyoblasts with round or elongated eosinophilic cytoplasm and a vesicular nucleus. Strap-like rhabdomyoblasts with intracytoplasmic cross striations were also present.

Leiomyoma

Leiomyomas are benign tumors of smooth muscle origin that are rare in the mediastinum (1,79,80).

In a recent review, Shaffer and associates (80) encountered only 11 mediastinal leiomyomata in the literature, including their own patient. The tumors were five times more frequent in female patients and arose from the esophagus, great vessels, or other mediastinal structures with smooth muscle walls. We recently encountered an additional patient with a well-circumscribed mediastinal leiomyoma. The tumor was well encapsulated and exhibited a whorled cut surface (Fig. 11-14). It was composed histologically of interlacing bundles of spindle cells with elongated nuclei exhibiting rounded ends and an ill-defined eosinophilic cytoplasm.

Leiomyosarcoma

Leiomyosarcomas are malignant tumors of smooth muscle origin that can originate from the wall of mediastinal vascular structures such as the superior vena cava and the pulmonary artery (81–86). They have also been described in the wall of a bronchial cyst (86).

Pulmonary artery leiomyosarcomas occur in adult patients of either sex, who present with signs and symptoms related to decreased pulmonary inflow (84,85). The tumors are usually intraluminal and grow from the base of the heart into both pulmonary arteries. Histologically, they are composed of interlacing bundles of large spindle cells with elongated hyperchromatic nuclei, abundant mitotic figures, and focal areas of necrosis (Fig. 11-15).

Superior vena cava leiomyosarcomas are detected in patients with the superior vena cava syndrome or presenting with chest pain and other nonspecific symptoms (82,87). Davis and associates (82) reported an instance of leiomyosarcoma in this location resected surgically and treated with postoperative radiotherapy with no evidence of recurrence 6½ years after the initial diagnosis.

TUMORS OF PLURIPOTENTIAL MESENCHYME

Mesenchymomas

Mesenchymomas are tumors composed of two or more unrelated differentiated tissue types such as smooth muscle, cartilage, bone, and others in addition to a

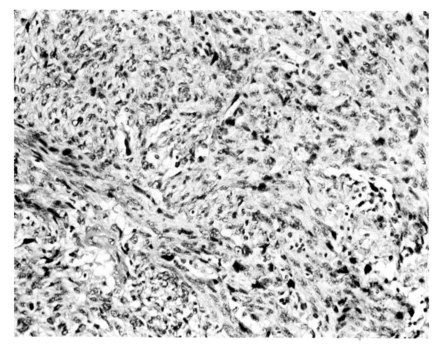

FIG. 11–15. Leiomyosarcoma composed of interlacing bundles of large spindle cells. (H&E × 100, original)

fibrous component (9). A few instances of benign and malignant mesenchymomas were encountered in the mediastinum by Pachter and Lattes (1). An additional example composed only of cartilage and adipose tissue and classified as a mediastinal chondrolipoma has been reported more recently by Lim (88).

Synovial Sarcoma

Synovial sarcomas are common, malignant soft tissue tumors that have only recently been recognized in the mediastinum (89,90). They are thought to originate from pluripotential mesenchymal cells that differentiate into a biphasic pattern of growth. They can be adherent to the pleura or pericardium without arising from these mesothelial-lined surfaces (90). Histologically, synovial sarcomas are composed of epithelial cells lining clefts and glandular spaces closely admixed with spindle mesenchymal cells with frequent papillary structure formation. The glandular lumina have PAS positive, diastase-resistant material. The epithelial cells exhibit immunoreactivity with antibodies to keratin, while the spindle cells stain with antibodies to vimentin (90). Mediastinal synovial sarcomas are difficult to differentiate from malignant mesotheliomas, thymomas, malignant nerve sheath tumors with glandular differentiation, and germ cell neoplasms (90).

TUMORS OF SKELETAL TISSUES

Chondroma

Widdowson and Lewis-Jones (91) recently described a patient with a large chondroma arising from the posterior mediastinum (91).

Osteogenic Sarcoma

Several extraskeletal osteogenic sarcomas have been reported in the mediastinum (Fig. 11-16) (92–96). The patient reported by Valderrama and associates (93) is of particular interest because the sarcoma probably arose from ectopic hamartomatous thymic tissue encountered at the periphery of the neoplasm (Fig. 11-17). This thymic tissue contained benign bone.

Catanese and associates (94) reported a patient with mediastinal osteogenic sarcoma arising as a second malignancy following treatment for Hodgkin's disease.

Chondrosarcoma

Chondrosarcomas rarely present initially as mediastinal tumors. They arise from the tracheobronchial tree (97,98). We have studied a myxoid chondrosarcoma pre-

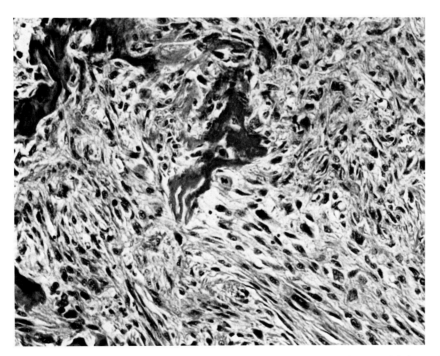

FIG. 11–16. Osteogenic sarcoma with malignant spindle cells with osteoid formation. (H&E × 100, original) (Courtesy of Dr. E. Valderrama, New York.)

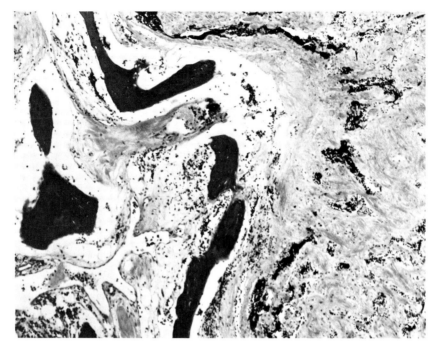

FIG. 11–17. Hamartomatous thymus with benign bone formation. (H&E × 40, original) (Courtesy of Dr. E. Valderrama, New York.)

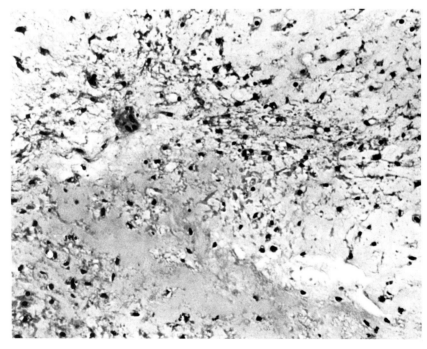

FIG. 11–18. Myxoid chondrosarcoma with malignant chondrocytes and myxoid stroma. (H&E × 100, original)

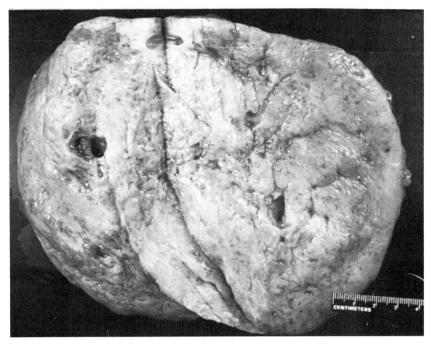

FIG. 11–19. Solitary fibrous tumor of the mediastinum. The tumor is well encapsulated, firm, gray–white, and has focal areas of hemorrhage.

senting as a posterior mediastinal mass and arising from the thoracic vertebrae (Fig. 11-18).

OTHER TUMORS AND TUMOR-LIKE CONDITIONS

Several other soft tissue neoplasms and tumor-like conditions have been described in the mediastinum as rare causes of mediastinal masses. They include instances of fibrous mesothelioma located entirely in the mediastinum without pleural and pericardial connections (Fig. 11-19), myxomas, meningiomas arising from the stellate ganglion, chordomas, histiocytosis X, granular cell tumors, and extramedullary hematopoiesis (1,99–106). Primary amyloidosis also can present as an isolated mediastinal mass (107,108).

REFERENCES

1. Pachter MR, Lattes R: Mesenchymal tumors of the mediastinum. I. Tumors of fibrous tissue, adipose tissue, smooth muscle and striated muscle. *Cancer* 1963;16:74–94.
2. Pachter MR, Lattes R: Mesenchymal tumors of the mediastinum. II. Tumors of blood vascular origin. *Cancer* 1963;16:95–107.
3. Pachter MR, Lattes R: Mesenchymal tumors of the mediastinum. III. Tumors of lymph vascular origin. *Cancer* 1963;16:108–117.
4. Conkle DM, Adkins RB Jr: Primary malignant tumors of the mediastinum. *Ann Thorac Surg* 1972;14:553–567.
5. Welch KJ, Tapper D, Vawter GP: Surgical treatment of thymic cysts and neoplasms in children. *J Pediatr Surg* 1979;14:691–698.

6. Luosto R, Koikkalainen K, Jyrala A, et al: Mediastinal tumours. A follow-up study of 208 patients. *Scand J Thorac Cardiovasc Surg* 1978;12:253–259.
7. Ovrum E, Birkeland S: Mediastinal tumours and cysts. A review of 91 cases. *Scand J Thorac Cardiovasc Surg* 1979;13:161–168.
8. Benjamin SP, McCormack LJ, Effler DB, et al: Primary tumors of the mediastinum. *Chest* 1972;62:297–303.
9. Enzinger FM, Weiss SW: *Soft tissue tumors*. CV Mosby, St. Louis, 2nd ed., 1988.
10. Sumner TE, Volberg FM, Kiser PE, et al: Mediastinal cystic hygroma in children. *Pediatr Radiol* 1981;11:160–162.
11. Bratu M, Brown M, Carter M, et al: Cystic hygroma of the mediastinum in children. *Am J Dis Child* 1970;119:348–351.
12. Hall ER Jr, Blades B: Lymphangioma of mediastinum. Report of 2 cases. *Dis Chest* 1957;32:207–213.
13. Thompson JE, Keiller VH: Lymphangioma of the neck. *Ann Surg* 1923;77:385–396.
14. Jahn C, Schmutz G, Wihlm JM, et al: Cystic lymphangioma of the mediastinum. Radiologic data apropos of 7 cases. *J Radiol* 1987;68:89–96.
15. Perkes EA, Haller JO, Kassner EG, et al: Mediastinal cystic hygroma in infants. Two cases with no extension into the neck. *Clin Pediatr* 1979;18:168–170.
16. Feng YF, Masterson JB, Riddell RH: Lymphangioma of the middle mediastinum as an incidental finding on a chest radiograph. *Thorax* 1980;35:955–956.
17. Feutz EP, Yune HY, Mandelbaum I, et al: Intrathoracic cystic hygroma. A report of three cases. *Radiology* 1973;108:61–66.
18. Brown LR, Reiman HM, Rosenow EC III, et al: Intrathoracic lymphangioma. *Mayo Clin Proc* 1986;61:882–892.
19. Ionescu GO, Tuleasca I, Gavrilita N, et al: Infantile giant mediastinal cystic hygroma. *J Pediatr Surg* 1976;11:469–470.
20. King DT, Duffy DM, Hirose FM, et al: Lymphangiosarcoma arising from lymphangioma circumscriptum. *Arch Dermatol* 1979;115:969–972.
21. Johnson DW, Klazynski PT, Gordon WH, et al: Mediastinal lymphangioma and chylothorax: the role of radiotherapy. *Ann Thorac Surg* 1986;41:325–328.
22. Watts MA, Gibbons JA, Aaron BL: Mediastinal and osseous lymphangiomatosis: case report and review. *Ann Thorac Surg* 1982;34:324–328.
23. Bell KA, Simon BK: Chylothorax and lymphangiomas of bone: unusual manifestations of lymphatic disease. *South Med J* 1978;71:459–460.
24. Berberich FR, Bernstein ID, Ochs HD, et al: Lymphangiomatosis with chylothorax. *J Pediatr* 1975;87:941–943.
25. Gilsanz V, Yeh HC, Baron MG: Multiple lymphangiomas of the neck, axilla, mediastinum and bones in an adult. *Radiology* 1976;120:161–162.
26. McCarty KS, Mossler JA, McLelland R, et al: Pulmonary lymphangiomyomatosis responsive to progesterone. *N Engl J Med* 1980;303:1461–1465.
27. Stovin PG: Pulmonary lymphangiomyomatosis syndrome. *J Pathol* 1973;109:7.
28. Steffelaar JW, Nijkamp DA, Hilvering C: Pulmonary lymphangiomatosis: demonstration of smooth muscle antigens by immunofluorescence technique. *Scand J Respir Dis* 1977;58:103–109.
29. Silverstein EF, Ellis K, Wolff M, et al: Pulmonary lymphangiomyomatosis. *Am J Roentgenol* 1974;120:832–850.
30. Vazquez JJ, Fernandez-Cuervo L, Fidalgo B: Lymphangiomyomatosis: morphogenetic study and ultrastructural confirmation of the histogenesis of the lung lesion. *Cancer* 1976;37:2321–2328.
31. Valensi QJ: Pulmonary lymphangiomyoma, a probable forme fruste of tuberous sclerosis. A case report and review of the literature. *Am Rev Respir Dis* 1973;108:1411–1415.
32. Wolff M: Lymphangiomyoma: clinicopathological study and ultrastructural confirmation of its histogenesis. *Cancer* 1973;31:988–1007.
33. Marchevsky AM, Hartman G, Ross D, et al: Lung transplantation: the pathologic diagnosis of pulmonary complications. *Mod Pathol* (in press).
34. Gindhart TD, Tucker WY, Choy SH: Cavernous hemangioma of the superior mediastinum. Report of a case with electron microscopy and computerized tomography. *Am J Surg Pathol* 1979;3:353–361.
35. Kings GLM: Multifocal hemangiomatous malformation: A case. *Thorax* 1975;30:485–488.
36. Kissin MW: Mediastinal cavernous hemangioma. *Br J Dis Chest* 1977;71:208–210.
37. Davis JM, Mark GJ, Greene R: Benign blood vascular tumors of the mediastinum. Report of four cases and review of the literature. *Radiology* 1978;126:581–587.
38. Kalicinski ZH, Joszt W, Perdzynski W, et al: Hemangioma of the superior caval vein. *J Pediatr Surg* 1982;17:178–179.
39. Kelley MJ, Mannes EJ, Ravin CE: Mediastinal masses of vascular origin. A review. *J Thorac Cardiovasc Surg* 1978;76:559–572.

40. Bedros AA, Munson J, Toomey FE: Hemangioendothelioma presenting as posterior mediastinal mass in a child. *Cancer* 1980;46:801–803.
41. Cohen AJ, Sbaschnig RJ, Hochholzer L, et al: Mediastinal hemangiomas. *Ann Thorac Surg* 1987;43:656–659.
42. Saada J, Almosni M, Bakdach H, et al: Benign mediastinal hemangiomas. *Rev Mal Respir* 1987;4:141–143.
43. Ceccanti JP, Chauvin G, Guendon R, et al: Giant tumoral hemangioma of the mediastinum. Apropos of a case. *Ann Chir* 1989;43:157–160.
44. Westra D: Vascular pseudo-tumours of the mediastinum in asymptomatic patients. A tomographic study. I. Arteries. *Radiol Clin (Basel)* 1978;47:100–113.
45. Westra D: Vascular pseudotumours of the mediastinum in asymptomatic patients. A tomographic study. II. Veins. *Radiol Clin (Basel)* 1978;47:169–181.
46. Wychulis AR, Payne WS, Clagett OT, et al: Surgical treatment of mediastinal tumors. A forty year experience. *J Thorac Cardiovasc Surg* 1971;62:379–392.
47. Benjamin SP, McCormack LJ, Effler DB, et al: Primary tumors of the mediastinum. *Chest* 1972;62:297–303.
48. Tarr RW, Page DL, Glick AG, et al: Benign hemangioendothelioma involving posterior mediastinum: CT findings. *J Comput Assist Tomogr* 1986;10:865–867.
49. Bortolani EM, Giorgetti PL, Ghilardi G: Mediastinal neoplasms of mesenchymal origin. *Minerva Chir* 1989;44:1163–1166.
50. Gibbs AR, Johnson NF, Giddins JC, et al: Primary angiosarcoma of the mediastinum: light and electron microscopic demonstration of factor VIII-related antigen in neoplastic cells. *Hum Pathol* 1984;15:687–691.
51. Toursarkissian B, O'Connor WN, Dillon ML: Mediastinal epithelioid hemangioendothelioma. *Ann Thorac Surg* 1990;49:680–685.
52. Barua NR, Patel AR, Takita H, et al: Fibrosarcoma of the mediastinum. *J Surg Oncol* 1979;12:11–17.
53. Baldwin RS: Hypoglycemia associated wtih fibrosarcoma of the mediastinum. Review of Doege's patient. *Ann Surg* 1964;160:975–977.
54. Walsh CH, Wright AD, Coore HG: Hypoglycemia associated with an intrathoracic fibrosarcoma. *Clin Endocrinol* 1975;4:393–398.
55. Ringertz N, Lidholm SO: Mediastinal tumors and cysts. *J Thorac Surg* 1956;31:458–487.
56. Thorbjarnarson B: Sarcomata at the New York Hospital. *Arch Surg* 1961;82:489–510.
57. Chen W, Chan CW, Mok CK: Malignant fibrous histiocytoma of the mediastinum. *Cancer* 1982;50:797–800.
58. Mills SA, Breyer RH, Johnston FR, et al: Malignant fibrous histiocytoma of the mediastinum and lung. A report of three cases. *J Thorac Cardiovasc Surg* 1982;84:367–372.
59. Natsuaki M, Yoshikawa Y, Itoh T, et al: Xanthogranulomatous malignant fibrous histiocytoma arising from posterior mediastinum. *Thorax* 1986;41:322–323.
60. Sarama RF, DiGiacomo WA, Safirstein BH: Primary mediastinal lipoma. *J Med Soc NJ* 1981;78:901–902.
61. Shub C, Parkin TW, Lie JT: An unusual mediastinal lipoma simulating cardiomegaly. *Mayo Clin Proc* 1979;54:60–62.
62. Politis J, Funahasi A, Gehlsen JA et al: Intrathoracic lipomas. Report of three cases and review of the literature with emphasis on endobronchial lipoma. *J Thorac Cardiovasc Surg* 1979;77:550–556.
63. Lee WJ, Fattal G: Mediastinal lipomatosis in simple obesity. *Chest* 1976;70:308–309.
64. Homer MJ, Wechsler RJ, Carter BL: Mediastinal lipomatosis. CT confirmation of a normal variant. *Radiology* 1978;128:657–661.
65. Drasin GF, Lynch T, Temes GP: Ectopic ACTH production and mediastinal lipomatosis. *Radiology* 1978;127:610.
66. Shukla LW, Katz JA, Wagner ML: Mediastinal lipomatosis: a complication of high dose steroid therapy in children. *Pediatr Radiol* 1988;19:57–58.
67. Vellios F, Baez J, Shumacker HB: Lipoblastomatosis: a tumor of fetal fat different from hibermoma. Report of a case with observations on the embryogenesis of human adipose tissue. *Am J Pathol* 1958;34:1140–1159.
68. Tabrisky J, Rowe JH, Christie SG, et al: Benign mediastinal lipoblastomatosis. *J Pediatr Surg* 1974;9:399–401.
69. Schweitzer DL, Aguam AS: Primary liposarcoma of the mediastinum. Report of a case and review of the literature. *J Thorac Cardiovasc Surg* 1977;74:83–97.
70. Standerfer RJ, Armistead SH, Paneth M: Liposarcoma of the mediastinum: report of two cases and review of the literature. *Thorax* 1981;36:693–694.
71. Lacey CJN, Petch MC: Primary liposarcoma of the pericardium. *Thorax* 1979;34:120–122.
72. Mendez G Jr, Isikoff MB, Isikoff SK, et al: Fatty tumors of the thorax demonstrated by CT. *Am J Radiol* 1979;133:207–212.

73. Enzinger FM, Winslow DJ: Liposarcoma. A study of 103 cases. *Virchows Arch [Pathol Anat]* 1962;335:367–388.
74. Shibata K, Koga Y, Onitsuka T, et al: Primary liposarcoma of the mediastinum—a case report and review of the literature. *Jpn J Surg* 1986;16:277–283.
75. Plukker JT, Joosten HJ, Rensing JB, et al: Primary liposarcoma of the mediastinum in a child. *J Surg Oncol* 1988;37:257–263.
76. McLean TR, Almassi GH, Hackbarth DA, et al: Mediastinal involvement by myxoid liposarcoma. *Ann Thorac Surg* 1989;47:920–921.
77. Grieger TA, Carl M, Liebert HP, et al: Mediastinal liposarcoma in a patient infected with the human immunodeficiency virus [letter]. *Am J Med* 1988;84:366.
78. Miller R, Kurtz SM, Powers JM: Mediastinal rhabdomyoma. *Cancer* 1978;42:1983–1988.
79. Suzuki T, Ishihara T, Yamazaki S, et al: Vascular-leiomyoma of the posterior mediastinum. A case report. *J Jpn Thor Dis Assoc* 1982;20:1075–1077.
80. Shaffer K, Pugatch RD, Sugarbaker DJL: Primary mediastinal leiomyoma. *Ann Thorac Surg* 1990;50:301–302.
81. Wang NS, Seemayer TA, Ahmed MN, et al: Pulmonary leiomyosarcoma associated with an arteriovenous fistula. *Arch Pathol* 1974;98:100–105.
82. Davis GL, Bergmann M, O'Kane H: Leiomyosarcoma of the superior vena cava. A first case with resection. *J Thorac Cardiovasc Surg* 1976;72:408–412.
83. Rasaretnam R, Panabokke RG: Leiomyosarcoma of the mediastinum. *Br J Dis Chest* 1975;69:63–69.
84. Hayes WL, Farha SJ, Brown RL: Primary leiomyosarcoma of the pulmonary artery. *Am J Cardiol* 1974;34:615–617.
85. Henrichs KJ, Wenisch HJC, Hofmann W, et al: Leiomyosarcoma of the pulmonary artery. A light and electronmicroscopical study. *Virchows Arch [Pathol Anat]* 1979;383:207–216.
86. Bernheim J, Griffel B, Versano S, et al: Mediastinal leiomyosarcoma in the wall of a bronchial cyst (letter). *Arch Pathol Lab Med* 1980;104:221.
87. Sunderrajan EV, Luger AM, Rosenholtz MJ, et al: Leiomyosarcoma in the mediastinum presenting as superior vena cava syndrome. *Cancer* 1984;53:2553–2556.
88. Lim YC: Mediastinal chondrolipoma. *Am J Surg Pathol* 1980;4:407–409.
89. Pulpeiro JR, Cruz R, Arenas A, et al: Para-oesophageal synovial sarcoma. *Eur J Radiol* 1988;8:120–121.
90. Witkin GB, Miettinen M, Rosai J: A biphasic tumor of the mediastinum with features of synovial sarcoma. A report of four cases. *Am J Surg Pathol* 1989;13:490–499.
91. Widdowson DJ, Lewis-Jones HG: A large soft-tissue chondroma arising from the posterior mediastinum. *Clin Radiol* 1988;39:333–335.
92. Ikeda T, Ishihara T, Yoshimatsu H, et al: Primary osteogenic sarcoma of the mediastinum. *Thorax* 1974;29:582–588.
93. Valderrama E, Kahn LB, Wind E: Extraskeletal osteosarcoma arising in an ectopic hamartomatous thymus. Report of a case and review of the literature. *Cancer* 1983;51:1132–1137.
94. Catanese J, Dutcher JP, Dorfman HD, et al: Mediastinal osteosarcoma with extension to lungs in a patient treated for Hodgkin's disease. *Cancer* 1988;62:2252–2257.
95. Tarr RW, Kerner T, McCook B, et al: Primary extraosseous osteogenic sarcoma of the mediastinum: clinical, pathologic, and radiologic correlation. *South Med J* 1988;81:1317–1319.
96. Greenwood SM, Meschter SC: Extraskeletal osteogenic sarcoma of the mediastinum. *Arch Pathol Lab Med* 1989;113:430–433.
97. McConnell TH: Bony and cartilagenous tumors of the heart and great vessels: report of an osteosarcoma of the pulmonary artery. *Cancer* 1970;25:611–617.
98. Daniels AC, Conner GH, Straus FH: Primary chondrosarcoma of the tracheobronchial tree. Report of a unique case and brief review. *Arch Pathol* 1967;84:615–624.
99. Wilson AJ, Ratliff JL, Lagios MD, et al: Mediastinal meningioma. *Am J Surg Pathol* 1979;3:557–562.
100. Kuten A, Jose B, O'Shea PA, et al: Superior vena cava syndrome secondary to histiocytosis-X in a child: case report. *Med Pediatr Oncol* 1979;7:225–228.
101. Jaituni S, Arkee MSK, Caterine JM: Mediastinal myxoma: a case report. *J Iowa Med Soc* 1974;64:107–110.
102. Elbers H, vd Stadt J, Wagenaar SS: Tumor-simulating thoracic extramedullary hematopoiesis. *Ann Thorac Surg* 1980;30:584–587.
103. Falappa P, Danza FM, Leone G, et al: Thoracic extramedullary hematopoiesis: evaluation by conventional radiology and computed tomography. *Diag Imaging* 1982;51:19–24.
104. Castellano GC, Johnston HW: Intrathoracic chordoma presenting as a posterior mediastinal tumor. *South Med J* 1975;68:109–112.
105. Aisner SC, Chakravarthy AK, Joslyn JN, et al: Bilateral granular cell tumors of the posterior mediastinum. *Ann Thorac Surg* 1988;46:688–689.

106. Witkin GB, Rosai J: Solitary fibrous tumor of the mediastinum. A report of 14 cases. *Am J Surg Pathol* 1989;13:547–557.
107. Osnoss KL, Harrell DD: Isolated mediastinal mass in primary amyloidosis. *Chest* 1980;78: 786–788.
108. Shaw P, Grossman R, Fernandes BJ: Nodular mediastinal amyloidosis. *Hum Pathol* 1984; 15:1183–1185.

12

Neurogenic Tumors of the Mediastinum

Intrathoracic neurogenic tumors account for 19% to 39% of mediastinal neoplasms (1–8). They occur most frequently in the posterior mediastinum, where they represent 75% of primary lesions of this compartment and arise from sympathetic ganglia, paraganglia, and peripheral nerves (sympathetic trunk, intercostals, vagus). They are less frequent in the anterior mediastinum.

Mediastinal neurogenic tumors are benign in most instances, with an overall incidence of malignancy ranging from 3% to 19% (2,9,10).

They can be classified according to their histogenesis into tumors of peripheral nerves, autonomic ganglia, paraganglia, and probable Schwann cell origin, as shown in Table 1. Over 70% of all mediastinal neurogenic tumors are benign peripheral nerve origin neoplasms (neurofibromas, schwannomas, and tumors with mixed features of both).

TUMORS OF PERIPHERAL NERVES

Schwannoma

Schwannoma (neurilemmoma, neurinoma) is the most frequent neurogenic tumor of the mediastinum (1–11). It affects patients of both sexes in their third and fourth decades of life (4). Both sides of the chest are involved equally (2).

Schwannomas are single in most instances but can be multiple in patients with von Recklinghausen's disease (neurofibromatosis).

Patients with schwannomas are asymptomatic in most instances and are found to have a mediastinal mass on chest roentgenograms but can present with chest pain, respiratory symptoms such as cough, dyspnea, or hemoptysis, and/or neurological manifestations (2,6,7). Respiratory symptoms are usually associated with large, bulky schwannomas. Neurologic symptoms do not necessarily indicate malignancy and include hoarseness resulting from recurrent nerve paralysis, Horner's syndrome, Pancoast's syndrome, and intercostal or brachial plexus neuralgias (6,7). Spinal cord compression or dysphagia caused by esophageal displacement by a large schwannoma is unusual (2).

Pathogenesis

Schwannomas arise from Schwann cells normally present in nerve sheaths and develop as slowly growing, well-encapsulated tumors located on the nerve of origin (12).

TABLE 1. *Neurogenic tumors of the mediastinum*

Tumors of peripheral nerves
  Benign
    Schwannoma (neurilemmoma)
    Melanotic schwannoma
    Neurofibroma
    Neurofibromatosis
    Pigmented neuroectodermal tumor
  Malignant
    Tumor of nerve sheath origin (malignant schwannoma)
    Malignant melanocytic schwannoma
Tumors of autonomic ganglia
  Benign
    Ganglioneuroma
  Malignant
    Neuroblastoma
    Ganglioneuroblastoma
Tumors of paraganglia
  Paraganglioma
  Pheochromocytoma
Tumors of probable Schwann cell origin
  Granular cell tumor
Tumors of neural tube remnants ependymoma

Roentgenologic Features

Schwannomas are round or oval masses of uniform density and sharp margins located in the posterior mediastinum, intercostal spaces, or, less frequently, the anterior mediastinum (2). They exhibit a characteristic D-shaped outline on lateral projections and may be focally calcified and/or cystic. Schwannomas seldom erode the ribs or vertebrae.

Computed tomographic (CT) scans are particularly useful to demonstrate the size and degree of mediastinal and thoracic wall involvement by the schwannomas (Fig. 12-1) and can demonstrate extrathoracic tumor extensions through intercostal or intervertebral spaces in a dumbbell fashion.

Pathologic Features

Schwannomas are well encapsulated, round or fusiform, and are closely associated with nerves (Fig. 12-2). They are usually single but can rarely be multiple or present in patients with von Recklinghausen's disease (12). They can reach a large size in the mediastinum (12).

On section, they are soft, white, yellow, or pink, with occasional areas of calcification and/or cystic degeneration. Their capsule is continuous with the epineurium, the most external nerve sheath.

Schwannomas are composed histologically of spindle cells with elongated, twisted nuclei with rounded borders and indistinct amphophilic cytoplasm arranged in various patterns that are classified as Antoni A and B areas (12). The tumor cells can have prominent vacuolar cytoplasmic degeneration.

Antoni A areas are characterized by cellular, compact, interlacing fascicles or short bundles of spindle cells (Fig. 12-3). Nuclear palisading and Verocay body for-

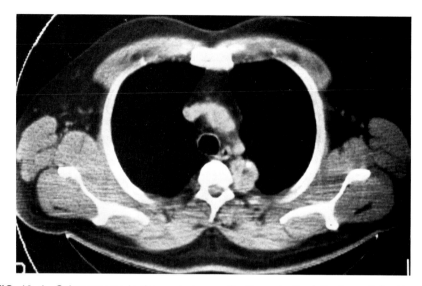

FIG. 12–1. Schwannoma in the posterior mediastinum to the left of a vertebral body.

mation are prominent in focal areas (Fig. 12-4). Verocay bodies are oval formations composed of two compact rows of well-aligned spindle tumor cells.

Antoni B areas are characterized by spindle or oval cells admixed with a loose, myxoid connective tissue stroma exhibiting prominent collagen fibers that stand out from the background (Fig. 12-5). These areas are hypocellular and have prominent microcystic degeneration as well as characteristic dilated vessels with tortuous lumina and focal thrombosis. Foci of calcification are also present. Mitotic figures are infrequent in benign schwannomas.

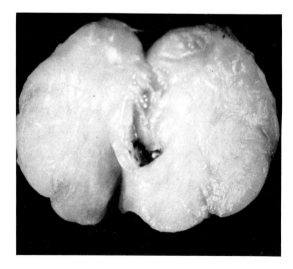

FIG. 12–2. Schwannoma. The tumor is well encapsulated, firm, tan–yellow, with a myxoid surface.

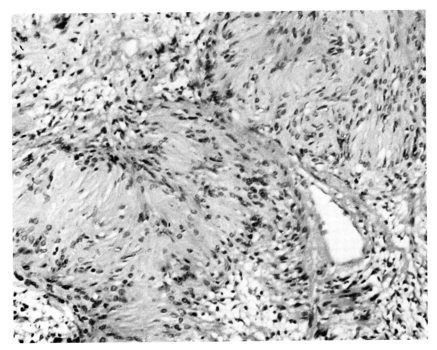

FIG. 12–3. Schwannoma. Antoni type A area with interlacing bundles of compact spindle cells. (H&E × 100, original)

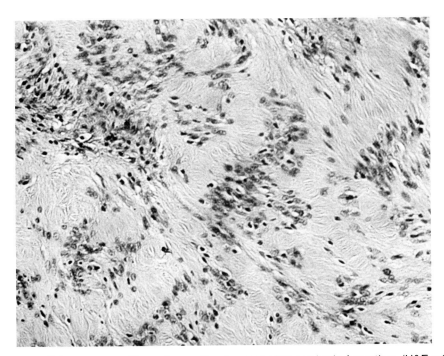

FIG. 12–4. Schwannoma with nuclear palisading and Verocay body formation. (H&E × 100, original)

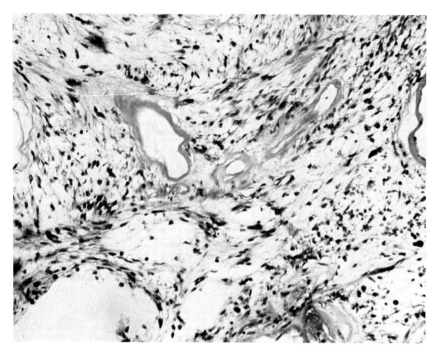

FIG. 12–5. Schwannoma. Antoni type B area with loose spindle cells in an edematous stroma with microcystic change. (H&E × 100, original)

Immunohistochemical Features

S-100 protein, an acidic nervous-system-specific protein, can be detected in the cytoplasm and nuclei of schwannoma tumor cells by staining paraffin sections with specific antisera and a PAP method (13).

S-100 protein is normally present in neurons and glial cells, where it may play a role in genomic regulation (14). It has also been demonstrated in various neoplasms of neural origin such as glioblastomas, astrocytomas, and ependymomas as well as in tumors of presumed neural or neuroectodermal origin such as malignant melanomas and granular cell tumors (15).

Schwannomas usually exhibit uniformaly intense S-100 protein immunoreactivity, in contrast with neurofibromas in which the staining tends to be variable and focal. They can also exhibit variable immunostaining with antibodies to myelin proteins (12).

S-100 protein has not been detected, however, in tumors that can be confused histologically with schwannomas such as leiomyomas, meningiomas, and fibrous histiocytomas.

Ultrastructural Features

Schwannomas have characteristic ultrastructural features that closely resemble those of normal Schwann cells (16–18). The tumor cells are elongated and have long

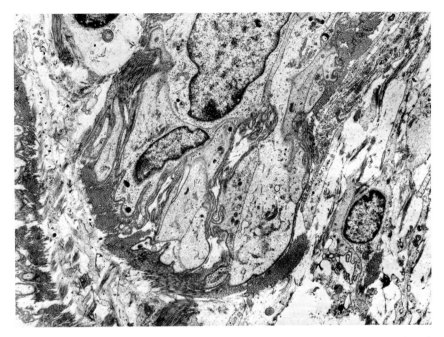

FIG. 12–6. Schwannoma with spindle cells showing complex interdigitating cytoplasmic processes enveloped by continuous basal lamina. ($\times$ 3,300, original)

cytoplasmic processes forming cytoplasmic layers adjacent to the cell body and are enveloped by a distinct continuous basal lamina (Fig. 12-6).

The cytoplasm contains microfilaments that are arranged at random and do not form fascicles or dense bodies as seen in smooth muscle cells. The nucleus is frequently convoluted. The stroma contains long-spacing collagen but no nerve fibers.

Prognosis and Treatment

Schwannomas are benign and are cured by surgical excision (1–4). They seldom become malignant. Indeed, in an extensive review of soft tissue tumors, Enzinger and Weiss (12) encountered only a single acceptable report of malignant transformation of a benign schwannoma (19).

Melanotic Schwannomas

A few cases of this unusual pigmented variant of schwannomas in the posterior mediastinum have been described (20–23). These tumors frequently extend into the spinal canal through the intervertebral foramina in a dumbbell fashion (spinothoracic melanotic schwannomas).

They are composed of spindle cells arranged in bundles, whorls, or palisades and containing variable amounts of intracytoplasmic brown granules that stain positively for melanin and negatively with iron stains. These granules have ultrastructural characteristics of melanosomes (20,21).

The tumor stroma can exhibit focal calcified spherules with features of psammoma bodies (22).

The origin of melanotic schwannomas is still controversial (20), and some investigators regard them as potentially malignant (22).

It has been postulated that the tumor cells either phagocytize melanin elaborated by adjacent melanoblasts or undergo melanocytic transformation and synthesize the pigment in their own cytoplasm (20,23). The latter hypothesis is more acceptable because of the common neural crest origin of Schwann cells and melanocytes and the difficulty in demonstrating melanosomes in melanotic schwannomas (20,23).

Neurofibromas

Neurofibromas are the second most frequent neurogenic tumors of the mediastinum, where they occur as isolated neoplasms or as multiple thoracic manifestations of neurofibromatosis (von Recklinghausen's disease) (24–27). In selected series of intrathoracic neural tumors, neurofibromas are the most frequent variant (2).

Neurofibromas occur most frequently in the posterior mediastinum of patients in the third and fourth decades of life. They have no sex predilection and develop as benign, slowly growing tumors that are usually discovered on routine chest roentgenograms. They can be symptomatic, however, and present with clinical manifestations similar to those of schwannomas (1–8,28).

Pathogenesis

Neurofibromas are nerve sheath tumors that share a common embryologic origin with schwannomas. Indeed, neurogenic tumors frequently have combined morphologic features of schwannomas and neurofibromas (2). However, neurofibromas result from the proliferation of perineural fibroblasts, Schwann cells, and neurites, whereas only Schwann cells contribute to the development of schwannomas.

Roentgenologic Features

Neurofibromas are indistinguishable radiologically from schwannomas and can masquerade as a developmental cyst on CT scans and magnetic resonance imaging (MRI) (29,30).

Pathologic Features

Neurofibromas are soft, well circumscribed, but not encapsulated, white–gray, and usually grow in the mediastinum within a nerve of origin, resulting in a fusiform mass (Fig. 12-7) (12).

They usually extend through the epineurium of the nerve of origin into the adjacent soft tissues and do not remain encapsulated. They lack the encapsulation, myxoid character, and/or cystic degeneration that are frequently present in schwannomas.

Neurofibromas are composed histologically of spindle cells with elongated, wavy nuclei and pointed ends dispersed in a loose connective tissue stroma containing "wire-like" strands of collagen, occasional nerve fibers, inflammatory cells, and

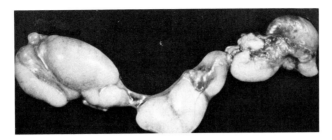

FIG. 12–7. Plexiform neurofibroma in patient with neurofibromatosis.

mast cells. The tumor cells occasionally become organized into whorls or storiform areas but lack the formation of Verocay bodies and the nuclear palisading seen in schwannomas. Benign neurofibromas can exhibit focal pleomorphism, but mitotic figures are infrequent.

Nerve fibers are demonstrated in silver-stained preparations (Bodian's stain). Mast cells are demonstrated with metachromatic stains (toluidine blue).

Occasionally, the stroma of neurofibromas is predominantly myxoid, resembling myxomas or myxoid liposarcomas. The neurogenic tumors have, however, a prominent vascular pattern, are more cellular than myxomas, and can have focal areas of neural differentiation with formation of nerve fascicles and specialized tactile structures (Wagner–Meissner bodies). Liposarcomas, on the other hand, exhibit characteristic malignant lipoblasts.

Neurofibromas also can exhibit other unusual features including the formation of pressure receptors (Pacini corpuscles), focal rosettes, mucin-producing glands, and epithelioid, melanin-containing, and/or granular cells (12).

Immunohistochemical Features

S-100 protein has been identified in neurofibromas (13). Acetylcholinesterase activity can be demonstrated in the nerve fibers of the tumor (31).

Ultrastructural Features

Ultrastructural studies demonstrate neurites, fibroblasts, Schwann cells, and mesoaxons enclosed in plasmalemmal invaginations in neurofibromas (11,31). Fibroblasts can be distinguished from Schwann cells by the lack of basal lamina, prominent cell projections, and microfilaments.

Schwannomas, by contrast, are composed of a homogeneous population of Schwann cells with prominent cytoplasmic projections that spiral around themselves, basal lamina, and intracytoplasmic microfilaments (12).

Prognosis and Treatment

Solitary neurofibromas are benign neoplasms that can be cured by surgical excision. They seldom recur or become malignant (32). These complications can occur as many as 13 years postoperatively (11).

Multiple intrathoracic neurofibromas in patients with neurofibromatoses can present, however, difficult clinical problems, as it is often impossible to resect them completely. Moreover, the lesions have a higher risk of malignant transformation (31,32).

Neurofibromatosis (Von Recklinghausen's Disease)

Neurofibromatosis is the most frequent variant of the phakomatoses or neurocutaneous syndromes. It affects approximately one in every 2,500 to 3,300 live births (32). It was first described by von Recklinghausen in 1882 (12).

Pathogenesis

Neurofibromatosis is a congenital disease inherited as an autosomal dominant trait with a high degree of penetrance (32). The gene responsible for the disease has been recently identified and localized to chromosome 17 (12). About half of the patients have a family history of the disease, whereas the others present with neurofibromatosis *de novo* as a result of new mutations (12). Indeed, the mutation rate of neurofibromatosis is considered one of the highest for diseases inherited as an autosomal dominant trait (12).

The pathogenesis of neurofibromatosis and the mechanisms by which the genetic defects result in the development of multiple neoplasms are still unclear. Biochemical studies of isoenzymes of glucose-6-phosphate dehydrogenase have demonstrated that both forms of the enzyme can be present in neurofibromas, indicating a probable polyclonal origin (33). However, when the tumors undergo malignant transformation the lesions exhibit monoclonality (12).

Other studies have demonstrated elevated circulating levels of a serum factor (nerve growth–stimulating activity) in patients with neurofibromatosis. This yet to be characterized substance may stimulate neural tissue growth in a manner similar to nerve growth factor (34).

Clinical Findings

Neurofibromatosis occurs in patients of all races and is more frequent in males (32). It presents with protean clinical manifestations that can be classified into two forms: peripheral and central neurofibromatosis (32). These variants of von Recklinghausen's disease do not usually overlap in a patient or in members of a family affected by the disorder.

Patients with the peripheral form of neurofibromatosis have areas of skin pigmentation (cafe-au-lait spots) and multiple neurofibromas. They can also have skeletal defects (scoliosis, intrathoracic meningocele, congenital bowing of bones with pseudoarthrosis, orbital malformations, and osteolytic lesions), megacolon, vascular lesions, disorders of sexual and mental development, pulmonary interstitial fibrosis, multiple tumors (nephroblastoma, schwannoma, pheochromocytoma, ganglioneuroma, lipoma, medullary carcinoma of the thyroid, and/or leukemia), and other systemic abnormalities (12,35–42).

Cafe-au-lait spots appear in childhood and are considered of diagnostic value when they are larger than 1.5 cm in diameter. Patients with more than six cafe-au-lait spots each larger than 1.5 cm in diameter are diagnosed as having neurofibromatosis. Cafe-au-lait spots increase in size and number with age (32).

Neurofibromas appear in childhood or adolescence, are multiple, and develop in any conceivable location including the skin, subcutaneous tissue, gastrointestinal tract, appendix, larynx, blood vessels, heart, and retroperitoneum. The mediastinum also can be involved (12). Indeed, in one series, as many as 30% of patients with mediastinal neurofibromas had neurofibromatosis (41). Rarely, these patients present with the superior vena cava syndrome and sleep apnea (25).

Patients with central neurofibromatosis present with nervous system tumors including neurilemmomas, astrocytomas, meningiomas, and/or ependymomas (42). They seldom have peripheral abnormalities and/or mediastinal neurofibromas (12).

Pathologic Features

Patients with neurofibromatosis can present with single or multiple mediastinal neurofibromas that have identical morphologic features to the solitary lesions already described. More characteristically, they present with plexiform neurofibromas involving major mediastinal nerves such as the vagus or the sympathetic chain (12,26,27,36). Plexiform neurofibromas are pathognomonic of neurofibromatosis (32). They appear as long, thick, convoluted masses that enlarge the nerve of origin. Indeed, they have been compared to a "bag of worms" (Fig. 12-7). Histologically, they consist of multiple tortuous enlarged nerve fibers admixed with a loose connective stroma containing Schwann cells and fibroblasts.

Prognosis and Treatment

The protean clinical problems of patients with von Recklinghausen's disease frequently are treated surgically. The lesions are resected when they become large or painful and/or compress vital structures (12). It is often not practical, however, to attempt to remove all multiple intrathoracic neurofibromas (2,6).

Patients with neurofibromatosis are at a high risk of developing malignancies, and up to 29% of cases can develop sarcomas (12). This estimate may be too high, and although it is difficult to determine the exact incidence of malignancy in neurofibromatosis, it is probably between 2% and 13% (32,43).

Patients usually develop malignant schwannomas when they have had neurofibromatosis for 10 years or longer. They have a poor prognosis, since fewer than 20% of cases survive 5 years (12,41).

Pigmented Neuroectodermal Tumor of Infancy (Melanotic Progonoma)

This unusual tumor of presumed neural crest origin presents as upper or lower jaw masses in infants but can infrequently involve the mediastinum, epididymis, brain, and anterior fontanelle (12,44,45).

Pigmented neuroectodermal tumors are dark gray or black and are composed histologically of irregular spaces lined by cuboidal cells containing intracytoplasmic melanin and ultrastructural features of epithelium and melanocytes. The tumors also have nests of smaller cells with round nuclei and scanty cytoplasm and neurofibrillary stromal material resembling neuroblastomas.

Pigmented neuroectodermal tumors of infancy were initially considered to be benign tumors (12). However, they are now considered malignant, as they are able to recur in 15% of cases and metastasize widely (44,46).

They may be difficult to distinguish histologically from pigmented neuroblastomas (21). The latter, however, lack the alveolar spaces lined by pigmented cells that are characteristic of melanotic progonomas.

D'Abrera and Burfitt-Williams (21) studied another unusual variant of mediastinal melanotic tumor composed exclusively of neuroepithelial and pigmented cells, which they considered a "one-sided" variant of teratoma.

Malignant Tumor of Nerve Sheath Origin (Malignant Schwannoma)

Malignant tumors of nerve sheath origin are the malignant counterparts of neurofibromas and schwannomas. They have been designated by various names, including malignant schwannoma, neurogenic sarcoma, and neurofibrosarcoma (12,47–57). Indeed, the term malignant "schwannoma" is probably a misnomer in some instances, as ultrastructural studies cannot always demonstrate Schwann cells in these tumors (53). The most general term, malignant tumor of nerve sheath origin, is more accurate.

These tumors are unusual in the mediastinum and account for only 0.5% to 7% of malignant neoplasms of the area (5–7,55). They are more frequent in the posterior mediastinum but can occur in the anterior compartment as well. Indeed, several studies have suggested that anterior mediastinal neurogenic tumors, although rare, are more likely to be malignant than their posterior counterparts (55,56).

Malignant tumors of nerve sheath origin affect patients of both sexes in the third through fifth decades of life. They appear as isolated mediastinal masses or as a manifestation of neurofibromatosis. Patients with neurofibromatosis and malignant schwannomas are usually males and younger than those lacking the systemic disease (12). They usually develop malignant neoplasms in the third decade of life (43). Malignant tumors of nerve sheath origin also can occur in patients who have received radiotherapy for the treatment of breast cancer or other malignancies (12).

Clinical and Radiologic Manifestations

Patients with malignant tumors of nerve sheath origin have similar clinical manifestations to those with other mediastinal tumors, including pain, dyspnea, hoarseness, dysphagia, spinal cord compression, Horner's and superior vena cava syndromes, hypoglycemia, and other symptoms. The neurogenic neoplasms are usually large and symptomatic at the time of initial diagnosis.

Radiologically, these neoplasms appear as round or oval masses that occupy a large portion of the thorax, displace adjacent structures such as the esophagus, invade adjacent bones, and/or extend through the intervertebral foramina.

Malignant neurogenic tumors also can extend into the neck (2).

Diagnostic Criteria

There has been controversy regarding which sarcomas should be designated malignant schwannomas (12). Therefore, it is important to define our diagnostic criteria for the diagnosis of malignant tumors of nerve sheath origin before describing the pathologic features of these neoplasms.

Stout (57) proposed to designate as neurogenic tumors only those neoplasms that clearly arise from a nerve or are present in patients with von Recklinghausen's disease. In his opinion, the histologic features of neurogenic sarcomas are otherwise indistinguishable from those of fibrosarcomas.

Enzinger and Weiss (12) adopted a more liberal approach and recognized that "certain histological features can be applied to diagnose these tumors in less typical settings." They classify as malignant schwannomas those tumors that exhibit nuclear palisading, tactoid differentiation, perivascular changes, and heterologous elements such as cartilage, bone, glands, or muscle as well as neoplasms with ultrastructural features of Schwann cell differentiation.

We prefer to utilize the more general term "malignant tumors of nerve sheath origin" for the diagnosis of these sarcomas because occasionally it is not possible to demonstrate with the electron microscope features of Schwann cell differentiation in neoplasms that are clearly neurogenic (i.e., arise from a nerve). We require the presence of at least one of the following criteria for the diagnosis of malignant tumor of nerve sheath origin: origin in a major nerve, origin in a nerve or soft tissues in a patient with neurofibromatosis, ultrastructural evidence of Schwann cell differentiation, or presence of S-100 protein in tumor cells.

Pathologic Features

Malignant tumors of nerve sheath origin are large, round, or fusiform, and usually measure more than 5 cm in diameter (Fig. 12-8). An origin from a major nerve can be frequently demonstrated. This nerve is usually larger than normal because of thickening of its perineural sheaths in areas adjacent to the tumor.

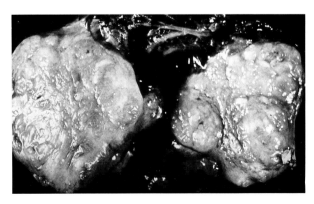

FIG. 12–8. Malignant tumor of nerve sheath origin. The tumor is partially circumscribed, soft, gray, myxoid, and invades the adjacent lung parenchyma.

The sarcomas are partially or completely encapsulated and have a soft, gray, yellow, or pink surface with extensive areas of necrosis, hemorrhage, and/or cystic degeneration.

Histologically, malignant tumors of nerve sheath origin are a group of neoplasms with protean morphologic manifestations and variable differentiation, ranging from well-differentiated lesions that retain Schwann cell or neural features to highly anaplastic sarcomas that cannot be identified as neurogenic unless they are present in a patient with neurofibromatosis. They are composed of spindle cells with irregular, wavy, or comma-shaped nuclei and indistinct cytoplasm arranged in fascicles with occasional areas exhibiting nuclear palisading and rudimentary tactoid differentiation (Fig. 12-9). Several other subtle yet characteristic morphologic features have been described in malignant tumors of nerve sheath origin, including hyaline bands, nodules, extensive perineural and intraneural invasion, subendothelial proliferation of tumor cells, epithelioid areas, focal rosettes, and heterologous elements such as islands of mature cartilage and/or bone, malignant skeletal muscle ("triton tumors"), mucin-secreting glands (Fig. 12-10), and squamous differentiation (12,58,59). In addition, malignant tumors of nerve sheath origin in patients with neurofibromatosis can, rarely, exhibit features of cellular neurofibromas that can be diagnosed as malignant only in the presence of prominent cellular pleomorphism and high mitotic activity ("malignant neurofibroma").

Ultrastructural Features

The cells of well-differentiated malignant tumors of nerve sheath origin exhibit ultrastructural features of schwannian differentiation including long interdigitating cytoplasmic processes that focally wrap around themselves in a manner similar to that seen in myelinated nerves, microtubules, neurofilaments that are not organized in dense bodies as in smooth muscle cells, and basal lamina (51,60–62).

In less-differentiated lesions, it is difficult to identify these features. Indeed, the cells of these tumors resemble fibroblasts or undifferentiated mesenchymal cells.

Immunocytochemical Features

Nakajima and associates (63) demonstrated S-100 protein immunoreactivity in the cytoplasm and nuclei of 10 of 14 neurogenic sarcomas. The intensity of immunoreactivity was less than that observed in benign schwannomas. Other malignant tumors that can be difficult to distinguish from malignant tumors of nerve sheath origin such as leiomyosarcomas, fibrosarcomas, and fibrous histiocytomas were negative.

Treatment and Prognosis

Malignant tumors of nerve sheath origin are aggressive neoplasms that tend to recur locally and metastasize to the lungs and other organs. The prognosis is worse in patients with neurofibromatosis, probably because of the tendency to develop poorly differentiated sarcomas with high mitotic activity in deep locations, where they are detected late and are more difficult to resect.

Patients with solitary malignant tumors of nerve sheath origin have a 75% 5-year

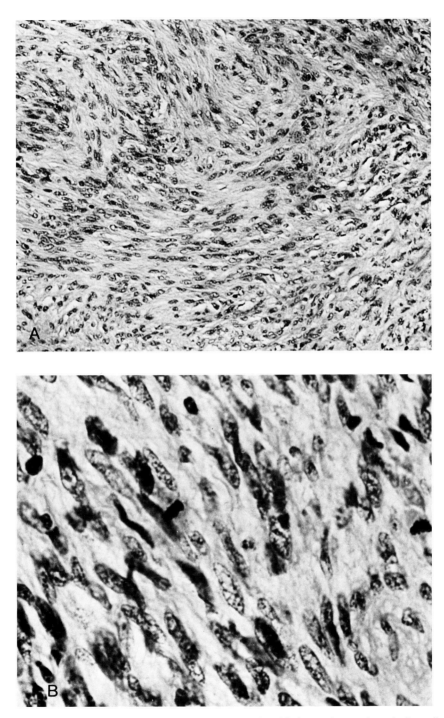

FIG. 12–9. A: Malignant tumor of nerve sheath origin with hyperchromatic spindle cells arranged in fascicles. (H&E × 100, original) **B:** Higher power of malignant spindle cells. (H&E × 400, original)

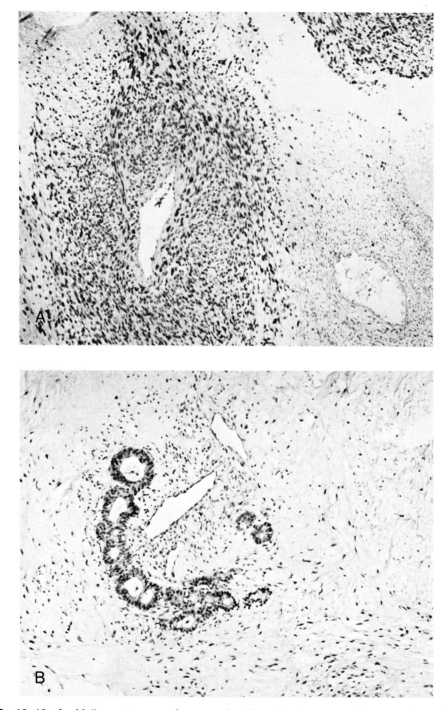

FIG. 12–10. A: Malignant tumor of nerve sheath origin in a neurofibromatosis patient. (H&E × 40, original) **B:** The same tumor has mucin-producing glands in an adjacent area (H&E × 40, original)

survival rate (49,64). Patients with neurofibromatosis and malignant tumors of nerve sheath origin have a 78% incidence of recurrences and 15% to 30% 5-year survival rates (41,50).

Malignant tumors of nerve sheath origin are treated with surgical resection. It has not yet been established whether radiotherapy or chemotherapy is an effective mode of adjuvant therapy (12).

TUMORS OF AUTONOMIC GANGLIA

A spectrum of benign and malignant tumors can arise from the sympathetic ganglia of the posterior mediastinum (8–12). They include *ganglioneuroblastomas*, malignant neoplasms that contain mature ganglion cells in addition to neuroblastomatous elements; neuroblastomas, poorly differentiated, highly malignant tumors composed of primitive neuroblast similar to those present in the fetal adrenal medulla; and *ganglioneuromas*, benign, well-differentiated tumors composed of mature ganglion and Schwann cells.

Ganglioneuromas

Ganglioneuromas are benign tumors that are predominantly found in the posterior mediastinum and retroperitoneum (65–70). They are a disease of children older than 3 to 4 years of age and young adults and are very infrequent in patients younger than 2 years old (65).

Ganglioneuromas usually appear *de novo* but may follow maturation of a neuroblastoma (71). Patients present with large posterior mediastinal masses that are usually symptomatic and present with clinical manifestations similar to those of other neurogenic tumors of the mediastinum. Occasionally, patients also have Horner's syndrome and heterochromia iridis as a result of sympathetic injury by a tumor invading the superior cervical ganglion (72). Ganglioneuromas can be familial (73).

Radiologic Features

Ganglioneuromas appear on chest roentgenograms as large, round or oval posterior mediastinal tumors with smooth contours and frequent areas of stippled calcification (74). They seldom have intraspinal extensions (dumbbell tumors) but can be associated with mild rib erosion resulting from the mass effect.

Pathologic Features

Ganglioneuromas are well-circumscribed, encapsulated, firm, gray to yellow tumors that frequently have a whorled, trabeculated surface that simulates a leiomyoma (Fig. 12-11). Histologically, they are composed of Schwann cells arranged in irregular fascicles, nerve fibers, and large ganglion cells (Fig. 12-12). The latter have large nuclei with prominent nucleoli and abundant cytoplasm with Nissl granules and occasional lightly eosinophilic inclusions that resemble Pick's bodies (Fig. 12-13). These inclusions as well as intracytoplasmic granules are argentaffinic (67). Ultra-

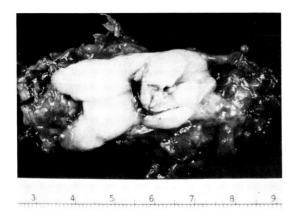

FIG. 12–11. Ganglioneuroma. The tumor is well circumscribed, firm, gray, with a lobulated cut surface.

structurally, these cells have variable numbers of neurofilaments, microtubules, and dense-core vesicles (65–68).

The ganglion cells of ganglioneuromas are very characteristic and can be identified in aspiration cytology specimens (75).

Prognosis and Treatment

Ganglioneuromas are benign tumors that are cured by complete surgical excision (65,69,70). However, occasionally regional lymph nodes contain islands of tumor.

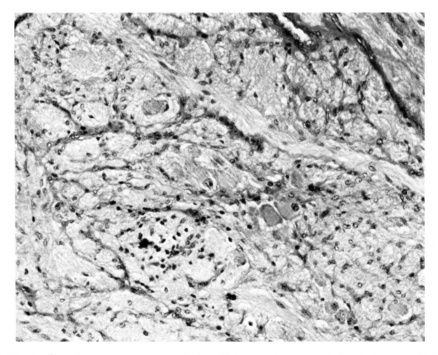

FIG. 12–12. Ganglioneuroma composed of multiple ganglion cells admixed with neurofibrillary material. (H&E × 100, original)

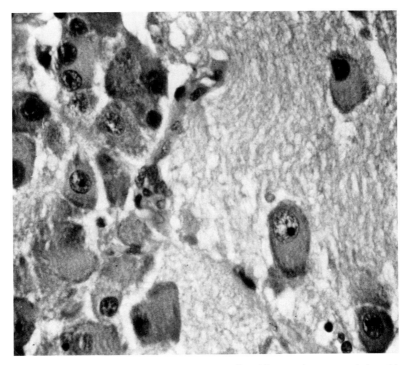

FIG. 12–13. Ganglioneuroma with large ganglion cells with round open nuclei and basophilic granular cytoplasm. (H&E × 400, original)

These "metastatic" ganglioneuromas are probably the result of foci of neuroblastomas that have matured into a benign neoplasm (12). Indeed, these patients do not subsequently develop metastatic disease.

Enzinger and Weiss (12) have described rare instances of malignant transformation of ganglioneuromas to malignant schwannomas.

Neuroblastoma

Neuroblastoma is the most common malignant tumor of early childhood and involves one per 10,000 live births and 9.6 (white) and 7.0 (black) per million children per year in the United States (76,77).

Half of these patients are younger than 2 years, and 90% are discovered to have neuroblastomas before the age of 5 years (12). The tumor is slightly more prevalent in males (78).

Neuroblastomas most frequently arise from the adrenal glands but can originate in extraadrenal sympathetic ganglia. They involve the mediastinum in 16% of cases, where they account for approximately 6% of all mediastinal neurogenic tumors (2,79). Neuroblastomas can be congenital and are occasionally associated with various chromosomal anomalies such as trisomies 13 and 18 (80). They also can be familial or occur in patients with neurofibromatosis (81–84). Cases associated with the fetal hydantoin syndrome also have been described (85).

Neuroblastomas are tumors of presumed neural crest origin and share multiple biochemical characteristics with amine precursor uptake and decarboxylation (APUD) cells (12).

Clinical Manifestations

Patients with mediastinal neuroblastomas are usually symptomatic at the time of initial diagnosis and present with signs and symptoms related to compression of various mediastinal structures as well as with Horner's syndrome, heterochromia iridis, failure to thrive, encephalopathy, myoclonus–opsoclonus–ataxia, cutaneous blanching, joint pain, Cushing's syndrome, myasthenia gravis, chronic diarrhea, Wiedemann–Beckwith syndrome, and various congenital anomalies (77,86–92). Their tumors are usually discovered at an early age (76,78).

Patients also have elevated plasma and urine levels of catecholamines (89). Elevated urine levels of vanillylmandelic acid (VMA), homovanillic acid (HVA), and 3-methoxy-4-hydroxyphenylglycol (MHPG) are present in 80% of patients and have diagnostic value (12).

Patients also can have elevated plasma levels of carcinoembryonic antigen (CEA), antismooth muscle antibodies, and ferritin (93,94).

Roentgenologic Features

Neuroblastomas appear on chest roentgenograms as large posterior mediastinal masses with ill-defined borders ("ghost-like") and frequent areas of finely stippled calcification (74,95,96). Rib erosion and displacement are frequent (74). The tumors can extend into the spinal canal in a dumbbell fashion. CT scans and MRI are very helpful to visualize the neurogenic tumors and may obviate the need for myelography (97).

Pathologic Features

Neuroblastomas are usually large, lobulated, and encapsulated with a soft, gray–red surface that frequently has multiple hemorrhagic areas (Fig. 12-14). Histologi-

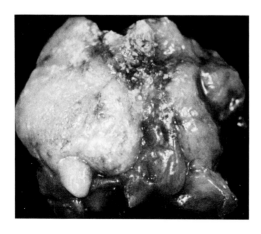

FIG. 12–14. Neuroblastoma. The tumor is well circumscribed, lobulated, soft, with areas of calcification and hemorrhage.

cally, they are composed of small cells with scanty cytoplasm devoid of glycogen and round to polygonal nuclei with a stippled-chromatin pattern ("salt and pepper") and inconspicuous nucleolus (Fig. 12-15). These cells are arranged in various patterns according to the degree of differentiation of the tumors.

Well-differentiated neuroblastomas have cell cords surrounded by a delicate fibrovascular stroma, abundant rosettes containing neurofibrillary material in their center, and occasional large cells with ganglionic differentiation (Fig. 12-16). Their stroma also has abundant neurofibrillary material (Fig. 12-17). Rarely, the tumor cells contain abundant intracytoplasmic neuromelanin (pigmented neuroblastomas) (45).

Poorly differentiated neuroblastomas are composed of solid sheets of small cells resembling the primitive sympathetic system anlage (Fig. 12-18) (12).

Foci of calcification are frequent in neuroblastomas.

Histochemical and Immunocytochemical Features

The tumor cells of neuroblastomas contain intracytoplasmic catecholamines that can be detected with formalin-induced fluorescence and argyrophilic stains (12). Their cytoplasm also contains neuron-specific enolase (NSE) and synaptophysin, markers of neuroendocrine tumors (98).

Ultrastructural Features

Neuroblastomas have fine intracytoplasmic neurofilaments measuring approximately 10 nm, microtubules, dense-core neurosecretory granules, and abundant extracellular neurofibrillary material (99). These ultrastructural features are useful to distinguish them from other round-cell tumors of childhood such as Ewing's sarcoma, rhabdomyosarcoma, and malignant lymphoma. Ewing's sarcomas lack these organelles and instead have abundant intracytoplasmic glycogen. Rhabdomyosarcomas exhibit intracytoplasmic myofibrils arranged in focal bands. Malignant lym-

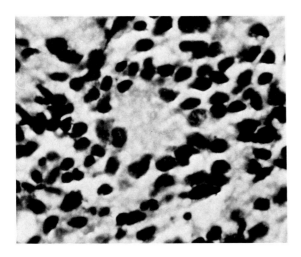

FIG. 12–15. Neuroblastoma composed of small round to oval cells with scanty cytoplasm and forming pseudorosette. The stroma has abundant fibrillary material. (H&E × 400, original)

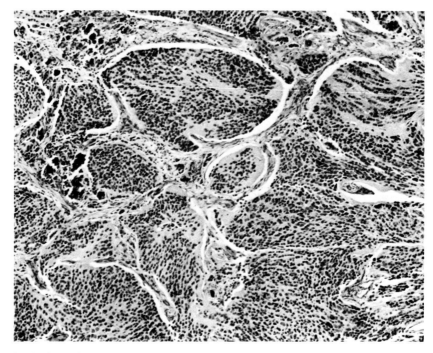

FIG. 12–16. Neuroblastoma with small tumor cells arranged in irregular nests separated by fibrovascular septa. The tumor is focally calcified. (H&E × 40, original)

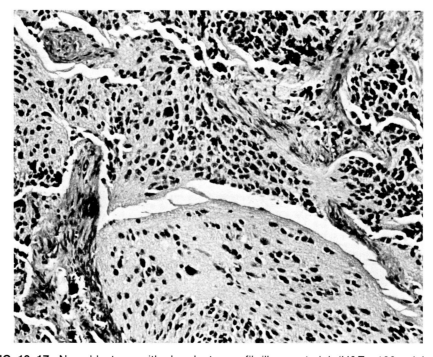

FIG. 12–17. Neuroblastoma with abundant neurofibrillary material. (H&E × 100, original)

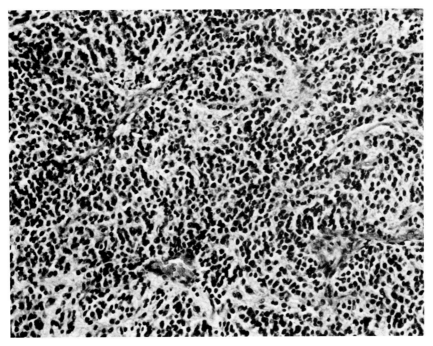

FIG. 12–18. Poorly differentiated neuroblastoma with compact solid sheets of small round cells. (H&E × 100, original)

phomas lack dense-core granules and filaments and may instead exhibit surface or intracytoplasmic immunoglobulins.

Prognosis and Treatment

Neuroblastomas are very aggressive neoplasms with an overall 2-year survival rate of 25% (77,100). The prognosis of patients with these neoplasms depends on various factors including the age of the child at the time of diagnosis, clinical stage of the disease, location of the tumor, and degree of histological differentiation (12).

Patients younger than 1 year of age have a better prognosis than older children and can be cured in 50% of instances. Frequently, their tumors are congenital and may be multiple but nondisseminated (101).

Patients with advanced neuroblastomas at the time of diagnosis have worse prognoses than those with tumors limited to the structure of origin. Evans and associates (76) proposed to stage these neoplasms into five groups: stages I (tumors limited to the structure of origin), II (tumor infiltrating beyond the structure of origin and/or regional lymph nodes on the ipsilateral side), III (tumors that extend beyond the midline), IV (tumors metastatic to remote sites such as bones, viscera, soft tissues, or distant lymph nodes), and IVS (tumors that would be classified as stage I or II but that present with liver, skin, or bone marrow involvement without radiological evidence of bone invasion). Survival rates vary from 4% for patients with stage IV disease to 80% for those with stage I neuroblastoma (102).

The location of the tumor is also important. Indeed, mediastinal neuroblastomas have a better prognosis than their adrenal counterparts (100).

Finally, the prognosis of patients with these tumors is related to the degree of differentiation. Lesions that contain abundant ganglionic elements, rosettes, and neurofibrillary material (grade I) have a better prognosis than less-differentiated tumors lacking these elements (grade III). Intermediate lesions (grade II) have a better prognosis than grade I neoplasms but worse than grade III tumors.

Rarely, neuroblastomas regress spontaneously and/or undergo maturation into ganglioneuromas (71). This process is more frequent in congenital tumors (12).

Patients are treated with surgery alone in stages I and II and receive adjuvant radiotherapy when the tumors cannot be completely excised or are more advanced. Stage IV neuroblastomas are treated with chemotherapy with poor results (2,6–8).

Recent studies have correlated the presence of high serum levels of NSE and/or amplification of the N-myc oncogene in the tumor with poor prognosis (103,104).

Ganglioneuroblastomas

Ganglioneuroblastomas are differentiating neuroblastomas that have abundant neurons at various stages of differentiation and prominent neurofibrillary extracellular material (Figs. 12-19 and 12-20) (12). These tumors have histologic features intermediate between those of neuroblastomas and ganglioneuromas and have a far better prognosis than less-differentiated neuroendocrine lesions (12).

Ganglioneuromas can be multiple and are rarely associated with adrenal tumors and congenital central hypoventilation syndrome, suggesting an origin from a maldeveloped neural crest (105).

TUMORS OF PARAGANGLIA

Paragangliomas and pheochromocytomas can occur in the posterior mediastinum (106–108). They have been described in Chapter 8.

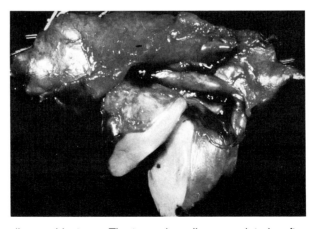

FIG. 12–19. Ganglioneuroblastoma. The tumor is well encapsulated, soft, gray, with a homogeneous cut surface.

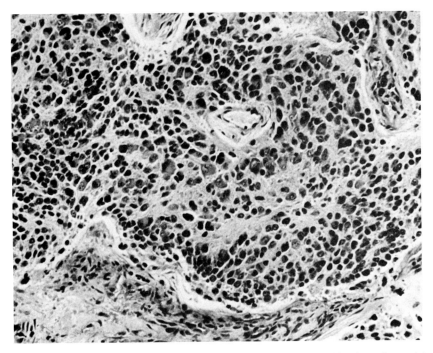

FIG. 12–20. Ganglioneuroblastoma composed of small round neuroblastic cells and larger ganglion cells. (H&E × 100, original)

TUMORS OF PROBABLE SCHWANN CELL ORIGIN

Granular Cell Tumor

Granular cell tumors (granular cell myoblastomas) have been described in the posterior mediastinum (109). These tumors, thought to derive from Schwann cells, are poorly circumscribed, soft, yellow or gray, and are composed histologically of round to polygonal uniform cells with central vesicular nuclei and coarsely granular eosinophilic cytoplasm. The tumor cells are usually arranged in ribbons or nests in the midst of a fibrous connective tissue stroma but can form large sheets without a characteristic pattern. Ultrastructurally, they exhibit abundant autophagic vacuoles containing cellular debris (12).

Granular cell tumors are benign neoplasms that are cured by resection. They seldom undergo malignant transformation (12,107).

TUMORS OF NEURAL TUBE REMNANTS

Ependymoma

Doglioni and associates (110) recently described a patient with a primary ependymoma of the posterior mediastinum that metastasized to adjacent lymph nodes. The tumor was composed of solid and papillary areas with elongated tubules and rosettes of ependymal type. The tumor cells had fibrillary cytoplasmic processes and exhibited intracytoplasmic glial-fibrillary acidic protein (GFAP) immunoreactivity. An origin in ependymal cell rests was suggested, although the possibility of a germ cell origin (monodermal teratoma) could not be ruled out.

REFERENCES

1. Chavez Espinosa JI, Chavez Fernandez JA, Hoyer OH, et al: Endothoracic neurogenic neoplasms (Analysis of 30 cases). *Rev Interam Radiol* 1980;5:49–54.
2. Davidson KG, Walbaum PR, McCormack RJM: Intrathoracic neural tumors. *Thorax* 1978; 33:359–367.
3. Strickland B, Wolverson MK: Intrathoracic vagus nerve tumors. *Thorax* 1974;29:215–222.
4. Gale AW, Jelihovsky T, Grant AF, et al: Neurogenic tumors of the mediastinum. *Ann Thorac Surg* 1974;17:434–443.
5. Benjamin SP, McCormack LJ, Effler DB, et al: Primary tumors of the mediastinum. *Chest* 1972;62:297–303.
6. Luosto R, Koikkalainen K, Jyrälä A, et al: Mediastinal tumours. A follow up study of 208 patients. *Scand J Thorac Cardiovasc Surg* 1978;12:253–259.
7. Ovrum E, Birkeland S: Mediastinal tumors and cysts. A review of 91 cases. *Scand J Thorac Cardiovasc Surg* 1979;13:161–168.
8. Ecker RR, Timmes JJ, Miscall L: Neurogenic tumors of the intrathoracic vagus nerve. *Arch Surg* 1963;86:222–229.
9. Blades B: Mediastinal tumors. Report of cases treated at Army Thoracic Surgery Centers in the United States. *Ann Surg* 1946;123:749–765.
10. Morrison IM: Tumours and cysts of the mediastinum. *Thorax* 1958;13:294–307.
11. Harjula A, Mattila S, Luosto R, et al: Mediastinal neurogenic tumours. Early and late results of surgical treatment. *Scand J Thorac Cardiovasc Surg* 1986;20:115–118.
12. Enzinger FM, Weiss SW: *Soft Tissue Tumors, Second Edition.* St. Louis, CV Mosby, 1988.
13. Steffansson K, Wollmann R, Jerkovic M: S100 protein in soft tissue tumors derived from Schwann cells and melanocytes. *Am J Pathol* 1982;106:261–268.
14. Bock E: Nervous system specific proteins. *J Neurochem* 1978;30:7–14.
15. Nakazato Y, Ishizeki J, Takahashi K, et al: Immunohistochemical localization of S-100 protein in granular cell myoblastoma. *Cancer* 1982;49:1624–1628.
16. Lassmann H, Jurecka W, Lassmann G, et al: Different types of benign nerve sheath tumors: light microscopy, electron microscopy and autoradiography. *Virchows Arch [Pathol Anat]* 1977; 375:197–210.
17. Sian CS, Ryan SF: The ultrastructure of neurilemmoma with emphasis on Antoni B tissue. *Hum Pathol* 1981;12:145–160.
18. Lazarus SS, Trombetta LD: Ultrastructural identification of a benign perineural cell tumor. *Cancer* 1978;41:1823–1829.
19. Carstens PHB, Schrodt GR: Malignant transformation of a benign encapsulated neurilemoma. *Am J Clin Pathol* 1969;51:144–149.
20. Paris F, Cabanes J, Muñoz C, et al: Melanotic spinothoracic schwannoma. *Thorax* 1979;34:243–246.
21. D'Abrera V St. E, Burfitt-Williams W: A melanotic neuroectodermal neoplasm of the posterior mediastinum. *J Pathol* 1973;111:165–172.
22. Katenkamp D, Filippowa N, Riakhlin NT: Melanocytic schwannoma. Light- and electron microscopic findings on the morphology, diagnosis, and differential diagnosis. *Zentralbl Allg Pathol* 1986;131:107–118.
23. Mandybur TI: Melanotic nerve sheath tumours. *J Neurosurg* 1974;41:187–192.
24. Chalmers AH, Armstrong P: Plexiform mediastinal neurofibromas. A report of two cases. *Br J Radiol* 1977;50:215–217.
25. Stradling JR, Huddart S, Arnold AG: Sleep apnea syndrome caused by neurofibromatosis and superior vena caval obstruction. *Thorax* 1981;36:634–635.
26. Sarin CL, Bennett MH, Jackson JW: Intrathoracic neurofibroma of the vagus nerve. *Br J Dis Chest* 1974;68:46–50.
27. Zorbas JA, Kreatsas GK: Neurofibroma of the intrathoracic vagus nerve in a man with Recklinghausen's disease: case report. *Milit Med* 1977;142:384–385.
28. Vasilakis D, Papaconstantinou C, Aletras H: Dumb-bell intrathoracic and intraspinal neurofibroma. Report of a case. *Scand J Thorac Cardiovasc Surg* 1986;20:171–173.
29. Shin MS, McElvein RB, Reeves RC, et al: Solitary neurofibroma of the vagus nerve in the aortopulmonary window masquerading as a developmental cyst. *J Comput Tomogr* 1988;12:57–60.

30. Ikezoe J, Sone S, Higashihara T, et al: CT of intrathoracic neurogenic tumours. *Eur J Radiol* 1986;6:266–269.
31. Kamata Y: Study on the ultrastructure and acetylcholinesterase activity in von Recklinghausen's neurofibromatosis. *Acta Pathol Jpn* 1978;28:393–410.
32. Crowe FW, Schull WJ, Neel JV: *A Clinical Pathological and Genetic Study of Multiple Neurofibromatosis*. Springfield, Ill, Charles C Thomas, 1956.
33. Fialkow PJ, Sagebiel RW, Gartler SM, et al: Multiple cell origin of hereditary neurofibromas. *N Engl J Med* 1971;284:298–300.
34. Schenkein I, Bueker ED, Helson L, et al: Increased nerve-growth stimulating activity in disseminated neurofibromatosis. *N Engl J Med* 1974;290:613–614.
35. Akwari OE, Payne WS, Onofrio BM, et al: Dumbbell neurogenic tumors of the mediastinum. *Mayo Clin Proc* 1978;53:353–358.
36. Dines DE, Payne WS, Howard PH Jr: Von Recklinghausen's neurofibromatosis with plexiform mediastinal involvement. Report of a case. *Dis Chest* 1966;50:437–439.
37. Raszkowski HJ, Hufner RF: Neurofibromatosis of the colon. A unique manifestation of von Recklinghausen's disease. *Cancer* 1971;27:134–142.
38. Salyer WR, Salyer DC: The vascular lesions of neurofibromatosis. *Angiology* 1974;25:510–519.
39. Stay EJ, Vawter G: The relationship between nephroblastoma and neurofibromatosis (von Recklinghausen's disease). *Cancer* 1977;39:2550–2555.
40. Webb WR, Goodman PC: Fibrosing alveolitis in patients with neurofibromatosis. *Radiology* 1977;122:289–293.
41. Reed JC, Hallet KK, Feigin DS: Neural tumors of the thorax: subject review from the AFIP. *Radiology* 1978;126:9–17.
42. Rodriguez HA, Berthrong M: Multiple primary intracranial tumors in von Recklinghausen's neurofibromatosis. *Arch Neurol* 1966;14:467–475.
43. Guccion JG, Enzinger FM: Malignant schwannoma associated with von Recklinghausen's neurofibromatosis. *Virchows Arch [Pathol Anat]* 1979;383:43–57.
44. Misugi K, Okajima H, Newton WA Jr, et al: Mediastinal origin of a melanotic progonoma or retinal anlage tumor: ultrastructural evidence for neural crest origin. *Cancer* 1965;18:477–484.
45. Stowens D, Lin TH: Melanotic progonoma of the brain. *Hum Pathol* 1974;5:105–113.
46. Williams AO: Melanotic ameloblastoma ("progonoma") of infancy showing osteogenesis. *J Pathol Bacteriol* 1967;93:545–548.
47. Krumerman MS, Stingle W: Synchronous malignant schwannomas in congenital neurofibromatosis. *Cancer* 1978;41:2444–2451.
48. Bambirra EA, Miranda D: Spontaneous aortic rupture in a malignant schwannoma. *South Med J* 1980;73:1533–1535.
49. D'Agostino AN, Soule EH, Miller RH: Primary malignant neoplasm of nerves (malignant neurilemmomas) in patients without manifestations of multiple neurofibromatosis (von Recklinghausen's disease). *Cancer* 1963;16:1003–1014.
50. D'Agostino AN, Soule EH, Miller RH: Sarcomas of the peripheral nerves and somatic soft tissues associated with multiple fibromatosis (von Recklinghausen's disease). *Cancer* 1963;16:1015–1027.
51. Stewart FW, Copeland MM: Neurogenic sarcoma. *Am J Cancer* 1931;15:1235–1320.
52. Storm FK, Eilber FR, Mirra J, et al: Neurofibrosarcoma. *Cancer* 1980;45:126–129.
53. Tsuneyoshi M, Enjoji M: Primary malignant peripheral nerve tumors (malignant schwannomas): a clinicopathologic and electron microscopic study. *Acta Pathol Jpn* 1979;29:363–375.
54. Conkle DM, Adkins RB Jr: Primary malignant tumors of the mediastinum. *Ann Thorac Surg* 1972;14:553–567.
55. Efskind L, Liavaag K: Intrathoracic neurogenic tumors. *J Thorac Surg* 1950;20:13–23.
56. Kent EM, Blades B, Valle AR, et al: Intrathoracic neurogenic tumors. *J Thorac Surg* 1944;13:116–161.
57. Stout AP: The malignant tumors of the peripheral nerves. *Am J Cancer* 1935;25:1–36.
58. Woodruff JM: Peripheral nerve tumors showing glandular differentiation (glandular schwannomas). *Cancer* 1976;37:2399–2413.
59. Woodruff JM, Chernik NL, Smith MC, et al: Peripheral nerve tumors with rhabdomyosarcomatous differentiation (malignant "triton" tumors). *Cancer* 1973;32:426–439.
60. MacKay B, Osborne BM: The contribution of electron microscopy to the diagnosis of tumors, in Ioachim HL (ed): *Pathobiology Annual*, vol. 8. New York, Raven Press, 1978, pp 359–405.
61. Chitale AR, Dickersin GR: Electron microscopy in the diagnosis of malignant schwannomas. A report of six cases. *Cancer* 1983;51:1448–1461.
62. Erlandson RA, Woodruff JM: Peripheral nerve sheath tumors: an electron microscopic study of 43 cases. *Cancer* 1982;49:273–287.
63. Nakajima T, Watanabe S, Sato Y, et al: An immunoperoxidase study of S-100 protein distribution in normal and neoplastic tissues. *Am J Surg Pathol* 1982;6:715–727.

64. Ghosh BC, Ghosh L, Huvos AG, et al: Malignant schwannoma: a clinicopathologic study. *Cancer* 1973;31:184–190.
65. Adam A, Hochholzer L: Ganglioneuroblastoma of the posterior mediastinum: a clinicopathologic review of 80 cases. *Cancer* 1981;47:373–381.
66. Pascaud JL, Le Goff JJ, Pascaud E, et al: Thoracic ganglioneuroma with intra-spinal prolongations in childhood. *Pediatr Radiol* 1980;9:109–110.
67. Bender BL, Ghatak NR: Light and electron microscopic observations on a ganglioneuroma. *Acta Neuropathol* 1978;42:7–10.
68. Yokoyama M, Okada K, Tokue A, et al: Ultrastructural and biochemical study of benign ganglioneuroma. *Virchows Arch [Pathol Anat]* 1973;361:195–209.
69. Hamilton JP, Koop CE: Ganglioneuromas in children. *Surg Gynecol Obstet* 1965;121:803–812.
70. Schweisguth O, Mathey J, Renault P, et al: Intrathoracic neurogenic tumors in infants and children. A study of 40 cases. *Ann Surg* 1959;150:29–41.
71. Aterman K, Schueller EF: Maturation of neuroblastoma to ganglioneuroma. *Am J Dis Child* 1970;120:217–222.
72. McRae D Jr, Shaw A: Ganglioneuroma, heterochromia iridis, and Horner's syndrome. *J Pediatr Surg* 1979;14:612–614.
73. Bergstrom JF, Long JM: Familial occurrence of ganglioneuromas. *Tex Med* 1974;70:62–65.
74. Bar-Ziv J, Nogrady MB: Mediastinal neuroblastoma and ganglioneuroma. The differentiation between primary and secondary involvement on the chest roentgenogram. *Am J Roentgenol Radium Ther Nucl Med* 1975;125:380–390.
75. Palombini L, Vetrani A: Cytologic diagnosis of ganglioneuroblastoma (letter). *Acta Cytol* 1976;20:286–289.
76. Evans AE, D'Angio GJ, Randolph J: A proposed staging for children with neuroblastoma. Children's Cancer Study Group A. *Cancer* 1971;27:374–378.
77. Evans AE, D'Angio GJ, Koop CE: Diagnosis and treatment of neuroblastoma. *Pediatr Clin North Am* 1976;23:161–170.
78. Kinnier-Wilson LM, Draper GJ: Neuroblastoma, its natural history and prognosis: a study of 487 cases. *Br Med J* 1974;3:301–307.
79. de Lorimier AA, Bragg KU, Linden G: Neuroblastoma in childhood. *Am J Dis Child* 1969;118:441–450.
80. Robinson MG, McCorquodale MM: Trisomy 18 and neurogenic neoplasia. *J Pediatr* 1981;99:428–429.
81. Chatten J, Voorhess ML: Familial neuroblastoma. Report of a kindred with multiple disorders, including neuroblastoma in four siblings. *N Engl J Med* 1967;277:1230–1236.
82. Wong KY, Hanenson IB, Lampkin BC: Familial neuroblastoma. *Am J Dis Child* 1971;121:415–416.
83. Feingold M, Gheradi GJ, Simons C: Familial neuroblastoma and trisomy 13. *Am J Dis Child* 1971;121:451.
84. Bolande RP, Towler WF: A possible relationship of neuroblastoma to von Recklinghausen's disease. *Cancer* 1970;26:162–175.
85. Pendergrass TW, Hanson JW: Fetal hydantoin syndrome and neuroblastoma. *Lancet* 1976;2:150.
86. Berg BO, Ablin AR, Wang W, et al: Encephalopathy asociated with occult neuroblastoma. *J Neurosurg* 1974;41:567–572.
87. Jaffe N, Cassady R, Filler RM, et al: Heterochromia and Horner's syndrome associated with cervical and mediastinal neuroblastoma. *J Pediatr* 1975;87:75–77.
88. Lucky AW, McGuire J, Komp DM: Infantile neuroblastoma presenting with cutaneous blanching nodules. *J Am Acad Dermatol* 1982;6:389–391.
89. Duckett JW, Koop CE: Neuroblastoma. *Urol Clin North Am* 1977;4:285–295.
90. Robinson MJ, Howard RN: Neuroblastoma, presenting as myasthenia gravis in a child aged 3 years. *Pediatrics* 1969;43:111–113.
91. Berry CL, Keeling J, Hilton C: Coincidence of congenital malformation and embryonic tumours of childhood. *Arch Dis Child* 1970;45:229–231.
92. Huber A, Gutjahr P: Mediastinal neuroblastoma in Wiedemann–Beckwith syndrome. *Monatsschr Kinderheilkd* 1989;137:243–244.
93. Wang JJ, Sinks LF, Ming Chu J: Carcinoembryonic antigen in patients with neuroblastoma. *J Surg Oncol* 1974;6:211–217.
94. Zauli D, Bianchi FB, Gardelli T, et al: Smooth-muscle antibodies in children with neuroblastoma. *Cancer* 1980;46:497–499.
95. Mullins JD: A pigmented differentiating neuroblastoma: a light and ultrastructural study. *Cancer* 1980;46:522–528.
96. Damgaard-Pedersen K: Neuroblastoma follow-up by computed tomography. *J Comput Assist Tomogr* 1979;3:274–275.
97. Siegel MJ, Jamroz GA, Glazer HS, et al: MR imaging of intraspinal extension of neuroblastoma. *J Comput Assist Tomogr* 1986;10:593–595.

98. Tapia FJ, Barbosa AJA, Marangos PJ, et al: Neuron-specific enolase is produced by neuroendocrine tumors. *Lancet* 1981;1:808–811.
99. Taxy JB: Electron microscopy in the diagnosis of neuroblastoma. *Arch Pathol Lab Med* 1980;104:355–360.
100. Fortner J, Nicastri A, Murphy ML: Neuroblastoma: Natural history and results of treating 133 cases. *Ann Surg* 1968;167:132–142.
101. Leape LL, Lowman JT, Loveland CG: Multifocal nondisseminated neuroblastoma. Report of two cases in siblings. *J Pediatr* 1978;92:75–77.
102. Evans AE, Chatten J, D'Angio GJ, et al: A review of 17 IV-S neuroblastoma patients at the Children's Hospital of Philadelphia. *Cancer* 1980;45:833–839.
103. Evans AE, D'Angio GL, Propert K, et al: Prognostic factors in neuroblastoma. *Cancer* 1987;59:1853–1859.
104. Brodeur GM, Seeger RC, Schwab M, et al: Amplification of N-myc in untreated human neuroblastomas correlate with advanced stage disease. *Science* 1984;224:1121–1124.
105. Swaminathan S, Gilsanz V, Atkinson J, et al: Congenital central hypoventilation syndrome associated with multiple ganglioneuromas. *Chest* 1989;96:423–424.
106. Reyes MG, Fresco R, Bruetman ME: Mediastinal paraganglioma causing spinal cord compression. *J Neurol Neurosurg Psychiatry* 1977;40:276–279.
107. Ogawa J, Inoue H, Koide S, et al: Functioning paraganglioma in the posterior mediastinum. *Ann Thorac Surg* 1982;33:507–510.
108. Routh A, Hickman BT, Hardy JD, et al: Malignant chemodectoma of posterior mediastinum. *South Med J* 1982;75:879–881.
109. Rosenbloom PM, Barrows GH, Kmetz DR, et al: Granular cell myoblastoma arising from the thoracic sympathetic nerve chain. *J Pediatr Surg* 1975;10:819–822.
110. Doglioni C, Bontempini L, Iuzzolino P, et al: Ependymoma of the mediastinum. *Arch Pathol Lab Med* 1988;112:194–196.

Subject Index